# The 4 Stages of Heart Failure

May, 2015

To Sharp Chula Vista,

With best wishes.

R E Fuller

# The 4 Stages of Heart Failure

## Brian E. Jaski, MD, FACC

Director of Clinical Research, San Diego Cardiac Center
Medical Director, Advanced Heart Failure and Cardiac Transplant
Sharp Memorial Hospital
San Diego, California

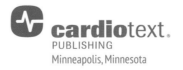

**cardio**text.
PUBLISHING
Minneapolis, Minnesota

Cardiotext Publishing, LLC
3405 W. 44th Street
Minneapolis, Minnesota 55410
USA

www.cardiotextpublishing.com

Any updates to this book may be found at:
www.cardiotextpublishing.com/4-stages-of-heart-failure

Comments, inquiries, and requests for bulk sales can be directed to the publisher
at: info@cardiotextpublishing.com.

Library of Congress Control Number: 2015932328

ISBN: 978-1-935395-30-0

Printed in the United States of America

# TABLE OF CONTENTS

# IN GRATITUDE

I am deeply grateful to many individuals who helped make this guide possible. I thank Dr. Sharon Hunt, who pioneered a paradigm of progressive stages of heart failure and Dr. Clyde Yancy, who advanced this construct. My present and past colleagues at the San Diego Cardiac Center and Sharp Memorial Hospital have served as a source of encouragement, knowledge, and inspiration. Dr. Kirk Peterson reviewed a draft of this book and provided wise counsel regarding both presentation and content. I thank the Sharp Foundation for its support.

This publication benefited from the tireless efforts of my research associates Bryan Ortiz, Christopher Grigoriadis, Jessica Alicdan, Justin Gibson, and Michelle Williamson. Their technical skills, insights, and optimism have buoyed me throughout the 4-year period of concept to product. I am indebted to the team at Cardiotext Publishing, especially Dr. Katharine Swenson, who as a former cardiology fellow of mine and a clinical cardiologist has been unique in her ability to edit and guide the final phases of this project.

I gratefully acknowledge the cardiology fellows from Balboa Naval Hospital. Over the last 25 years, during their Heart Failure rotations at Sharp Memorial hospital, I honed the principles and practices put forth in this book, demonstrating the proverb "by learning you will teach; by teaching you will learn."

I dedicate this book to my patients whose courage, resilience, and humility have served as both *raison d'être* and model for my professional life.

Finally, to "my girls"—my wife Cindy and our daughter KC: The joy you have brought to my life makes everything else possible.

—Brian E. Jaski, MD
San Diego Cardiac Center
January 2015

# ABOUT THE AUTHOR

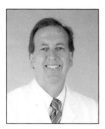 **Brian E. Jaski, MD, FACC,** is a clinical cardiologist, researcher, and medical educator. After earning undergraduate degrees in electrical engineering and biology from MIT, he graduated from Harvard Medical School, Harvard-MIT Division of Health Sciences Technology, where he subsequently also completed a cardiology fellowship at the Brigham and Women's Hospital. Since 1985, when he joined the San Diego Cardiac Center, he has served as Medical Director of the Advanced Heart Failure and Cardiac Transplant program at Sharp Memorial Hospital. He publishes in the areas of cardiac pathophysiology, pharmacology, circulatory support devices, and cardiac transplant. He is board certified in the subspecialties of Advanced Heart Failure and Cardiac Transplant and Interventional Cardiology. He founded Heart Failure Online (www.heartfailure.org) in 1996. He enjoys family, travel, and running half marathons.

# FOREWORD

In my recent role as President of the World Heart Federation, I became acutely aware and concerned that the world's increasing and aging population, globalization, and rapid urbanization have fundamentally changed disease patterns. Noncommunicable diseases, of which cardiovascular disease accounts for nearly half, have overtaken communicable diseases as leading causes of death and disability in the world. Cardiovascular disease remains the number 1 global cause of death, accounting for 17.3 million deaths per year, a number that is expected to grow to 23.6 million by 2030. As a Past President of the American Heart Association, I know too well that in the United States, heart failure is a major cause of morbidity and mortality, and for more than a decade has been the leading cause for hospital admissions in the Medicare population.

Significant advances have occurred in our understanding and management of heart failure. In particular, an expanded view of origins ranging from environmental to genetic cardiovascular risk factors has emerged. Once the stage is set for structural heart disease, the progression to more advanced heart failure may unfold gradually or rapidly. Detailed guidelines have been published and widely distributed to address the need for diagnosis and treatment of heart failure, and since 2010, Advanced Heart Failure and Cardiac Transplant has assumed subspecialty status within the American Board of Internal Medicine. But the challenge remains when interpreting new guidelines in clinical situations: when should recommendations be applied and for whom?

I first met, and subsequently recruited, Brian Jaski to join the San Diego Cardiac Center when he was a third-year cardiology fellow at the Brigham and Women's Hospital. I was impressed by his background in scientific principles, which he utilized in the practice of clinical cardiology, and by his strong clinical abilities and devotion to patient care. In the thirty years since we first met, my respect for him has only grown.

In addition to developing a highly successful, internationally recognized advanced heart failure program in San Diego, Brian has participated in and chaired data and safety monitoring and adverse event adjudication committees for both drug and device multicenter trials. His many publications reflect the breadth of his knowledge and contributions.

After three decades of practice, research, and teaching, Brian's cumulative experience and clinical acumen is distilled and presented in this book using the model of the 4 stages of heart failure as a backbone. His book is unique in its single-author coordination, yet reflects Brian's multiple perspectives.

This book will be valuable to all training and practicing clinicians. The latest therapies are detailed with practical tips for application. His book is beautifully color illustrated with summary diagrams and key data graphics that will guide day-to-day practice. He writes as if you and he are both completing patient rounds together. Brian is to be commended for capturing the essence of treating this formidable clinical challenge and demystifying the stages of heart failure. I learned from reading this book and know you will, too.

—Sidney C. Smith, Jr., MD, FACC, FAHA, FESC, FACP
Professor of Medicine, University of North Carolina at Chapel Hill
Past President, American Heart Association
Past President, World Heart Federation

I have written this book to enable the reader to craft solutions for patients to breathe comfortably, reclaim their previous lifestyles, and forestall premature death. Whereas many textbooks cull diverse expert opinions, my intent is to provide a balanced perspective that concisely "separates the wheat from the chaff." For the trainee, a familiarity with these fundamentals can provide a basis for future practice; for the experienced practitioner, this book may inspire patient care beyond a previous standard.

The pandemic of heart failure parallels an unprecedented extension of the human lifespan over the last century. While heart failure can occur at any age, those who live longer are more likely to succumb to the culmination of a lifetime of cardiovascular insults. Fortunately, advances have occurred. Modifiable risks have been identified. Widely available diagnostic tools allow early intervention. Multiple pharmacologic agents have achieved class I guideline treatment recommendations. Medical devices have demonstrated surprising efficacy. Applications derived from molecular biology have entered the medical arena.

In 2001, the American College of Cardiology and the American Heart Association defined 4 progressive stages of heart failure:

**A:** Risk factors for heart failure.

**B:** Asymptomatic ventricular dysfunction.

**C:** Clinical heart failure.

**D:** Advanced heart failure.

These 4 stages were most recently expanded and refined in 2013. This book emphasizes the understanding of these stages as a continuum and provides a scaffold to build tailored approaches to treatment and improve individual outcomes.

—Dr. Brian E. Jaski

| | | | |
|---|---|---|---|
| AA | amyloid A protein | ATTR | amyloidosis transthyretin-related |
| ACCF | American College of Cardiology Foundation | AV | atrioventricular |
| ACE | angiotensin converting enzyme | $\Delta$AVO$_2$ | arteriovenous oxygen difference* (difference between arterial and venous oxygen concentration) |
| ACEI | angiotensin converting enzyme inhibitor | | |
| ACLS | advanced cardiac life support | BiPAP | biphasic positive airway pressure |
| ADA | American Diabetes Association | BMI | body mass index (kg/m$^2$) |
| ADH | antidiuretic hormone (vasopressin) | BNP | b-type natriuretic peptide |
| | | BSA | body surface area |
| ADHF | acute decompensated heart failure | BUN | blood urea nitrogen |
| | | Ca$^{2+}$ | calcium |
| AHA | American Heart Association | CABG | coronary artery bypass graft |
| AHFS | acute heart failure syndrome | CAD | coronary artery disease |
| AKI | acute kidney injury | cAMP | cyclic adenosine monophosphate |
| AL | amyloid light-chain protein | CBC | complete blood count |
| ALT | alanine transaminase (also called SGPT) | CCr | creatinine clearance rate |
| ALVD | asymptomatic left ventricular dysfunction | CDC | Centers for Disease Control |
| AMPK | adenosine monophosphate-activated protein kinase | cGMP | cyclic guanosine monophosphate |
| | | CHF | congestive heart failure |
| ANP | atrial natriuretic peptide | CKD | chronic kidney disease |
| ARB | angiotensin II receptor blocker | CMR | cardiac magnetic resonance |
| | | CNP | c-type natriuretic peptide |
| AST | aspartate aminotransferase (also called SGOT) | CPAP | continuous positive airway pressure |
| | | CPS | cardiopulmonary support |
| AT | anaerobic threshold | CR | creatinine |
| ATP | adenosine triphosphate | CRS | cardiorenal syndrome |

*See Chapter 2 for formula and calculation.

| | | | | |
|---|---|---|---|---|
| CRT | cardiac resynchronization therapy | | HF-pEF | heart failure with preserved ejection fraction |
| CSA | central sleep apnea | | HF-rEF | heart failure with reduced ejection fraction |
| CT | computed tomography | | | |
| CTCA | computed tomography coronary angiography | | HFE | gene and protein that regulate iron absorption |
| cTn | cardiac troponin | | HLVH | hypertensive left ventricular hypertrophy |
| CVP | central venous pressure | | HOCM | hypertrophic obstructive cardiomyopathy |
| CysC | cystatin C | | | |
| Cyt | cytoplasm | | HR | heart rate |
| CXR | chest x-ray | | HTN | hypertension |
| DBP | diastolic blood pressure | | IABP | intra-aortic balloon pump |
| DIAS | diastolic | | ICD | implantable cardioverter-defibrillator |
| DNA | deoxyribonucleic acid | | | |
| DPTI | diastolic pressure–time index | | IHSS | idiopathic hypertrophic subaortic stenosis |
| DT | deceleration time | | INR | international normalized ratio |
| ECG | electrocardiography | | | |
| ECLS | extracorporeal life support | | IVD | intravenous diuretics |
| ECMO | extracorporeal membrane oxygenation | | IV | intravenous |
| | | | J-G | juxtaglomerular |
| EF | ejection fraction | | LA | left atrial |
| eGFR | estimated glomerular filtration rate | | LAMP2 | lysosomal-associated membrane protein 2 |
| EMB | endomyocardial biopsy | | LV | left ventricle / left ventricular |
| ESR | erythrocyte sedimentation rate | | | |
| | | | LVAD | left ventricular assist device |
| FM | fulminant myocarditis | | | |
| GFR | glomerular filtration rate | | LVDP | left ventricular diastolic pressure |
| GGT | gamma-glutamyl transferase | | LVEF | left ventricular ejection fraction |
| GLA | α-Galactosidase A | | | |
| GTP | guanosine triphosphate | | LVH | left ventricular hypertrophy |
| HCM | hypertrophic cardiomyopathy | | LVOT | left ventricular outflow tract |
| HF | heart failure | | LVSD | left ventricular systolic dysfunction |

| | | | |
|---|---|---|---|
| MCS | mechanical circulatory support | RCM | restrictive cardiomyopathy |
| MDRD | modification of diet in renal disease | RDA | recommended dietary allowance |
| MI | myocardial infarction | RER | respiratory exchange ratio |
| mPTP | mitochondrial permeability transition pores | RNA | ribonucleic acid |
| MR | magnetic resonance | RV | right ventricular |
| MRA | mineralocorticoid receptor antagonist | S-ICD | subcutaneous implantable cardioverter-defibrillator |
| MRI | magnetic resonance imaging | SBP | systolic blood pressure |
| mRNA | messenger ribonucleic acid | SCD | sudden cardiac death |
| NCEP | National Cholesterol Education Program | SCr | serum creatinine |
| NE | norepinephrine | Scys | serum cystatin C |
| NEP | neutral endopeptidase | SDB | sleep-disordered breathing |
| NGAL | neutrophil gelatinase-associated lipocalin | SERCA2a | sacro(endo)plasmic reticulum calcium transport ATPase 2a |
| NIH | National Institutes of Health | SGOT | serum glutamic oxaloacetic transaminase |
| NT-proBNP | N-terminal pro-B-type natriuretic peptide | SGPT | serum glutamic pyruvic transaminase |
| NYHA | New York Heart Association | SIRS | systemic inflammatory response syndrome |
| OSA | obstructive sleep apnea | SPECT | single-photon-emission computed tomography |
| PCWP | pulmonary capillary wedge pressure | SR | sarcoplasmic reticulum |
| PET | positron-emission tomography | STEMI | ST-elevation myocardial infarction |
| PND | paroxysmal nocturnal dyspnea | SYS | systolic |
| | | SV | stroke volume |
| PPVO$_2$ | percent predicted peak oxygen consumption | TAVR | transcatheter aortic valve replacement |
| PUF | peripheral ultrafiltration | TDI | tissue Doppler imaging |
| RAAS | renin-angiotensin-aldosterone system | TEE | transesophageal echocardiogram |
| rAAV | recombinant adeno-associated virus | TIMI | thrombolysis in myocardial infarction |
| | | TMEM43 | transmembrane protein 43 |
| | | TSH | thyroid stimulating hormone |

| | | | |
|---|---|---|---|
| **TTI** | tension-time index | **VO₂** | oxygen consumption |
| **TTR** | transthyretin | **VT** | ventricular tachycardia |
| **UO** | urine output | **W-IHM** | wireless implantable hemodynamic monitoring |
| **VAD** | ventricular assist device | | |
| **VHD** | valvular heart disease | **WHF** | worsening heart failure |
| | | **WRF** | worsening renal function |

# Introduction

## Definitions of Heart Failure

Heart failure is not a single diagnosis, but rather a syndrome of multiple etiologies. Like fever or jaundice, heart failure mandates an investigation into specific causes to permit effective therapies. Unlike these other maladies, heart failure may evolve insidiously and initially elude detection. Comorbidities commonly complicate assessment.

Beyond causing symptoms of vascular congestion, heart failure also threatens life through pump dysfunction and sudden death. In contrast to myocardial infarction where atherothrombosis is an accepted mechanism,[1] the pathophysiology of the heart failure syndrome is more diverse in initiation and progression. The 2013 ACCF/AHA Heart Failure Guidelines defined heart failure as "a complex clinical syndrome that results from any structural or functional impairment of ventricular filling or ejection of blood."[2]

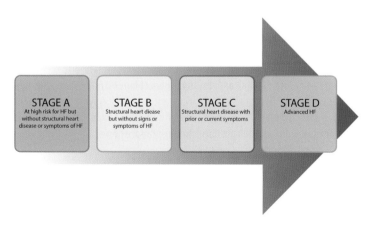

**FIGURE 1    The 4 stages of heart failure designated by the ACCF/AHA including those describing the risks for and those associated with manifest clinical heart failure.** A patient maintains his most advanced stage status even if symptoms improve.

*The 4 Stages of Heart Failure* © 2015 Brian E. Jaski. Cardiotext Publishing, ISBN: 978-1-935395-30-0.      1

# Clinical Definition of Heart Failure

In clinical practice, the following simplified definition can serve as an orientation for the 4 Stages of Heart Failure.

## HEART PUMP INSUFFICIENCY RESULTING IN SYMPTOMS

**Heart Pump:**
A complete description of the heart includes vascular, electrical, hormonal, and structural components. For heart failure to be present, however, there must be impairment of the heart to move blood in the circulation. A way to define impaired heart pump function is the inability of the heart to supply blood flow to meet the needs of the body either at rest or with activity, or to do so with increased left or right ventricular filling pressures. Of importance, this may occur with either a reduced or preserved ventricular ejection fraction.

**Insufficiency:**
The word "failure" implies a cessation of function, as in patients with "renal failure" who are either on or in imminent need of dialysis. In heart failure, heart pump insufficiency does not, in general, require complete replacement therapy. This semantic difference may be important to emphasize to patients or families with a new diagnosis of "heart failure."

**Resulting In:**
Risk factors or asymptomatic cardiac dysfunction often precede the first symptoms of heart failure. Advances in understanding neurohumoral mechanisms that impel this progression over time have led to significant therapies for heart failure with reduced ejection fraction.

**Symptoms:**
Stages A and B of the American College of Cardiology/American Heart Association classification of heart failure are asymptomatic and considered pre-heart failure.[2] A clinical definition of heart failure, however, is confined to Stages C and D, characterized by current or previous symptoms associated with heart pump insufficiency. Common symptoms are shortness of breath associated with lung congestion and peripheral edema.

# References

1. Nabel EG, Braunwald E. A tale of coronary artery disease and myocardial infarction. *N Engl J Med.* 2012;366(1):54-63.

2. Yancy CW, et al. 2013 ACCF/AHA guideline for the management of heart failure: a report of the American College of Cardiology Foundation/American Heart Association Task Force on Practice Guidelines. *J Am Coll Cardiol.* 2013;62(16):e147-e239.

# CHAPTER 1

# Heart Failure Diagnosis and Epidemiology

## FAST FACTS

- Heart failure diagnosis is usually based on Framingham criteria: either two major, or one major and two minor criteria. Less severe heart failure can manifest without fulfilling these criteria.

- The ACCF/AHA 4 Stages (A, B, C, D) and the New York Heart Association functional classifications of heart failure (I–IV) are complementary.

### In the United States:

- Heart failure annual incidence increased from 250,000 cases in 1970 to 825,000 cases in 2010, contributing to a prevalence of 5.1 million individuals ≥ 20 years of age.

- Lifetime risk for developing heart failure at the age of 40 years and greater is 1 in 5 in both men and women.

- Between 1979 and 2010, annual heart failure hospitalization rates tripled, with 1,023,000 hospital discharges in 2010.

- In the Medicare population, heart failure is the most common cause for hospitalization.

- After heart failure discharge, readmission rates for recurrent heart failure or other causes are 24% within the first month and 50% within the first 6 months.

- In 2012, direct and indirect medical costs associated with heart failure were $30.7 billion.

- One in 9 deaths includes heart failure on the death certificate.

*"The prime candidates for the development of heart failure are patients with hypertension in whom death from stroke has been prevented by antihypertensive therapy and survivors of acute myocardial infarction who have been spared death from arrhythmia."*

—Eugene Braunwald, Shattuck Lecture 1997[1]

## Heart Failure Recognition

The diagnosis of heart failure may emerge from history, physical examination, or laboratory data.

### CLINICAL CRITERIA OF HEART FAILURE

The Framingham study defined useful clinical criteria to identify patients with heart failure (Table 1.1). Patients not fulfilling the Framingham criteria can still have heart failure, albeit less severe disease, if they have symptoms of dyspnea or fatigue associated with structural or functional left ventricular abnormalities.[2] Specifically, heart failure may be present when an individual has physical limitations at rest or with activity due to inadequate cardiac output or increased left or right ventricular filling pressures. Blood levels of biomarkers, such as B-type natriuretic peptide (BNP), supplement clinical findings to characterize the presence and severity of heart failure.

### HEART FAILURE CLASSIFICATION

In 1928, the New York Heart Association (NYHA) functional classification was proposed to classify the severity of heart failure based on symptoms.[3] In this system, severity ranges from no limitation of functional activity (Class I), slight limitation of functional activity (Class II), marked limitation of functional activity (Class III), to the presence of symptoms at rest (Class IV). Although useful, to characterize a patient's functional impairment at any point in time and provide an index that correlates with prognosis, the system is limited by the potential for a patient's class to either worsen or improve rapidly in response to acute exacerbations or treatments (Figure 1.1).

**TABLE 1.1   Framingham diagnostic criteria for heart failure.** The diagnosis of heart failure, in the Framingham heart failure study, required two major or one major and two concurrent minor criteria. Minor criteria cannot be attributed to another medical condition.[4] *Source:* Adapted from the *New England Journal of Medicine,* with permission.

| MAJOR CRITERIA | MINOR CRITERIA |
| --- | --- |
| Acute pulmonary edema | Dyspnea on exertion |
| Paroxysmal nocturnal dyspnea or orthopnea | Night cough |
| Neck-vein distention | Tachycardia (> 120 beats/min) |
| Rales | Pleural effusion |
| $S_3$ gallop | Hepatomegaly |
| Abdominojugular reflux | Ankle edema |
| Cardiomegaly on chest x-ray | Vital capacity decrease (1/3 from max) |
| Increased venous pressure (> 16 cm $H_2O$) | Weight loss* |
| Weight loss* | |

*Weight loss > 4.5 kg 5 days into treatment can be classified as a major or minor criterion

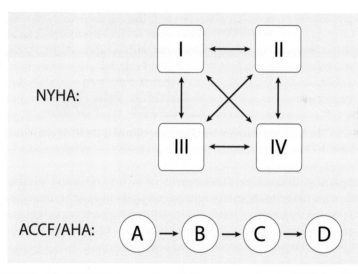

**FIGURE 1.1   The ACCF/AHA stages of heart failure compared to the NYHA classification.** Whereas NYHA functional class can wax and wane, the ACCF/AHA Stages (A–D) can only advance, usually with greater underlying structural and functional cardiac impairment.

Partly to address this potential for fluctuation in NYHA patient classification, in 2001 the American College of Cardiology Foundation and the American Heart Association published a four-component staging of heart failure in which progression occurs in only one direction encompassing risk factors (Stage A) to end-stage heart disease (Stage D).[5] This classification was most recently updated in 2013.[6] The previous New York Heart Association functional class, based solely on symptoms, can still describe the current functional status of a patient in Stages B through D. Especially in Stage C, however, any of the three symptomatic NYHA classifications (Class II, III, or IV) may repeatedly arise, resolve, and recur (Figure 1.2).

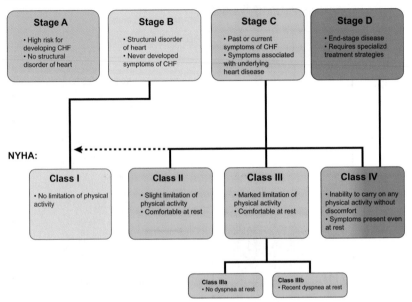

**FIGURE 1.2    The ACCF/AHA stages of heart failure compared to the NYHA classification.** With treatment, a heart failure patient can become asymptomatic, but will remain Stage C.

Stage B is defined as development of structural heart disease in patients who never manifest symptoms or signs of heart failure.[5] Most patients with a diagnosis of heart failure with either past or current symptoms are considered Stage C. Approximately 1% of patients with heart failure have progressed to an advanced Stage D.[2]

# Epidemiology

Heart failure is increasing, particularly as a disease of aging. The prevalence also varies by race and ethnicity.

## PANDEMIC OF HEART FAILURE

As patients survive the progression of acute and chronic cardiovascular disease, the subsequent development of heart failure accompanied by chronic, maladaptive ventricular remodeling becomes more common.[7,8] Insults to the kidneys and peripheral vasculature contribute to this progression. Since 1970, in the United States, heart failure annual incidence has increased markedly (Figure 1.3).

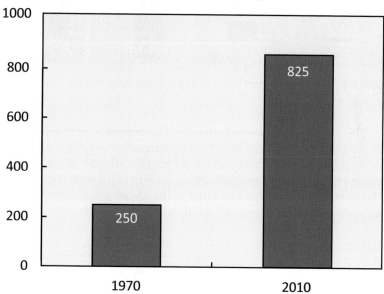

New Patients with Heart Failure (Thousands)

FIGURE 1.3    Increase in incidence of heart failure in United States since 1970.[9,10]

## HEART FAILURE AS A DISEASE OF AGING

After the age of 20, the prevalence of heart failure approximately doubles with each decade of life (Figure 1.4). In 2010, an estimated 5.1 million Americans ≥20 years of age had heart failure.[10] In a community cross-sectional study, 10% of individuals greater than 80 years had heart failure. In those with heart failure, 88% were greater than 65 years, and 49% were older than 80 years.[11]

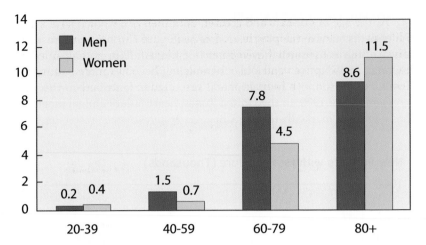

**FIGURE 1.4    Prevalence of heart failure by age in United States.**[10] *Source:* Adapted from *Circulation,* with permission.

The population that is over the age of 65 is rapidly increasing (Figure 1.5). By the year 2030, the U.S. Census Bureau projects that 22% of the U.S. population will be over age 65; worldwide estimates include 24% in Europe and 12% in Asia and Latin America.[12] Thus, in part, the pandemic of heart failure is attributed to aging of the global population, reflecting success in preventing premature death from other causes.[13]

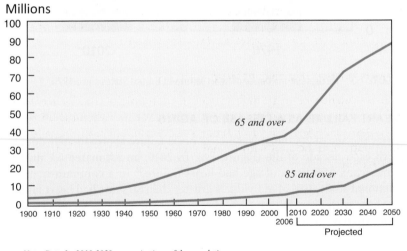

*Note: Data for 2010-2050 are projections of the population.*
*Reference population: These data refer to the resident population.*

**FIGURE 1.5    Numbers of individuals by age group in the United States.** Data for 2010–2050 are projections of the population.[13] *Source:* Adapted from *The Bridge: National Academy of Engineering,* with permission.

At the age of 40 years and greater, both men and women have a 1 in 5 lifetime risk for developing heart failure (Figure 1.6).[14] Even when heart failure due to myocardial infarction is excluded, lifetime risk of heart failure is 1 in 9 for men and 1 in 6 for women. By 2030, the absolute number of individuals with heart failure is projected to increase by 46%.[15]

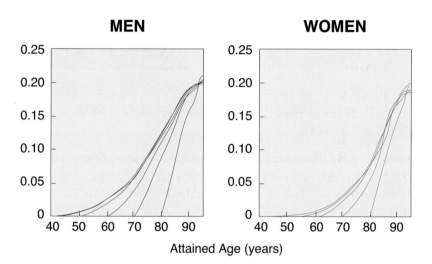

## Cumulative Risk

FIGURE 1.6 **Lifetime risk for developing heart failure.** At ages 40 and greater, the remaining lifetime risk for developing heart failure is 20%, but the risk increases the most in the last decade of life.[14] *Source:* Adapted from *Circulation,* with permission.

### HEART FAILURE AMONG ETHNIC GROUPS

The prevalence of heart failure varies by ethnicity. Blacks are most affected and have a predicted rise in prevalence over the next 20 years, from 2.8% to 3.6% (Figure 1.7). Increased prevalence among certain ethnic groups is associated with higher incidence of hypertension, obesity, and diabetes.

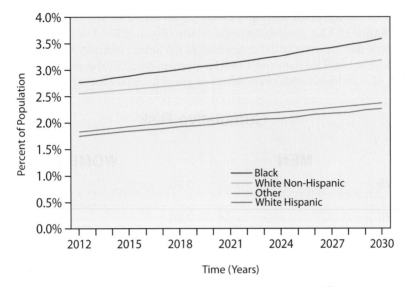

**FIGURE 1.7    Projected prevalence of heart failure increasing among different ethnic groups.**[16] *Source:* Adapted from *Circulation: Heart Failure,* with permission.

# Hospital Admissions and Readmission

Admissions for decompensated heart failure are disruptive and potentially life-threatening events that present a financial burden to society. Since 1970, overall hospitalization rates for heart failure have increased markedly, with a slight decrease noted since 2000 (Figure 1.8).

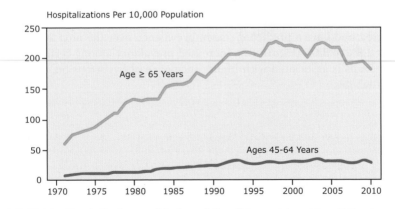

**FIGURE 1.8    Hospitalization trend for heart failure.**[17] *Source:* Adapted from National Institutes of Health: National Heart Lung and Blood Institute, with permission.

In the United States in 2010, admissions for heart failure numbered 1,023,000.[10] Excluding admissions related to uncomplicated pregnancy and delivery, heart failure was second in frequency only to pneumonia. In the Medicare population, heart failure was the leading cause of hospitalization, accounting for over 5% of total admissions.[18] Within 30 days after discharge, following any medical or surgical cause for hospital admission, heart failure was the most common reason for *readmission*, accounting for 8.6% of events.[19]

After hospital discharge for heart failure, subsequent readmission rates are also high. In patients hospitalized for heart failure, all-cause readmission rates are 24% within the first month, and 50% within 6 months.[20,21] Annema and coworkers found the causes of post-heart failure readmissions within 30 days related to recurrent heart failure in 32%, other cardiac causes (non-heart failure) in 32%, and non-cardiac causes in 36%.[22]

When adjusted for age, however, rates for heart failure as a primary or secondary diagnosis since the mid-1990s have plateaued or even decreased in some populations (Figure 1.9). Since patients with heart failure are commonly admitted for other conditions, including respiratory diseases such as pneumonia and chronic obstructive pulmonary disease, rates for hospitalizations with heart failure as a secondary or associated condition are approximately three times those as a primary diagnosis.[23]

Age-Adjusted Hospitalization Rates (per 100,000)

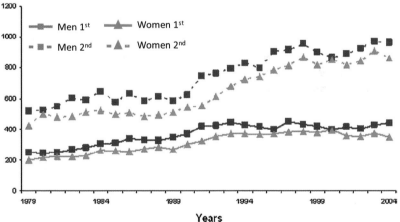

**FIGURE 1.9   Annual age-adjusted hospitalization rates in men and women between 1979 and 2004.** Hospitalization for heart failure as a primary diagnosis (1st) or as an additional diagnosis (2nd).[24] *Source:* Adapted from the *Journal of the American College of Cardiology,* with permission.

# Heart Failure Mortality

In the United States in 2010, heart failure contributed to 279,098 deaths, and for 57,757 cases, was the primary cause of death.[10] According to the Framingham database, after the onset of heart failure, the 30-day, 1-year, and 5-year age-adjusted mortality rates after onset of heart failure declined in the 1980s and 1990s (in both men and women), compared to the two previous decades. In men in the Framingham study, in the period from 1990 through 1999, mortality after heart failure onset was 11% at 30 days, 28% at 1 year, and 59% at 5 years.[25] This decline possibly reflects increased use of evidence-based therapies after heart failure diagnosis (Figure 1.10).[25]

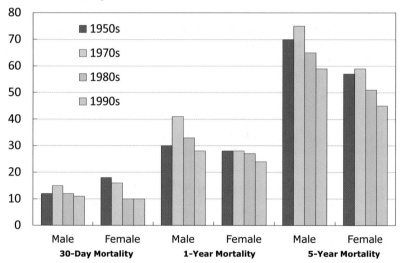

**FIGURE 1.10    Mortality rates after onset of heart failure.** Age-adjusted 30-day, 1-year, and 5-year mortality percentages (years 1950 to 1999) after onset of heart failure in Framingham heart study. Onset of heart failure determined when 2 major, or 1 major and 2 minor, Framingham criteria were met.[25] *Source:* Adapted from the *New England Journal of Medicine,* with permission.

Heart failure mortality varies by U.S. region (Figure 1.11), similar to the geographic distribution of diabetes and obesity (see Chapter 3).

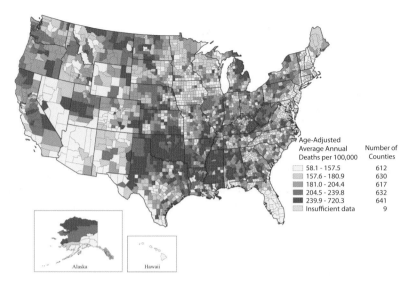

| Age-Adjusted Average Annual Deaths per 100,000 | Number of Counties |
|---|---|
| 58.1 - 157.5 | 612 |
| 157.6 - 180.9 | 630 |
| 181.0 - 204.4 | 617 |
| 204.5 - 239.8 | 632 |
| 239.9 - 720.3 | 641 |
| Insufficient data | 9 |

Alaska       Hawaii

**FIGURE 1.11    Regional heart failure death rates between 2007–2009 in adults age ≥ 35.**[26] *Source:* Adapted from the Centers for Disease Control, National Vital Statistics System and the U.S. Census Bureau, with permission.

## ALL-CAUSE IN-HOSPITAL MORTALITY

An observational study of Medicare fee-for-service patients hospitalized for heart failure between 1993 and 2005 reported that all-cause in-hospital mortality rate decreased from 8.2% to 4.5% (Figure 1.12).[27]

**All-cause In-hospital Mortality (%)**

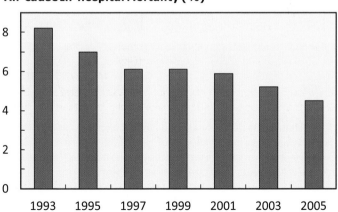

**FIGURE 1.12    All-cause in-hospital mortality rates with heart failure diagnosis.** In-hospital mortality in Medicare fee-for-service patients hospitalized for heart failure between 1993 and 2005.[27] *Source:* Adapted from the *Journal of American Medical Association,* with permission.

## IN-HOSPITAL MORTALITY AND RENAL FUNCTION

Renal function predicts in-hospital mortality from heart failure. In 2003, analysis of the Acute Decompensated Heart Failure National Registry (ADHERE) evaluated the risk for in-hospital mortality (Figure 1.13).[28] Three clinical variables at the time of admission were independently associated with in-hospital mortality: blood urea nitrogen (BUN), systolic blood pressure, and serum creatinine. Thus, 2 of 3 determinants of in-hospital death for heart failure patients were related to kidney dysfunction (see Chapter 10).

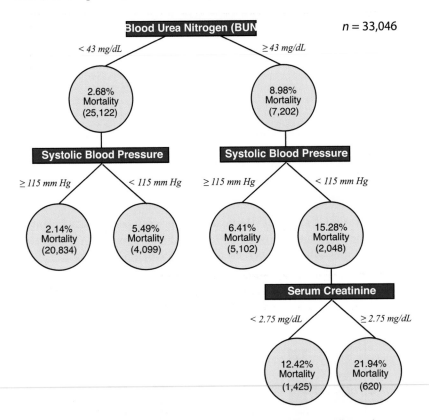

**FIGURE 1.13  Multivariate risk analyses for in-hospital mortality.** Overall mortality in the study was 4%, but ranged in subgroups from 2.1% to 21.9%. *Patient number in each subgroup based on available data such that sums may be less than total.[28] *Source:* Adapted from the *Journal of the American Medical Association*, with permission.

# Costs of Heart Failure

The total costs of heart failure (direct and indirect) are expected to increase from $30.7 billion to $69.7 billion by 2030, in part due to rising total hospitalization and readmission rates (Figure 1.14).[16] To obtain optimal outcomes and reduce preventable hospitalizations, coordination of care and social support are critical for heart failure patients.[29,30]

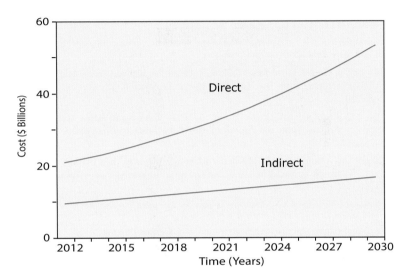

**FIGURE 1.14    Cost of medical care for heart failure.** The projected increase of direct and indirect costs of medical care attributed to heart failure in the United States from 2012 to 2030.[16] *Source:* Adapted from *Circulation: Heart Failure,* with permission.

# References

1.  Braunwald E. Shattuck lecture—cardiovascular medicine at the turn of the millennium: triumphs, concerns, and opportunities. *N Engl J Med.* 1997;337(19):1360-1369.

2.  Ammar KA, Jacobsen SJ, Mahoney DW, et al. Prevalence and prognostic significance of heart failure stages: application of the American College of Cardiology/American Heart Association heart failure staging criteria in the community. *Circulation.* 2007;115(12):1563-1570.

3.  Taichman DB, McGoon MD, Harhay MO, et al. Wide variation in clinicians' assessment of New York Heart Association/World Health Organization functional class in patients with pulmonary arterial hypertension. *Mayo Clinic Proc.* 2009;84(7): 586-592.

4.  McKee PA, Castelli WP, McNamara PM, Kannel WB. The natural history of congestive heart failure: the Framingham study. *N Engl J Med.* 1971;285(26): 1441-1446.

5.  Hunt SA, Abraham WT, Chin MH, et al. ACC/AHA 2005 Guideline Update for the Diagnosis and Management of Chronic Heart Failure in the Adult: a report of the American College of Cardiology/American Heart Association Task Force on Practice Guidelines (Writing Committee to Update the 2001 Guidelines for the Evaluation and Management of Heart Failure): developed in collaboration with the American College of Chest Physicians and the International Society for Heart and Lung Transplantation: endorsed by the Heart Rhythm Society. *Circulation.* 2005;112(12):e154-e235.

6.  Velagaleti RS, Pencina MJ, Murabito JM, et al. Long-term trends in the incidence of heart failure after myocardial infarction. *Circulation.* 2008;118(20):2057-2062.

7.  Braunwald E. Heart failure. *JCHF.* 2013;1(1):1-20.

8.  Burchfield JS, Xie M, Hill JA. Pathological ventricular remodeling: mechanisms: part 1 of 2. *Circulation.* 2013;128(4):388-400.

9.  Roger VL, Go AS, Lloyd-Jones DM, et al. Heart Disease and Stroke Statistics—2012 Update: a report from the American Heart Association. *Circulation.* 2012;125(1): e2-e220.

10. Go AS, Mozaffarian D, Roger VL, et al. Heart disease and stroke statistics—2014 update: a report from the American Heart Association. *Circulation.* 2014;129(3): e28-e292.

11. Senni M, Tribouilloy CM, Rodeheffer RJ, et al. Congestive heart failure in the community: trends in incidence and survival in a 10-year period. *Arch Intern Med.* 1999;159(1):29-34.

12. Vincent GK, Velkoff VA, U.S. Census Bureau. *The next four decades : the older population in the United States : 2010 to 2050.* Washington, D.C.: U.S. Dept. of Commerce, Economics and Statistics Administration, U.S. Census Bureau; 2010.

13. Czaja SJ, Sharit J. The Aging of the Population: Opportunities and Challenges for Human Factors Engineering. *The Bridge: National Academy of Engineering.* 2009; 39(1):34-40.

14. Lloyd-Jones DM, Larson MG, Leip EP, et al. Lifetime risk for developing congestive heart failure: the Framingham Heart Study. *Circulation.* 2002;106(24): 3068-3072.

15. Go AS, Mozaffarian D, Roger VL, et al. Heart disease and stroke statistics—2013 update: a report from the American Heart Association. *Circulation.* 2013;127(1): e6-e245.

16. Heidenreich PA, Albert NM, Allen LA, et al. Forecasting the impact of heart failure in the United States: a policy statement from the American Heart Association. *Circ Heart Fail.* 2013;6(3):606-619.

17. Fact Book: Fiscal Year 2012. *National Institutes of Health: National Heart Lung and Blood Institute.* 2012.

18. Wier LM, Andrews RM. The National Hospital Bill: The Most Expensive Conditions by Payer, 2008. *Healthcare Cost and Utilization Project Statistical Brief.* 2008:1-12.

19. Jencks SF, Williams MV, Coleman EA. Rehospitalizations among patients in the Medicare fee-for-service program. *N Engl J Med.* 2009;360(14):1418-1428.

20. Ross JS, Chen J, Lin Z, et al. Recent national trends in readmission rates after heart failure hospitalization. *Circ Heart Fail.* 2010;3(1):97-103.

21. Desai AS, Stevenson LW. Rehospitalization for heart failure: predict or prevent? *Circulation.* 2012;126(4):501-506.

22. Annema C, Luttik ML, Jaarsma T. Reasons for readmission in heart failure: perspectives of patients, caregivers, cardiologists, and heart failure nurses. *Heart Lung.* 2009;38(5):427-434.

23. Brown AM, Cleland JG. Influence of concomitant disease on patterns of hospitalization in patients with heart failure discharged from Scottish hospitals in 1995. *Eur Heart J.* 1998;19(7):1063-1069.

24. Fang J, Mensah GA, Croft JB, Keenan NL. Heart failure-related hospitalization in the U.S., 1979 to 2004. *J Am Coll Cardiol.* 2008;52(6):428-434.

25. Levy D, Kenchaiah S, Larson MG, et al. Long-term trends in the incidence of and survival with heart failure. *N Engl J Med.* 2002;347(18):1397-1402.

26. Heart Failure Fact Sheet. *CDC: Division for Heart Disease and Stroke Prevention* 2013; http://www.cdc.gov/dhdsp/data_statistics/fact_sheets/fs_heart_failure.htm.

27. Bueno H, Ross JS, Wang Y, et al. Trends in length of stay and short-term outcomes among Medicare patients hospitalized for heart failure, 1993–2006. *JAMA.* 2010; 303(21):2141-2147.

28. Fonarow GC, Adams KF, Jr., Abraham WT, Yancy CW, Boscardin WJ. Risk stratification for in-hospital mortality in acutely decompensated heart failure: classification and regression tree analysis. *JAMA.* 2005;293(5):572-580.

29. Shah NB, Der E, Ruggerio C, Heidenreich PA, Massie BM. Prevention of hospitalizations for heart failure with an interactive home monitoring program. *Am Heart J.* 1998;135(3):373-378.

30. Fonarow GC, Stevenson LW, Walden JA, et al. Impact of a comprehensive heart failure management program on hospital readmission and functional status of patients with advanced heart failure. *J Am Coll Cardiol.* 1997;30(3):725-732.

# CHAPTER 2

# Heart Failure Presentations and Functional Types

## FAST FACTS

- Heart failure occurs with either a reduced (HF-rEF) or preserved (HF-pEF) left ventricular ejection fraction.

- Impaired ventricular contraction (systolic dysfunction) reduces ejection fraction; impaired ventricular filling (diastolic dysfunction) occurs with a preserved or reduced ejection fraction.

- Clinical presentations vary depending on whether heart failure is new onset or chronic and compensated or decompensated.

- Coronary artery disease and left ventricular pressure or volume overload are common causes of cardiac insufficiency.

- Heart failure reduces peak oxygen consumption with exercise by multiple mechanisms.

- Measurement of the biomarkers BNP or NT-proBNP can help "rule in" or "rule out" the presence of heart failure.

*"Symptoms, as a rule, precede signs. Breathlessness is the most important and generally the earliest evidence of heart failure . . . it is necessary to rule out other causes, such as those of a functional and pulmonary nature, before regarding breathlessness as due entirely to the heart. In hypertension, aortic and coronary cases, dyspnea may first appear at night, while in other cases it is first noted on effort. Cheyne-Stokes breathing, especially during sleep, almost always means heart failure. Even before dyspnea occurs, most cardiac patients complain of fatigue, 'lack of pep', restlessness, insomnia, and nervousness."*

—Samuel Levine, MD, from *Clinical Heart Disease,* 1951[1]

## Heart Failure Designation Based on Left Ventricular Systolic Function

The four stages of heart failure are based on the progression of structural heart disease and development of symptoms. Identifying the presence or absence of systolic dysfunction is another important distinction.

### LEFT VENTRICULAR EJECTION FRACTION IN HEART FAILURE

Heart failure occurs with either a reduced (≤ 40%) or preserved (> 40%) left ventricular ejection fraction (EF). Individual center,[2] multicenter registry,[3] and randomized trial data,[4] demonstrate bimodal distributions in left ventricular ejection fraction with nadirs between 40% and 50% (Figure 2.1). The demographics and clinical etiology of patients with reduced (HF-rEF) or preserved (HF-pEF) ejection fraction also differ (Table 2.1). Nevertheless, significant overlap of these 2 groups exists.[5] The 2013 ACCF/AHA guidelines define patients with EF between 41% and 49% as borderline HF-pEF with clinical findings similar to those with EF ≥ 50%.[6]

Published cutoff values for HF-rEF versus HF-pEF range from 40% to 55%.[6-8] **In this book, HF-rEF will be defined as an ejection fraction of less than or equal to 40%** because of the common use of this value for entry into trials of therapies found effective in patients with systolic dysfunction.

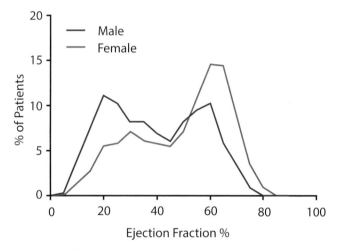

HFrEF    HFpEF

Hospital Based Sample (*n*=4910)

— Male
— Female

% of Patients

Ejection Fraction %

FIGURE 2.1    Bimodal distributions in left ventricular ejection fraction in patients admitted with heart failure at Mayo Clinic (*n* = 4910).[2] *Source:* Adapted from Borlaug & Redfield, *Circulation.* 2011;123(18):2006-2013; discussion 2014, with permission.

## PRESERVATION OF RESTING STROKE VOLUME

Until the late stages of heart failure, resting stroke volume is usually pre-served in both HF-rEF and HF-pEF. In a patient with HF-rEF, a decreased ejection fraction is associated with an increased end-diastolic volume. With HF-pEF, a noncompliant left ventricle is associated with an increased diastolic filling pressure to maintain end-diastolic volume.

TABLE 2.1    Hospitalized heart failure patient demographics with EF < 50% or ≥ 50% (Mean ± SD).[9]

| CHARACTERISTICS | EJECTION FRACTION < 50% (N = 2429) | EJECTION FRACTION ≥ 50% (N = 2167) | P VALUE |
|---|---|---|---|
| Age (yr) | 71.7 ± 12.1 | 74.4 ± 14.4 | < 0.001 |
| Male sex (% of patients) | 65.4 | 44.3 | < 0.001 |
| Body-mass index (kg/m²) | 28.6 ± 7.0 | 29.7 ± 7.8 | 0.002 |
| Serum creatinine on admission (mg/dL) | 1.6 ± 1.0 | 1.6 ± 1.1 | 0.31 |
| Hemoglobin on admission (g/dL) | 12.5 ± 2.0 | 11.8 ± 2.1 | < 0.001 |
| Hypertension (% of patients) | 48.0 | 62.7 | < 0.001 |
| Coronary artery disease (% of patients) | 63.7 | 52.9 | < 0.001 |
| Atrial fibrillation (% of patients) | 28.5 | 41.3 | < 0.001 |
| Diabetes (% of patients) | 34.3 | 33.1 | 0.42 |
| Substantial valve disease (% of patients) | 6.5 | 2.6 | < 0.001 |
| Ejection fraction (%) | 29 ± 10 | 61 ± 7 | < 0.001 |

Source: Adapted from Owan et al., N Engl J Med. 2006;355(3):251-259, with permission.

## ROLE OF DIASTOLIC DYSFUNCTION IN HF-pEF

> HF-rEF always implies systolic dysfunction; HF-pEF *often, but not always* includes diastolic dysfunction.

Doppler echocardiographic characterization of patterns of blood or tissue velocities during ventricular filling has been used to define abnormal filling patterns, diastolic dysfunction, and estimation of left atrial pressure (see Chapter 7). Diastolic dysfunction, however, is not equivalent to HF-pEF. Approximately one-third of patients with HF-pEF do not have identifiable diastolic dysfunction by echocardiography.[10] In addition, patients with a reduced ejection fraction may also have diastolic abnormalities, highlighting the linked relationship between the hemodynamics of systole and diastole.[11]

Finally, some individuals may have the echocardiographic findings of diastolic dysfunction without any past or present clinical syndrome of heart failure.[10]

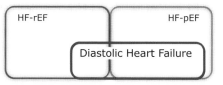

Therefore, in the presence of a left ventricular ejection fraction greater than 40%, the diagnosis of HF-pEF depends on the clinical findings consistent with an elevated left ventricular filling pressure (e.g., pulmonary edema) supported by echocardiographic findings or catheter pressure measurements. The HF-pEF patient typically will have elevated blood levels of brain natriuretic peptide (BNP) (see the Biomarkers section below, and Chapter 5), although not generally as high as in HF-rEF.[12]

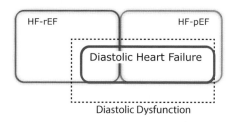

Diastolic Dysfunction

## WHEN TO TREAT HF-pEF LIKE HF-rEF

Two subgroups of patients with HF-pEF should be considered for pharmacologic therapies validated for HF-rEF. The first are those with a borderline EF of 40% to 50% with clinical features of either HF-rEF or HF-pEF. The second subgroup includes patients who previously had an EF ≤ 40% who now have recovered to a higher EF. Depending on the etiology of the previous reduced EF, this subgroup may be prone to relapses of reduced EF and therefore will benefit from long-term preventive therapy.[13]

# Acute and Chronic Presentations of Heart Failure

In addition to the treatment of symptoms and restoring hemodynamic stability, different presentations of heart failure have potentially different therapeutic goals.

### NEW-ONSET HEART FAILURE

If new in onset, then determining the etiology of heart failure is a priority. In the presence of acute pulmonary edema (Figure 2.2), an aggressive approach is necessary, and improvement of symptoms will follow amelioration of abnormal hemodynamics. In heart failure with acute ischemic syndromes, revascularization improves outcomes.[14,15]

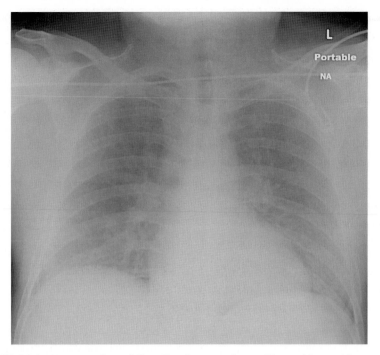

**FIGURE 2.2    New-onset heart failure.** This chest x-ray shows a 49-year-old man with acute anterior myocardial infarct and new-onset heart failure. Pulmonary congestion is present with a relatively normal-sized cardiac silhouette. Urgent percutaneous coronary revascularization and diuretics led to improvement.

## COMPENSATED CHRONIC HEART FAILURE

In a patient with compensated heart failure, there are few active symptoms by definition; after treating causes of cardiac dysfunction, the priority may be to delay or reverse progression of structural heart disease by blunting neurohumoral activation. These patients may have either newly recognized or known chronic left ventricular dysfunction without overt resting findings (Figure 2.3). Symptoms, however, may appear with activity.

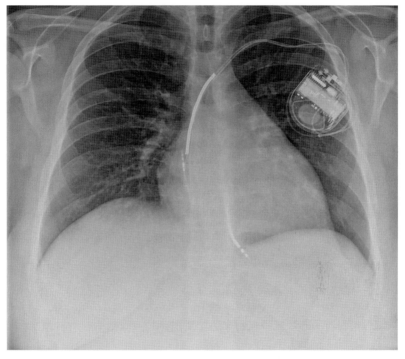

**FIGURE 2.3    Compensated chronic nonischemic cardiomyopathy.** In this 24-year-old man, heart size is increased, but lung fields are clear. An implantable cardioverter-defibrillator (ICD) device is present with leads in the right atrium and right ventricle.

## ACUTE-ON-CHRONIC HEART FAILURE

In a patient with a history of heart failure who presents in a decompensated state, the priority is less to make a diagnosis of the etiology of heart failure (this is usually known) and more to identify the precipitating factors for the decompensation (see Chapter 9). A patient may have pulmonary edema, systemic congestion, or both (Figures 2.4 and 2.5). Findings of low cardiac output, including fatigue, poor mentation, hypotension, and hepatic and renal dysfunction, may coexist.

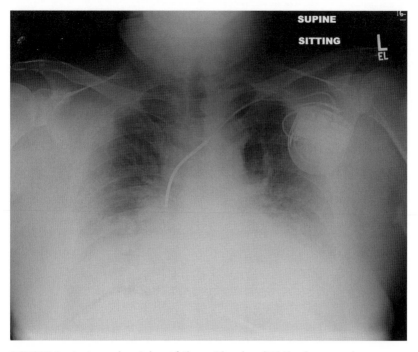

**FIGURE 2.4    Acute-on-chronic heart failure with reduced EF.** The chest x-ray shows a 60-year-old man with history of ischemic cardiomyopathy, moderate renal insufficiency, and increasing shortness of breath. Marked cardiomegaly is obscured by pulmonary congestion and bilateral pleural effusions.

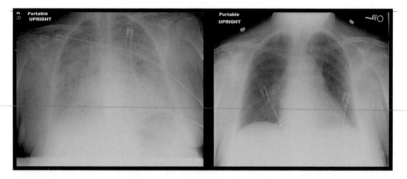

**FIGURE 2.5    Acute-on-chronic heart failure with preserved EF.** This x-ray shows a 79-year-old female presenting with acute shortness of breath and atrial fibrillation with rapid ventricular response associated with history of previous HF-pEF, coronary artery bypass surgery, hypertension, and diabetes. Left ventricular ejection fraction was 70%. Diuresis and slowing of heart rate led to resolution of pulmonary edema in 3 days.

# Common Causes of Heart Failure

Hemodynamic features of heart failure with circulatory congestion or inadequate tissue perfusion may be similar regardless of the etiology of heart pump insufficiency. HF-rEF with systolic dysfunction usually predominates following myocardial infarction, chronic volume overload, or dilated cardiomyopathy. HF-pEF with diastolic dysfunction typically develops with hypertension and diastolic dysfunction, myocardial ischemia without infarction, aortic stenosis, and with hypertrophic or restrictive cardiomyopathies (Figure 2.6).[16]

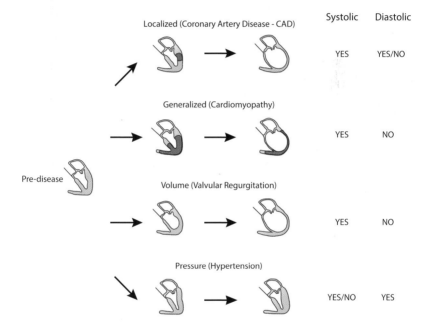

| | | Systolic | Diastolic |
|---|---|---|---|
| Localized (Coronary Artery Disease - CAD) | | YES | YES/NO |
| Generalized (Cardiomyopathy) | | YES | NO |
| Volume (Valvular Regurgitation) | | YES | NO |
| Pressure (Hypertension) | | YES/NO | YES |

**FIGURE 2.6 Secondary remodeling and heart failure.** Examples of types of heart failure with a primary insult progressing via secondary remodeling.[16] *Source:* Reproduced with permission from Gorlin R., *Circulation.* 1987;75(suppl IV):108-111.

## HEART FAILURE CAUSED BY CORONARY ARTERY DISEASE AND MYOCARDIAL INFARCTION

In patients with recent or remote myocardial infarctions, the severity of the associated heart failure correlates with the extent of left ventricular muscle volume replaced by necrosis or fibrosis.[17] In a meta-analysis of population-based versus clinical trial studies, the mean in-hospital incidence of heart failure after acute myocardial infarction was 37% in population-based studies compared to 18% in clinical trials, likely reflecting the exclusion of some high-risk patients in clinical trials.[18] Compared to those with uncomplicated myocardial infarction, patients with myocardial infarction and heart failure had up to a five-fold increase in 1-year mortality.[18] In a multicenter trial of reperfusion for acute ST-elevation myocardial infarction, the profound heart failure state of cardiogenic shock was present in less than 1% of patients at the time of admission, but developed in 6.4% during hospital admission.[19] The later development of cardiac pump failure may be mediated by time-dependent neurohumoral activation, fluid retention, myocardial remodeling, or reinfarction.[20]

### Cardiogenic Shock
Heart failure with severe systemic hypoperfusion, usually with hypotension and pulmonary edema.

Alternatively, coronary artery disease (CAD) without infarction but with global myocardial ischemia may also lead to heart failure. Abrupt onset (or "flash") pulmonary edema may be the initial presentation of diffuse atherosclerosis or left main CAD (Figure 2.7).[21] Especially in diabetics, this may occur without symptoms of angina.[22] Revascularization may improve prognosis in these groups.[23]

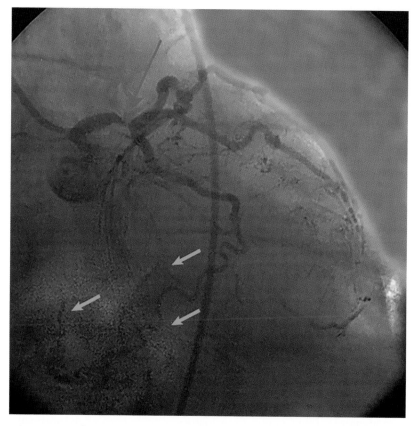

FIGURE 2.7    **Left main stenosis and heart failure.** Angiogram from patient with HF-pEF manifest as flash pulmonary edema due to coronary artery disease. **Upper arrow:** High grade distal left main coronary lesion. **Lower arrows:** Collateral left coronary artery filling of occluded branch of right coronary artery.

## HEART FAILURE CAUSED BY HYPERTENSION AND VALVULAR HEART DISEASE

The left ventricle responds to either pressure or volume overload with characteristic changes in morphology.

Chronic left ventricular *pressure* overload due to hypertension or aortic valve stenosis can lead to concentric hypertrophy of the left ventricle, with increases in left ventricular mass and wall thickness relative to internal chamber dimension.[24] Impaired diastolic filling and HF-pEF may result. Systolic function and EF are, at least initially, preserved. If pressure overload is sustained, however, eccentric (dilated) hypertrophy may gradually develop and result in HF-rEF.

Left ventricular *volume* overload due to valvular regurgitation or high output states can initially be associated with a normal or increased ejection fraction. Over time, however, progressive eccentric hypertrophy of the left ventricle is associated with a progressive decrease in ejection fraction.[24] Ultimately, a dilated left ventricle with poor systolic function can result (see Chapter 4).[25]

# Heart Failure Blunts Exercise Capacity

Reductions in both physical activity and peak oxygen consumption are characteristic findings associated with heart failure.

## CARDIAC HEMODYNAMICS

Abnormal hemodynamics at rest or with exertion can limit the ability of an individual with heart failure to perform aerobic activity.[25,26] Basic parameters of cardiac output, pulmonary capillary wedge pressure, and systemic vascular resistance differ between normal and heart failure patients (Figure 2.8).

Hemodynamics ("Blood Movement")
The study of the forces or mechanisms involved in the flow of blood and the circulation.

Clinical findings can indicate patient volume status and cardiac hemodynamics (see Chapter 6). A history of orthopnea or dyspnea with exertion, as well as physical exam findings of edema, neck vein distension, or abdominojugular reflux, imply circulatory congestion due to increased venous and ventricular filling pressures. Asthenia or poor mentation, a reduced pulse pressure, and renal or hepatic dysfunction without a non-cardiac cause can suggest a low cardiac output.

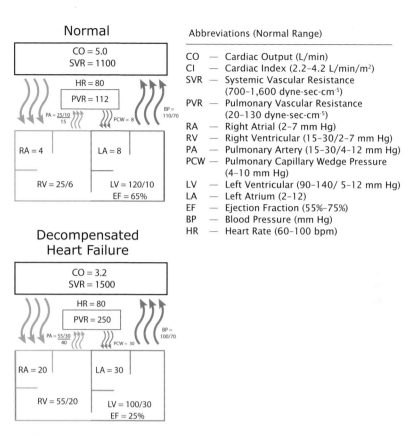

**Normal**

Abbreviations (Normal Range)

| | |
|---|---|
| CO | — Cardiac Output (L/min) |
| CI | — Cardiac Index (2.2–4.2 L/min/m²) |
| SVR | — Systemic Vascular Resistance (700–1,600 dyne·sec·cm⁻⁵) |
| PVR | — Pulmonary Vascular Resistance (20–130 dyne·sec·cm⁻⁵) |
| RA | — Right Atrial (2–7 mm Hg) |
| RV | — Right Ventricular (15–30/2–7 mm Hg) |
| PA | — Pulmonary Artery (15–30/4–12 mm Hg) |
| PCW | — Pulmonary Capillary Wedge Pressure (4–10 mm Hg) |
| LV | — Left Ventricular (90–140/ 5–12 mm Hg) |
| LA | — Left Atrium (2–12) |
| EF | — Ejection Fraction (55%–75%) |
| BP | — Blood Pressure (mm Hg) |
| HR | — Heart Rate (60–100 bpm) |

**Decompensated Heart Failure**

**FIGURE 2.8  Examples of hemodynamic parameters.** Normal values and values in decompensated heart failure.[27] *Source:* Adapted with permission from Jaski BE, *Basics of Heart Failure.* Springer Science + Business Media B.V.; 2000: 26.

## FACTORS CONTRIBUTING TO REDUCED OXYGEN CONSUMPTION

Peak oxygen consumption is determined by both the capacity of the heart to deliver oxygenated blood and the ability of the tissues to extract oxygen. Reasons for reduced peak oxygen consumption with activity include insufficient cardiac output (heart rate multiplied by stroke volume), anemia, pulmonary congestion, skeletal muscle deconditioning, or orthopedic limitations. In heart failure, the normal ability to increase cardiac output and oxygen consumption with exercise is reduced (Figure 2.9).

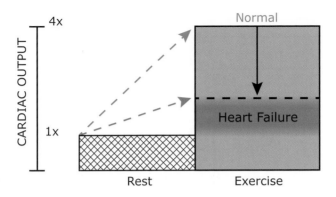

**FIGURE 2.9** Heart failure reduces exercise cardiac output and maximum oxygen consumption.

## ESTIMATING OXYGEN CONSUMPTION

Oxygen consumption ($VO_2$) equals the circulating cardiac output multiplied by the tissue oxygen extraction or $\Delta AVO_2$—the difference between the arterial oxygen concentration delivered to the body tissues minus the remaining oxygen concentration in the venous circulation after capillary exchange. Cardiac output equals the heart rate (HR) multiplied by the stroke volume (SV) ejected by the left ventricle with each beat.

$O_2$ consumption = cardiac output × $\Delta AVO_2$

$O_2$ consumption = (HR × SV) × $\Delta AVO_2$

## PHYSICAL ACTIVITY AND OXYGEN CONSUMPTION IN A NORMAL INDIVIDUAL

Normal individuals can increase oxygen consumption twelve-fold with exercise compared to standing at rest.[26] This is accomplished by an average twofold increase in heart rate (HR), a twofold increase in ventricular stroke volume (SV), and a threefold increase in tissue oxygen extraction ($\Delta AVO_2$) defined as the difference between arterial and venous blood oxygen concentration (Figure 2.10). An average 20-year-old man will have a maximum $VO_2$ of 45 mL/kg/min. Maximum oxygen utilization decreases with age such that an average 60-year-old man will have one-third less capacity.[26] On average, women will have a maximum $VO_2$ that is 20% less than men's. This is attributed to less muscle mass, lower hemoglobin and circulating blood volume, and smaller stroke volume in women.[26] Understanding an individual's hemodynamic basis for activity limitation can help target specific therapies, as well as gauge the severity of their impairment.

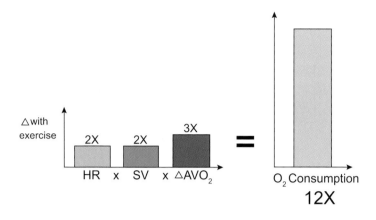

FIGURE 2.10 **Exercise increases oxygen consumption.** Increase in oxygen utilization from standing at rest to maximum exercise in an average 25 year old man weighing 80 kg.[26] Abbreviations: HR, heart rate; SV, stroke volume; $\Delta AVO_2$ (tissue extraction), arterial minus venous oxygen concentration.

## RESPIRATORY EXCHANGE RATIO

The respiratory exchange ratio (RER) is the ratio of carbon dioxide produced to oxygen consumed. RER can be used to determine whether an individual exceeds the anaerobic threshold with peak activity. At rest, the amount of oxygen an individual consumes is greater than the amount of carbon dioxide he or she produces (meaning, the RER is less than 1.0). When activity is limited by cardiac output reserve, the anaerobic threshold will be exceeded, and RER should then exceed 1.0. If peak $VO_2$ during exercise testing is measured as part of a heart failure evaluation, then RER should also be assessed. When RER at peak exercise remains less than 1.0 and anaerobic threshold is not exceeded, it may indicate that noncardiac factors limit physical activity.

## LIMITATIONS IN EXERCISE CAPACITY WITH HEART FAILURE

In patients with heart failure, the normal increase in oxygen consumption with exercise can be limited by inability to increase heart rate, stroke volume, or tissue oxygen extraction, or any combination of all three factors. For example, compared with a normal individual, a patient with heart failure and a fixed stroke volume will have an impaired increase of cardiac output with activity. This could limit the maximum potential increase in oxygen consumption with exercise to only sixfold when heart rate and tissue extraction of oxygen ($\Delta AVO_2$) have reached their maximum (Figure 2.11). An impaired increase in heart rate can also limit exercise (Figure 2.12). Alternatively, a patient with heart failure and either perceived dyspnea without hypoxia or skeletal muscle deconditioning will stop exercise before achieving a maximum tissue extraction of oxygen ($\Delta AVO_2$ of only 2X instead of 3X) (Figure 2.13).

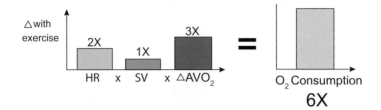

**FIGURE 2.11    Oxygen consumption limited by stroke volume.** Example of a fixed left ventricular stroke volume limiting oxygen utilization with exercise in heart failure.[27] *Source:* Adapted with permission from Jaski BE, *Basics of Heart Failure.* Springer Science + Business Media B.V.; 2000: 28.

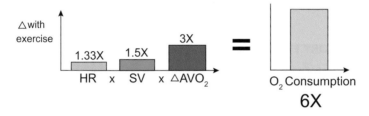

**FIGURE 2.12    Limitation by blunted heart rate rise.** Example of oxygen utilization limited by inadequate increases in heart rate and stroke volume with activity in heart failure.

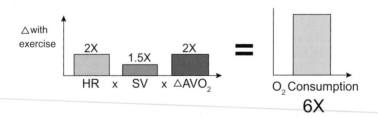

**FIGURE 2.13    Limitation in tissue oxygen extraction ($\Delta AVO_2$).** Example of oxygen utilization limited by perceived dyspnea without hypoxia or skeletal muscle deconditioning in heart failure patients with exercise, before maximum tissue extraction of oxygen is achieved. Typically, RER will not exceed 1.0.[27] *Source:* Adapted with permission from Jaski BE, *Basics of Heart Failure.* Springer Science + Business Media B.V.; 2000: 28.

# The Role of Biomarkers BNP and NT-proBNP When Heart Failure Is Suspected

B-type natriuretic peptide (BNP) functions in maintaining cardiovascular homeostasis by acting as a vasodilator and promoter of sodium excretion by the kidney. BNP is structurally and functionally similar to ANP (atrial natriuretic peptide) and CNP (C-type natriuretic peptide).

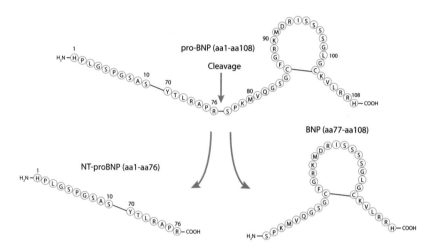

**FIGURE 2.14    Enzymatic cleavage and products of pro-BNP.** Pro-BNP from cardiac ventricular myocytes is cleaved into two molecules: inactive NT-proBNP (76 amino acids) and the biologically active BNP (32 amino acids).

Ventricular myocytes under increased volume or pressure load increase transcription and translation of the precursor protein pro-BNP.[12] Intracellular pro-BNP is enzymatically cleaved by proteases corin and furin into active (BNP) and inactive (NT-proBNP) molecules (Table 2.2), which are subsequently released by the myocyte in equimolar amounts (Figure 2.14).[28,29] While circulating BNP is cleared by receptors located in the liver, lungs, kidneys, and vascular endothelium, NT-proBNP is more exclusively cleared by the kidneys.[28] Measurement of an elevated blood level of BNP or NT-proBNP may signal the presence of clinical heart failure and help gauge its severity.[30]

**TABLE 2.2   BNP versus NT-proBNP.**

|  | BNP | NT-proBNP |
|---|---|---|
| SIZE (AMINO ACID) | 32AA | 76AA |
| ACTIVITY | Bioactive | Inactive |
| NORMAL RANGE | 5-50 pg/mL | 7-160 pg/mL |
| TYPICAL UPPER VALUE OF ASSAY | 3,000 pg/mL | 35,000 pg/mL |
| PLASMA HALF-LIFE | ~ 22 minutes | ~ 60-120 minutes |
| TIME TO REFLECT HEMODYNAMIC CHANGE | ~ 2 hours | ~ 12 hours |
| RENAL CLEARANCE | < 5% | > 90% |

## BNP TO DIAGNOSE OR RULE OUT HEART FAILURE

For patients who initially presented with acute dyspnea, The Breathing Not Properly study found that using a BNP level of 100 pg/mL or higher resulted in an 83.4% diagnostic accuracy (defined as the sum of true positive and true negative divided by total number of samples) for recognizing the presence of heart failure.[31] In the N-terminal PRIDE study (for **PR**o-**BNP** **I**nvestigation of **D**yspnea in the **E**mergency Department), NT-proBNP similarly had a high sensitivity and specificity for the diagnosis of acute heart failure in patients who presented with dyspnea.[32] An observed age-dependent relationship between NT-proBNP and the respective values for sensitivity and specificity, led to age-dependent optimal cutoff points for this biomarker (Figure 2.15).

## INTERPRETATION OF NATRIURETIC PEPTIDE LEVELS

Heart failure may not be the only reason for elevated BNP and NT-proBNP levels. In patients with renal insufficiency, measured natriuretic peptide levels may be high due to increased production, decreased clearance, or both (Figure 2.16, A–C). In general, however, the higher the level of BNP or NT-proBNP, the more likely it is that left ventricular dysfunction is present.[28]

## Heart Failure Biomarker Cutoffs

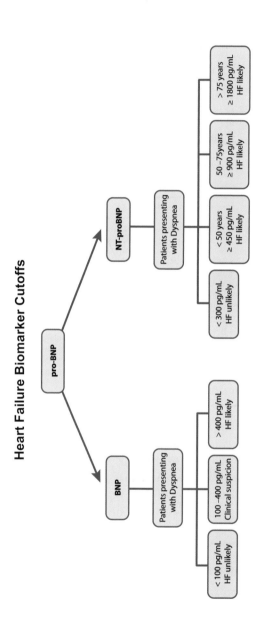

**FIGURE 2.15** "Rule in" values for heart failure biomarkers. Interpretation is independent of age for BNP levels (left arm). NT-proBNP levels (right arm) depend on patient age. Measurements of both peptide levels have similar sensitivities of >90% and specificities of >70%.[31,33]

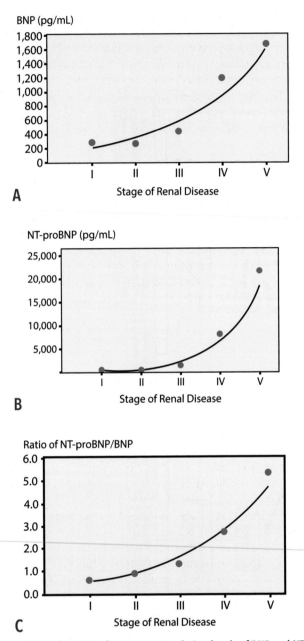

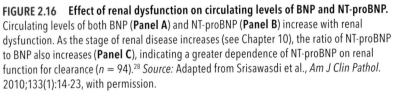

**FIGURE 2.16   Effect of renal dysfunction on circulating levels of BNP and NT-proBNP.**
Circulating levels of both BNP (**Panel A**) and NT-proBNP (**Panel B**) increase with renal
dysfunction. As the stage of renal disease increases (see Chapter 10), the ratio of NT-proBNP
to BNP also increases (**Panel C**), indicating a greater dependence of NT-proBNP on renal
function for clearance ($n = 94$).[28] *Source:* Adapted from Srisawasdi et al., *Am J Clin Pathol.*
2010;133(1):14-23, with permission.

Other conditions with increased natriuretic peptide levels include right ventricular dysfunction, pulmonary hypertension, chronic obstructive pulmonary disease, pneumonia, and pulmonary embolism.[34] Obesity may be inversely related to circulating levels of BNP and NT-proBNP. This is attributed to increased receptor-based clearance with increased body size.[35] In order to compensate for this relationship, it has been suggested to use lower cut-off values such as BNP <50 pg/mL when measuring levels in patients with a body mass index >35 kg/m².[34]

### MEASURED VERSUS ACTIVE ENDOGENOUS BNP

BNP and NT-proBNP are measured immunologically and elevated levels are strong indicators of heart failure. However, these assays may measure multiple forms of these peptides. These altered molecules, nicknamed "junk BNP," are immunoreactive, but minimally hormonally active.[36] In heart failure, the predominant altered form is uncleaved pro-BNP, suggesting that the precursor peptide can be released without cleavage into a hormonally active form. A decrease in the enzymatic activity of corin in patients with heart failure may be a reason for increased levels of detected but inactive pro-BNP.[37,38]

# Other Heart Failure Biomarkers

Other biomarkers may be useful as diagnostic and prognostic tools for heart failure. Cardiac troponin (cTn) is a sensitive and specific marker for cardiac injury resulting from ischemia or stress to the myocardium and is an independent risk factor for death in chronic heart failure.[35,39] Two other biomarkers produced by ventricular myocytes are ST2, which is released with stretch, and galectin-3, which is associated with myocardial fibrosis; both biomarkers are increased in patients with heart failure.[39-42] Although BNP and NT-proBNP may be superior in diagnosing heart failure, elevations of ST2 and galectin-3 may be more robust predictors for 60-day and 1-year mortality.[42] In the future, a panel of peptides may permit more personally tailored therapies based on a heart failure patient's phenotype (Figure 2.17).

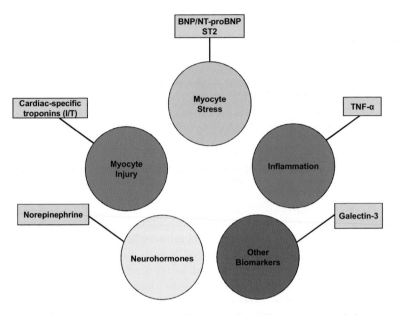

**FIGURE 2.17   Biomarkers linked to heart failure etiology.** These markers may help characterize pathogenesis, diagnosis, prognosis and potential therapeutic targets.

# EUGENE BRAUNWALD, MD
## (1929–PRESENT)

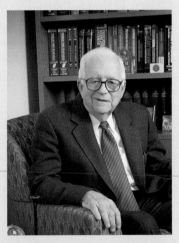

*"The best book of cardiology is the patient itself."*

A heart attack is a progressive event where coronary reperfusion may limit myocardial cell damage. Although this may seem to be an accepted fact, it is due in part to the work of Dr. Eugene Braunwald that this is now understood, among countless other aspects of cardiovascular medicine. In the field of heart failure, he has performed and published scientific clinical investigations of valvular, myocardial, and ischemic causes of cardiac impairment. Dr. Braunwald's publication of more than 1000 articles has guided the process of translating research into improved patient care. For decades he held the Distinguished Hersey Professor of Medicine at Harvard Medical School and chaired the Thrombolysis in Myocardial Infarction (TIMI) Study Group at Brigham and Women's Hospital. He has served as editor of both *Braunwald's Heart Disease* and *Harrison's Principles of Internal Medicine.* Dr. Braunwald's work, along with that of the many other cardiologists he has trained, has served as a catalyst for progress in the field of cardiovascular medicine.

# References

1. Levine SA. Nature and treatment of congestive heart failure. *Clinical Heart Disease.* 4 ed. Philadelphia: WB Saunders; 1951:291.

2. Borlaug BA, Redfield MM. Diastolic and systolic heart failure are distinct phenotypes within the heart failure spectrum. *Circulation.* 2011;123(18):2006-2013; discussion 2014.

3. Fonarow GC, Stough WG, Abraham WT, et al. Characteristics, treatments, and outcomes of patients with preserved systolic function hospitalized for heart failure: a report from the OPTIMIZE-HF Registry. *J Am Coll Cardiol.* 2007;50(8): 768-777.

4. Gaasch WH, Delorey DE, Kueffer FJ, Zile MR. Distribution of left ventricular ejection fraction in patients with ischemic and hypertensive heart disease and chronic heart failure. *J Am Coll Cardiol.* 2009;104(10):1413-1415.

5. Bronzwaer JG, Paulus WJ. Diastolic and systolic heart failure: different stages or distinct phenotypes of the heart failure syndrome? *Curr Heart Fail Rep.* 2009;6(4): 281-286.

6. Yancy CW, Jessup M, Bozkurt B, et al. 2013 ACCF/AHA Guideline for the Management of Heart Failure: a report of the American College of Cardiology Foundation/American Heart Association Task Force on Practice Guidelines. *J Am Coll Cardiol.* 2013;62(16):e147-e239.

7. Lindenfeld J, Albert NM, Boehmer JP, et al. HFSA 2010 Comprehensive Heart Failure Practice Guideline. *J Card Fail.* 2010;16(6):e1-e194.

8. Sanderson JE. HFNEF, HFpEF, HF-PEF, or DHF What is in an acronym? *JACC. Heart Fail.* 2014;2(1):93-94.

9. Owan TE, Hodge DO, Herges RM, Jacobsen SJ, Roger VL, Redfield MM. Trends in prevalence and outcome of heart failure with preserved ejection fraction. *N Engl J Med.* 2006;355(3):251-259.

10. Yu CM, Lin H, Yang H, Kong SL, Zhang Q, Lee SW. Progression of systolic abnormalities in patients with "isolated" diastolic heart failure and diastolic dysfunction. *Circulation.* 2002;105(10):1195-1201.

11. Brutsaert DL, Rademakers FE, Sys SU. Triple control of relaxation: implications in cardiac disease. *Circulation.* 1984;69(1):190-196.

12. Maeder MT, Mariani JA, Kaye DM. Hemodynamic determinants of myocardial B-type natriuretic peptide release: relative contributions of systolic and diastolic wall stress. *Hypertension.* 2010;56(4):682-689.

13. Yancy CW, Jessup M, Bozkurt B, et al. 2013 ACCF/AHA guideline for the management of heart failure: a report of the American College of Cardiology Foundation/American Heart Association Task Force on Practice Guidelines. *J Am Coll Cardiol.* 2013;62(16):e147-239.

14. Braunwald E, Kloner RA. The stunned myocardium: prolonged, postischemic ventricular dysfunction. *Circulation.* 1982;66(6):1146-1149.

15. Sjoblom J, Muhrbeck J, Witt N, Alam M, Frykman-Kull V. Evolution of left ventricular ejection fraction after acute myocardial infarction: implications for implantable cardioverter-defibrillator eligibility. *Circulation.* 2014;130(9):743-748.

16. Gorlin R. Treatment of congestive heart failure: where are we going? *Circulation.* 1987;75(5 Pt 2):IV108-IV111.

17. Page DL, Caulfield JB, Kastor JA, DeSanctis RW, Sanders CA. Myocardial changes associated with cardiogenic shock. *N Engl J Med.* 1971;285(3):133-137.

18. Hellermann JP, Jacobsen SJ, Gersh BJ, Rodeheffer RJ, Reeder GS, Roger VL. Heart failure after myocardial infarction: a review. *Am J Med.* 2002;113(4):324-330.

19. Holmes DR, Jr., Bates ER, Kleiman NS, et al. Contemporary reperfusion therapy for cardiogenic shock: the GUSTO-I trial experience. The GUSTO-I Investigators. Global Utilization of Streptokinase and Tissue Plasminogen Activator for Occluded Coronary Arteries. *J Am Coll Cardiol.* 1995;26(3):668-674.

20. Weisman HF, Healy B. Myocardial infarct expansion, infarct extension, and reinfarction: pathophysiologic concepts. *Prog Cardiovasc Dis.* 1987;30(2):73-110.

21. Lim MJ, Goldstein JA. In: Kern MJ, ed. *Hemodynamic Rounds: Interpretation of Cardiac Pathophysiology from Pressure Waveform Analysis.* Vol 3: Wiley-Blackwell; 2009:452.

22. Stern S. Symptoms other than chest pain may be important in the diagnosis of "silent ischemia," or "the sounds of silence." *Circulation.* 2005;111(24):e435-e437.

23. Jessup M, Abraham WT, Casey DE, et al. 2009 focused update: ACCF/AHA Guidelines for the Diagnosis and Management of Heart Failure in Adults: a report of the American College of Cardiology Foundation/American Heart Association Task Force on Practice Guidelines: developed in collaboration with the International Society for Heart and Lung Transplantation. *Circulation.* 2009;119(14):1977-2016.

24. Popescu BA, Beladan CC, Calin A, et al. Left ventricular remodelling and torsional dynamics in dilated cardiomyopathy: reversed apical rotation as a marker of disease severity. *Eur J Heart Fail.* 2009;11(10):945-951.

25. Ammar KA, Jacobsen SJ, Mahoney DW, et al. Prevalence and prognostic significance of heart failure stages: application of the American College of Cardiology/American Heart Association heart failure staging criteria in the community. *Circulation.* 2007;115(12):1563-1570.

26. Mitchell JH, Blomqvist G. Maximal oxygen uptake. *N Engl J Med.* 1971;284(18): 1018-1022.

27. Jaski BE. *Basics of Heart Failure: A Problem Solving Approach.* Boston: Kluwer Academic Publishers; 2000.

28. Srisawasdi P, Vanavanan S, Charoenpanichkit C, Kroll MH. The effect of renal dysfunction on BNP, NT-proBNP, and their ratio. *Am J Clin Pathol.* 2010;133(1):14-23.

29. Hawkridge AM, Heublein DM, Bergen HR, III, Cataliotti A, Burnett JC, Jr., Muddiman DC. Quantitative mass spectral evidence for the absence of circulating brain natriuretic peptide (BNP-32) in severe human heart failure. *Proc Natl Acad Sci U.S.A.* 2005;102(48):17442-17447.

30. Felker GM, Hasselblad V, Hernandez AF, O'Connor CM. Biomarker-guided therapy in chronic heart failure: a meta-analysis of randomized controlled trials. *Am Heart J.* 2009;158(3):422-430.

31. Maisel AS, Krishnaswamy P, Nowak RM, et al. Rapid measurement of B-type natriuretic peptide in the emergency diagnosis of heart failure. *N Engl J Med.* 2002; 347(3):161-167.

32. Januzzi JL, Jr., Camargo CA, Anwaruddin S, et al. The N-terminal Pro-BNP investigation of dyspnea in the emergency department (PRIDE) study. *Am J Cardiol.* 2005; 95(8):948-954.

33. Januzzi JL, van Kimmenade R, Lainchbury J, et al. NT-proBNP testing for diagnosis and short-term prognosis in acute destabilized heart failure: an international pooled

analysis of 1256 patients: the International Collaborative of NT-proBNP Study. *Eur Heart J.* 2006;27(3):330-337.

34. Maisel A, Mueller C, Adams K, Jr., et al. State of the art: using natriuretic peptide levels in clinical practice. *Eur J Heart Fail.* 2008;10(9):824-839.

35. Jaffe AS, Babuin L, Apple FS. Biomarkers in acute cardiac disease: the present and the future. *J Am Coll Cardiol.* 2006;48(1):1-11.

36. Hobbs RE, Mills RM. Endogenous B-type natriuretic peptide: a limb of the regulatory response to acutely decompensated heart failure. *Clin Cardiol.* 2008;31(9):407-412.

37. Chen S, Sen S, Young D, Wang W, Moravec CS, Wu Q. Protease corin expression and activity in failing hearts. *Am J Physiol Heart Circ Physiol.* 2010;299(5):H1687-H1692.

38. Xu-Cai YO, Wu Q. Molecular forms of natriuretic peptides in heart failure and their implications. *Heart.* 2010;96(6):419-424.

39. Braunwald E. Biomarkers in heart failure. *N Engl J Med.* 2008;358(20):2148-2159.

40. de Boer RA, Yu L, van Veldhuisen DJ. Galectin-3 in cardiac remodeling and heart failure. *Curr Heart Fail Rep.* 2010;7(1):1-8.

41. van Kimmenade RR, Januzzi JL, Jr., Ellinor PT, et al. Utility of amino-terminal pro-brain natriuretic peptide, galectin-3, and apelin for the evaluation of patients with acute heart failure. *J Am Coll Cardiol.* 2006;48(6):1217-1224.

42. Januzzi JL, Jr., Peacock WF, Maisel AS, et al. Measurement of the interleukin family member ST2 in patients with acute dyspnea: results from the PRIDE (Pro-Brain Natriuretic Peptide Investigation of Dyspnea in the Emergency Department) study. *J Am Coll Cardiol.* 2007;50(7):607-613.

# CHAPTER 3

# Stage A: Patients at Risk for Developing Structural Heart Disease

*"The superior physician prevents sickness."*

—Chinese proverb

## Major Risk Factors and Increasing Prevalence of Heart Failure

Attention to the modifiable risk factors for heart failure, which are present in Stage A, may help reduce the increasing prevalence of heart failure as the population ages.

### COMMON ETIOLOGIES OF HEART FAILURE

The Framingham Study prospectively determined the etiologies of heart failure in 534 patients (Figure 3.1).[1] Overall, coronary artery disease was the most common principal cause of heart failure, even though hypertension was a frequent comorbidity.

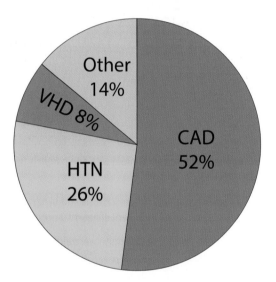

FIGURE 3.1    **Primary etiology of heart failure.** Primary etiology of heart failure at time of onset in the Framingham Heart Study (*n* = 534). Abbreviations: CAD, coronary artery disease; HTN, hypertension; VHD, valvular heart disease. Other, includes nonischemic cardiomyopathies.[1] *Source:* Adapted from Lee et al., *Circulation.* 2009;119(24):3070-3077, with permission.

Alternative causes of heart failure include valvular heart disease and cardiomyopathy. Valvular disease as a cause of heart failure is important to identify because valve correction (surgical or percutaneous) can improve cardiac performance and patient outcome. Hypertension was more frequent in patients with higher ejection fractions (Figure 3.2).

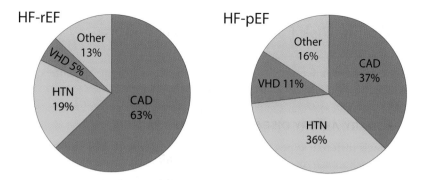

**FIGURE 3.2   HF-rEF versus HF-pEF in Framingham Heart Study.** Etiology of heart failure divided by ejection fraction. **Left panel:** LVEF ≤ 45%, n = 314; 59% of total. **Right panel:** LVEF > 45%, n = 220; 41% of total. Abbreviations: Same as Figure 3.1.[1] *Source:* Adapted from Lee et al., *Circulation.* 2009;119(24):3070-3077, with permission.

## PREVALENCE OF RISK FACTORS FOR HEART FAILURE

The common risk factors for developing heart failure (coronary artery disease, hypertension, and diabetes) are associated with aging and obesity (Figure 3.3). When these conditions coexist, the incidence rate of heart failure markedly increases.[4]

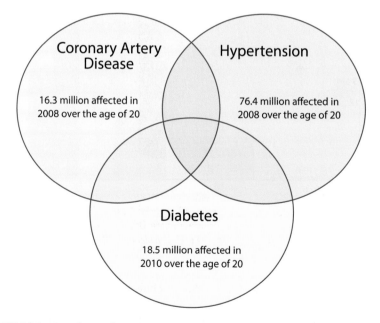

**FIGURE 3.3   Prevalence of coronary artery disease, hypertension, and diabetes in the United States.**[2,3] *Source:* Adapted from Roger et al., *Circulation.* 2012;125(1):e2-e220 and Centers for Disease Control and Prevention, 2011, with permission.

## Treatable Risk Factors for Heart Failure

Many of the risk factors for heart failure have treatment guidelines that reduce the morbidity and mortality of this syndrome.

### CORONARY ARTERY DISEASE AND HEART FAILURE

Although different types of coronary artery disease (CAD) can occur at any age, atherosclerotic CAD is a disease of aging (Figure 3.4).[5] In 2010, in age groups < 45, 45–64, and ≥ 65 years, the prevalence of CAD increased from 1.2% to 7.1% to 19.8%, respectively.[6] However, between 2006 and 2010, the overall age-adjusted prevalence of CAD in the United States decreased from 6.7% to 6.0%.[6] Although age-adjusted rates declined, coronary artery disease still accounted for one-third of all deaths in individuals over the age of 35 and was the primary cause of death in 405,309 cases in 2008.[7]

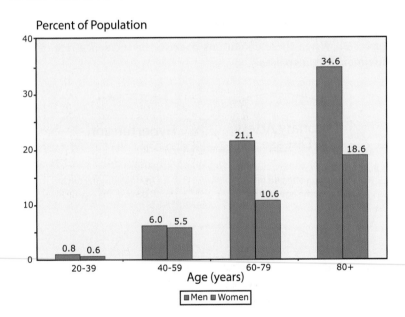

FIGURE 3.4  **Prevalence of coronary heart disease by age group.** Data from 2007-2010.[8]
*Source:* Adapted from Go et al., *Circulation.* 2013;127(1):e6-e245, with permission.

*Prevention of Heart Failure by Treating Lipids in Patients with CAD*

In the Scandinavian Simvastatin Survival Study (4S) trial, individuals with CAD without evidence of heart failure were treated with simvastatin versus placebo. Statin-treated patients had a lower risk of developing heart failure over a median follow-up of 5.4 years (relative risk = 0.79, $P < 0.015$).[9] In the same trial, the simvastatin-treated patients also had a reduced likelihood of developing a decline in kidney function (relative risk 0.68, $P = 0.01$), highlighting the importance of preservation of multi-organ function to achieve the goal of prevention of heart failure.[10]

## HYPERTENSION AND HEART FAILURE

Like CAD, hypertension incidence increases with age (Figure 3.5).[11] Within any given age group over the past decade, the prevalence of hypertension, defined as having a blood pressure of $\geq 140/90$ or on antihypertensive therapy, has remained steady (Figure 3.6).[12]

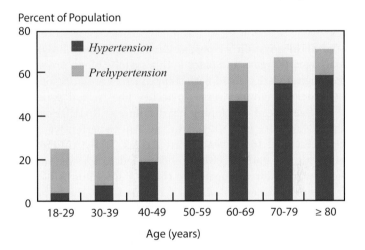

FIGURE 3.5 **Prevalence of hypertension by age in the United States.** Definitions: *Hypertension* is defined as systolic BP $\geq 140$ mm Hg, or diastolic BP $\geq 90$ mm Hg, or on medication. *Prehypertension* is defined as systolic BP 120–139 mm Hg or diastolic BP 80–89 mm Hg.[11] *Source:* Adapted from the *National Heart, Lung, and Blood Institute Chart Book 2012,* with permission.

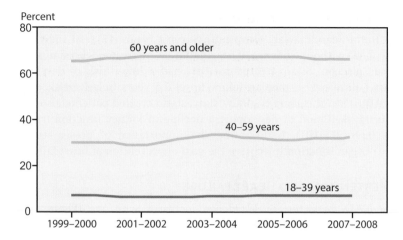

**FIGURE 3.6    Prevalence of hypertension by age group has remained steady over time.**[12]
*Source:* Adapted from the Centers for Disease Control and Prevention, with permission.

## Prevention of Heart Failure by Treating Hypertension

In the SHEP (Systolic Hypertension in the Elderly Program) trial, individuals aged 60 years and older with a systolic blood pressure of 160 mm Hg or higher were treated with stepped care consisting of a diuretic, then beta-blocker therapies versus placebo. The treated patients had a reduced relative risk of developing heart failure (RR = 0.51) over a mean follow-up of 4.5 years ($P < 0.001$).[13] In the Antihypertensive and Lipid-Lowering Treatment to Prevent Heart Attack Trial (ALLHAT), initial treatment with the diuretic chlorthalidone led to a lower incidence of subsequent heart failure compared to the ACE inhibitor lisinopril or the calcium channel blocker amlodipine.[14] In this study, the importance of prevention of heart failure in hypertension was confirmed. After the development of heart failure, high 10-year all-cause mortality rates were similar among those with HF-rEF and with HF-pEF (84% and 81% respectively), with no significant differences among patients initially treated with diuretics, ACE inhibitors, or calcium channel blockers.[15]

In patients who may also have CAD, diabetes, valvular heart disease, or cardiomyopathy, 75% who develop heart failure have a history of hypertension as either a primary or secondary etiology.[8] The Eighth Joint National Committee on treatment of high blood pressure recommended treating blood pressure to a goal of less than 140/90 mm Hg in those less than 60 years of age or with diabetes or chronic kidney disease at any age.[16] In those 60 years or older, a systolic goal of less than 150 mm Hg was recommended. The European Society of Cardiology made a systolic goal of < 140 mm Hg the treatment target for all individuals less than 80 years.[17] In those 80 years or older with an initial systolic blood pressure ≥ 160 mm Hg, a goal of < 150 mm Hg was recommended.

## DIABETES AND HEART FAILURE

Since 1990, the age-adjusted prevalence of diabetes in the United States has increased by more than 60%, affecting 10.9 million people over the age of 65 in 2008 (Figure 3.7).[3,18] In diabetics compared to normoglycemic controls, the risk of development of heart failure is increased two-fold in men and fivefold in women.[18,19]

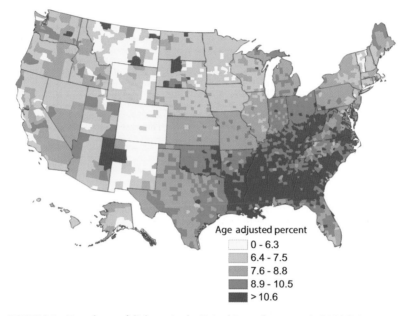

**FIGURE 3.7    Prevalence of diabetes in the United States by county in 2008.**[20] *Source:* Adapted from the Centers for Disease Control and Prevention, with permission.

Diabetes as a risk factor for the development of heart failure may be due to myocardial, metabolic, and vascular changes induced by chronic hyperglycemia.[21] In diabetic patients with normal systolic function, exercise is associated with a blunted increase of left ventricular contractility and impairment in sympathetic innervation.[21] Obesity and diabetes occur frequently in patients with both preserved and reduced ejection fraction.[22] In people with diabetes ≥ 65 years of age, the development of heart failure portends a significantly worse prognosis. A higher mortality rate was found for diabetic patients with heart failure compared with diabetic patients who were free of heart failure (32.7 per 100 person–years versus 3.7 per 100 person–years, respectively).[23]

## OBESITY AND HEART FAILURE

Obesity is associated with diabetes, but also independently with the development of heart failure (Figure 3.8).[24] Increasing baseline weight correlates with subsequent higher mean serum glucose and heart failure onset frequency (Figure 3.9).[25]

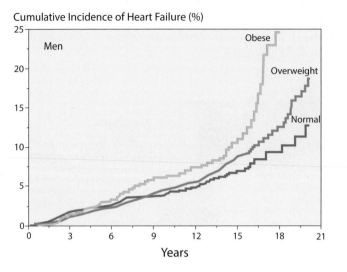

**FIGURE 3.8   Incidence of heart failure with increased levels of obesity in men in The Framingham Study (*n* = 2,704).** The associated incidence of heart failure in normal (BMI 18.5–24.9), overweight (BMI 25.0–29.9), and obese (BMI ≥ 30.0) men, was 10.2%, 14.2%, and 15.5%, respectively. Similar trends were present in women. BMI: Body Mass Index (kg/m²).[24] *Source:* Adapted from Kenchaiah et al., *N Engl J Med.* 2002;347(5):305-313, with permission.

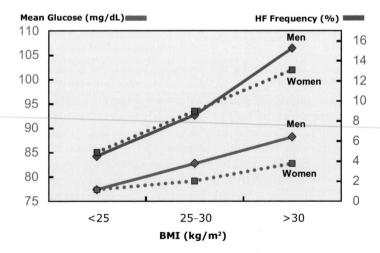

**FIGURE 3.9   Correlation between body mass index (BMI) and heart failure frequency.** Baseline BMI in patients without diabetes predicts subsequent glucose levels and heart failure over a follow-up of 13 ± 8 years.[25] *Source:* Adapted from Thrainsdottir et al., *Eur J Heart Fail.* 2007;9(10):1051-1057, with permission.

Over a 20-year period, obesity, defined as a body mass index (BMI) $\geq 30$ kg/m$^2$, has increased to a prevalence of more than 20% throughout the entire United States, and in some states more than 30% (Figure 3.10).[26] This phenomenon is not confined to the United States. A recent worldwide study documented an average BMI increase of 0.4 kg/m$^2$ per decade between 1980 and 2008.[27]

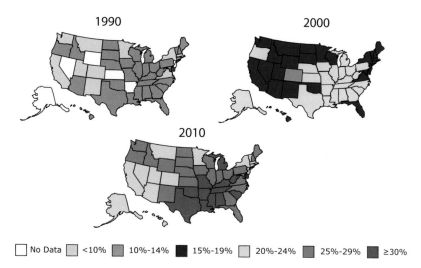

FIGURE 3.10  **Prevalence of obesity (%) in the United States by state.** Obesity defined as BMI > 30 kg/m$^2$. Behavioral Risk Factor Surveillance System.[26] *Source:* Adapted from the Centers for Disease Control and Prevention, with permission.

After the development of heart failure, surprisingly, increasing body surface area predicts better subsequent survival in both acute and chronic heart failure.[28,29] This has been called the "obesity paradox." The reasons for this are uncertain, but may include beneficial endocrine effects of adipose tissue. Alternatively, obesity may unmask cardiac insufficiency at an earlier stage in the natural history of heart failure.

## Goals for the Management of Heart Failure Risk Factors

National healthcare organizations have developed specific goals for managing risk factors associated with developing heart failure (Table 3.1).

TABLE 3.1    Goals for management of risk factors for the development of heart failure.[30]

| RISK FACTORS | POPULATION | TREATMENT |
|---|---|---|
| HYPERTENSION | Everyone with hypertension | < 140/90 mm Hg, depending on age (see text)<br>Limit sodium to ≤ 1500 mg/day |
| DIABETES | See American Diabetes Association (ADA) Guidelines[31] | |
| HYPERLIPIDEMIA | See ACC/AHA Guideline on the treatment of blood cholesterol[32] | |
| PHYSICAL INACTIVITY | Everyone | Sustained aerobic activity 20–30 minutes, 3–5 times weekly |
| OBESITY | BMI > 30 | Evidence-based weight-control program to achieve BMI < 30 |
| EXCESSIVE ALCOHOL INTAKE | Men | Limit alcohol intake to 1-2 drink equivalents per day |
| | Women | 1 drink equivalent |
| | Those with propensity to abuse alcohol or who have alcoholic cardiomyopathy | Abstention |
| SMOKING | Everyone | Cessation |
| VITAMIN/MINERAL DEFICIENCY | Everyone | Diet high in $K^+$, calcium |
| POOR DIET | Everyone | 4 or more servings of fruit and vegetables per day; 1 or more servings of breakfast cereal per week |

# References

1. Lee DS, Gona P, Vasan RS, et al. Relation of disease pathogenesis and risk factors to heart failure with preserved or reduced ejection fraction: insights from the framingham heart study of the national heart, lung, and blood institute. *Circulation.* 2009;119(24):3070-3077.

2. Roger VL, Go AS, Lloyd-Jones DM, et al. Heart disease and stroke statistics—2012 update: a report from the American Heart Association. *Circulation.* 2012;125(1): e2-e220.

3. *2011 National Diabetes Fact Sheet.* Centers for Disease Control and Prevention. 2011;1-12. Available from: http://www.cdc.gov/diabetes/pubs/factsheet11.htm.

4. Yancy CW, Jessup M, Bozkurt B, et al. 2013 ACCF/AHA Guideline for the Management of Heart Failure: a report of the American College of Cardiology Foundation/

American Heart Association Task Force on Practice Guidelines. *J Am Coll Cardiol.* 2013;62(16):e147-e239.

5.  Gheorghiade M, Bonow RO. Chronic heart failure in the United States: a manifestation of coronary artery disease. *Circulation.* 1998;97(3):282-289.

6.  Fang J, Shaw KM, Keenan NL. Prevalence of coronary heart disease—United States, 2006-2010. *MMWR Morb Mortal Wkly Rep.* 2011;60(40):1377-1381.

7.  Jessup M, Abraham WT, Casey DE, et al. 2009 Focused update: ACCF/AHA Guidelines for the diagnosis and management of heart failure in adults: a report of the American College of Cardiology Foundation/American Heart Association Task Force on Practice Guidelines: developed in collaboration with the International Society for Heart and Lung Transplantation. *Circulation.* 2009;119(14):1977-2016.

8.  Go AS, Mozaffarian D, Roger VL, et al. Heart disease and stroke statistics—2013 update: a report from the American Heart Association. *Circulation.* 2013;127(1): e6-e245.

9.  Kjekshus J, Pedersen TR, Olsson AG, Faergeman O, Pyörälä K. The effects of simvastatin on the incidence of heart failure in patients with coronary heart disease. *J Card Fail.* 1997;3(4):249-254.

10. Huskey J, Lindenfeld J, Cook T, et al. Effect of simvastatin on kidney function loss in patients with coronary heart disease: findings from the Scandinavian Simvastatin Survival Study (4S). *Atherosclerosis.* 2009;205(1):202-206.

11. *Morbidity and Mortality: 2012 Chart Book on Cardiovascular, Lung, and Blood Diseases.* National Institutes of Health: National Heart Lung and Blood Institute. 2012.

12. Yoon SS, Ostchega Y, Louis T. Recent trends in the prevalence of high blood pressure and its treatment and control, 1999–2008. *NCHS Data Brief.* 2010;(48):1-8.

13. Kostis JB, Davis BR, Cutler J, et al. Prevention of heart failure by antihypertensive drug treatment in older persons with isolated systolic hypertension. SHEP Cooperative Research Group. *JAMA.* 1997;278(3):212-216.

14. The ALLHAT Officers and Coordinators for the ALLHAT Collaborative Research Group. Major outcomes in high-risk hypertensive patients randomized to angiotensin-converting enzyme inhibitor or calcium channel blocker vs diuretic: the Antihypertensive and Lipid-Lowering Treatment to Prevent Heart Attack Trial (ALLHAT). *JAMA.* 2002;288(23):2981-2997.

15. Piller LB, Baraniuk S, Simpson LM, et al. Long-term follow-up of participants with heart failure in the antihypertensive and lipid-lowering treatment to prevent heart attack trial (ALLHAT). *Circulation.* 2011;124(17):1811-1818.

16. James PA, Oparil S, Carter BL, et al. 2014 Evidence-based guideline for the management of high blood pressure in adults: Report from the panel members appointed to the Eighth Joint National Committee (JNC 8). *JAMA.* 2014;311(5):507-520.

17. Mancia G, Fagard R, Narkiewicz K, et al. 2013 ESH/ESC Guidelines for the management of arterial hypertension: the Task Force for the management of arterial hypertension of the European Society of Hypertension (ESH) and of the European Society of Cardiology (ESC). *J Hypertens.* 2013;31(7):1281-1357.

18. Horwich TB, Fonarow GC. Glucose, obesity, metabolic syndrome, and diabetes relevance to incidence of heart failure. *J Am Coll Cardiol.* 2010:55(4):283-293.

19. Nichols GA, Gullion CM, Koro CE, Ephross SA, Brown JB. The incidence of congestive heart failure in type 2 diabetes: an update. *Diabetes Care.* 2004;27(8):1879-1884.

20. *Prevalence and Trends Data: Nationwide (States and DC)—2008*. CDC: Behavioral Risk Factor Surveillance System 2008. 2008; Available from: http://apps.nccd.cdc.gov/brfss/page.asp?yr=2008&state=UB&cat=DB#DB

21. Scognamiglio R, Avogaro A, Casara D, et al. Myocardial dysfunction and adrenergic cardiac innervation in patients with insulin-dependent diabetes mellitus. *J Am Coll Cardiol.* 1998;31(2):404-412.

22. Pieske B. Heart failure with preserved ejection fraction—a growing epidemic or "The Emperor's New Clothes?" *Eur J Heart Fail.* 2011;13(1):11-13.

23. Bertoni AG, Hundley WG, Massing MW, Bonds DE, Burke GL, Goff DC Jr. Heart failure prevalence, incidence, and mortality in the elderly with diabetes. *Diabetes Care.* 2004;27(3):699-703.

24. Kenchaiah S, Evans JC, Levy D, et al. Obesity and the risk of heart failure. *N Engl J Med.* 2002;347(5):305-313.

25. Thrainsdottir IS, Aspelund T, Gudnason V, et al. Increasing glucose levels and BMI predict future heart failure experience from the Reykjavik Study. *Eur J Heart Fail.* 2007;9(10):1051-1057.

26. Prevalence and Trends Data. *CDC: Behavioral Risk Factor Surveillance System 2012.* Accessed January 9, 2012; Available from: http://www.cdc.gov/brfss/

27. Finucane MM, Stevens GA, Cowan MJ, et al. National, regional, and global trends in body-mass index since 1980: systematic analysis of health examination surveys and epidemiological studies with 960 country-years and 9.1 million participants. *Lancet.* 2011;377(9765):557-567.

28. Fonarow GC, Srikanthan P, Costanzo MR, Cintron GB, Lopatin M; ADHERE Scientific Advisory Committee and Investigators. An obesity paradox in acute heart failure: analysis of body mass index and inhospital mortality for 108,927 patients in the Acute Decompensated Heart Failure National Registry. *Am Heart J.* 2007;153(1):74-81.

29. Curtis JP, Selter JG, Wang Y, Rathore SS, et al. The obesity paradox: body mass index and outcomes in patients with heart failure. *Arch Intern Med.* 2005;165(1):55-61.

30. Heart Failure Society of America, Lindenfeld J, Albert NM, et al. HFSA 2010 Comprehensive Heart Failure Practice Guideline. *J Card Fail.* 2010;16(6): e1-e194.

31. National Diabetes Education Initiative. *American Diabetes Association (ADA) 2014 Guidelines.* 2014 Accessed April 16, 2014; Available from: http://www.ndei.org/ADA-2014-guidelines-diabetes-diagnosis-A1C-testing.aspx

32. Stone NJ, Robinson JG, Lichtenstein AH, et al. 2013 ACC/AHA Guideline on the Treatment of Blood Cholesterol to Reduce Atherosclerotic Cardiovascular Risk in Adults: A Report of the American College of Cardiology/American Heart Association Task Force on Practice Guidelines. *J Am Coll Cardiol.* 2014;63(25 Pt B): 2889-2934.

# CHAPTER 4

# Structural Heart Disease and Progression to Failure: Stages B, C, and D

## FAST FACTS

- Structural, biochemical, and functional abnormalities in the heart and other body systems progress throughout the stages of heart failure.

- Cardiac sarcomere proteins undergo constant turnover. Biochemical and mechanical signaling can modulate progression or regression of ventricular remodeling, including concentric and eccentric hypertrophy.

- Neurohumoral responses to impaired cardiac performance are initially adaptive, but become maladaptive if sustained.

- Decreased SERCA2a protein levels impair myocyte calcium trafficking.

- Autophagy, apoptosis, and necrosis are three processes that influence cell survival in response to cellular stress.

- Gene mutations can lead to hypertrophic, dilated, or restrictive cardiomyopathies. Less common genetic myopathies include left ventricular noncompaction and arrhythmogenic right ventricular cardiomyopathy.

*"DNA neither cares nor knows. DNA just is. And we dance to its music."*

—Richard Dawkins,
*River Out of Eden: A Darwinian View of Life*[1]

*The 4 Stages of Heart Failure* © 2015 Brian E. Jaski. Cardiotext Publishing, ISBN: 978-1-935395-30-0.

# Morphologic Changes in Heart Failure

Initiation and progression of disease is the product of genetic predisposition, environment, and chance. Following a primary injury to the heart, altered mechanical loading and neurohumoral signals orchestrate a secondary transition in cardiovascular phenotype. In part, this manifests as a reinitiation of a fetal repertoire of gene expression. Over time, qualitative and quantitative changes in proteins regulating myocyte contractility and calcium homeostasis contribute to impaired systolic and diastolic ventricular function.

## HEART SIZE

Initial structural heart damage progresses to chronic heart failure associated with increases in heart mass and size (Figure 4.1). Although this progression is mostly due to increases in preexisting myocyte size, proliferation of resident endogenous and circulating exogenous stem cells may contribute to this process.[2] The different phenotypes of hypertrophy depend on the inciting factors for growth (Figure 4.2). Patients with HF-pEF, compared to normal controls and hypertensive patients without heart failure, exhibit an average 33% increase in left ventricular mass and wall thickness, but without change in end-diastolic chamber volume.[3] Patients with HF-rEF, compared to controls, demonstrate more than twofold increases in left ventricular mass and end-diastolic chamber volume.[4]

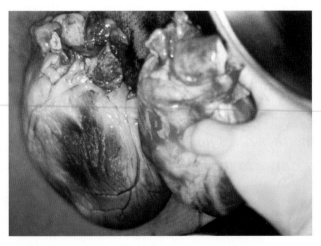

**FIGURE 4.1    Heart size.** Markedly enlarged heart removed from patient with end-stage heart failure due to ischemic cardiomyopathy (**left**) versus normal sized donor heart about to be transplanted (**right**).

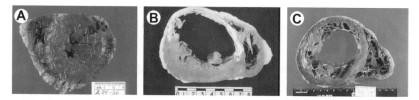

**FIGURE 4.2    Common pathologies of heart failure remodeling.** Postmortem examples: **Panel A:** Hypertensive hypertrophic cardiomyopathy. **Panel B:** Dilated ischemic cardiomyopathy. **Panel C:** Dilated nonischemic cardiomyopathy. The pathology shown in Panel A is associated with HF-pEF, whereas those in Panels B and C are associated with HF-rEF.[5] *Source:* Adapted from Konstam, *J Card Fail.* 2003;9(1):1-3, with permission.

## VENTRICULAR REMODELING

The heart is often viewed as a structurally stable, mechanical tissue pump that adjusts its performance in response to changes in loading conditions or inotropic state. When viewed by electron microscopy, repeating sarcomere units appear to be permanent, crystalline structures. In fact, the heart is a dynamic biologic structure with ongoing turnover of its intracellular contracting components associated with the continuous assembly and degradation of specific sarcomere proteins. On average, troponin subunits (T/I/C) have a half-life of 3 to 5 days; actin and tropomyosin 7 to 10 days; and myosin 5 to 8 days.[6] Thus, the heart, while cyclically generating force and motion, is an organ with potential for great plasticity that is primed for cellular and structural modulation when changes in mechanical and molecular signals occur.

Myocardial injury alters the loading and biochemical environment of both impaired and uninjured cardiac cells. Biochemical signals, whether endocrine (coming from an external source), paracrine (acting on neighboring cells), autocrine (acting on the same cell), or intracrine (acting internally on the same cell without extracellular secretion), can all contribute to a subsequent net biologic response.[7] As in other tissues, these mediators in part reinitiate fetal growth repertoires of transcription and translation.[8] Over time, characteristic patterns of heart morphology emerge associated with different effects on ventricular filling or ejection of blood (Figure 4.2).

Cell proliferation, apoptosis, hypertrophy, and atrophy modify the physical characteristics of the heart—a process referred to as *ventricular remodeling.*[8] While remodeling may initially represent a reparative response to abnormal myocardial conditions, if sustained, it can ultimately contribute to ventricular dysfunction. This paradox may in part be explained by a limited set of mechanisms in response to transient cellular stress that have not evolved in the face of the current major causes of persistent adult cardiac disability, such as coronary artery disease and hypertension.

# Patterns of Maladaptive Hypertrophy

Ventricular dysfunction occurs in part because of maladaptive hypertrophy. The loading conditions on the left ventricle and the extracellular environment both contribute to the processes of remodeling that result in two main classifications of hypertrophy.

## CONCENTRIC VERSUS ECCENTRIC HYPERTROPHY

The normal left ventricle surrounds a rotated ellipse or football-shaped chamber with end-diastolic wall thickness ≤ 11 mm and chamber diameter ≤ 56 mm. During systolic wall thickening and ejection of blood, the base of the left ventricle, including the mitral and aortic valves, moves toward a relatively stationary apex.[9] The return motion of the base during early ventricular filling can be measure by echocardiography to assess diastolic function (see Chapter 7, Figure 7.3).

> **RELATIVE WALL THICKNESS**
> Ratio of left ventricular wall thickness to left ventricular internal chamber dimension at end-diastole.

### Concentric Hypertrophy

Concentric hypertrophy can develop in response to a sustained increase in left ventricular systolic pressure (e.g., hypertension or aortic stenosis). In response, end-diastolic wall thickness and relative wall thickness (wall thickness/chamber dimension) increase.[10] This increase in wall thickness by the Laplace relation results in a decrease in afterload wall stress (pressure × radius/wall thickness) at end-systole, which means that ejection fraction and stroke volume may initially be maintained. A left ventricle subjected to long-standing pressure overload, however, can progress to a dilated ventricle with eccentric hypertrophy, reduced ejection fraction, and decreased stroke volume (Figure 4.3).

### Eccentric Hypertrophy (Dilated Left Ventricle)

Eccentric hypertrophy can follow myocardial injury (e.g., infarction, genetic cardiomyopathy, or myocarditis), a chronic volume overload (e.g., aortic or mitral valve regurgitation), or a decompensated state of concentric hypertrophy (Figure 4.3). For example, initially after myocardial infarction, passive stretch will help maintain a forward stroke volume via the Frank-Starling mechanism. Thinning and elongation of the fibrous infarcted segment further increase heart size (Figure 4.4).[10] Eventually, increased wall stress and neurohumoral activation effect ventricular remodeling of the infarcted and noninfarcted myocardium, increasing chamber size, decreasing relative wall thickness, and decreasing ejection fraction.

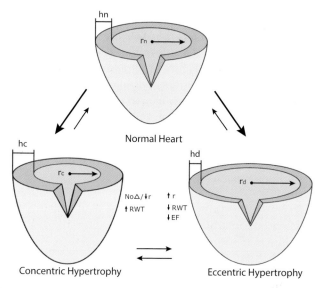

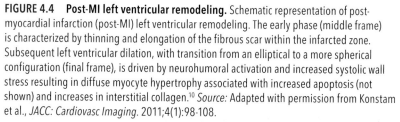

**FIGURE 4.3** **Concentric and eccentric hypertrophy.** Abbreviations: r, chamber radius; h, wall thickness; σ, wall stress (force/area of muscle); EF, ejection fraction; RWT, relative wall thickness.[11] *Source:* Adapted with permission from Jaski BE, *Basics of Heart Failure.* Springer Science + Business Media B.V.; 2000: 61.

## POST-MI REMODELING

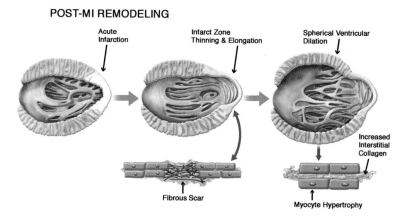

**FIGURE 4.4** **Post-MI left ventricular remodeling.** Schematic representation of post-myocardial infarction (post-MI) left ventricular remodeling. The early phase (middle frame) is characterized by thinning and elongation of the fibrous scar within the infarcted zone. Subsequent left ventricular dilation, with transition from an elliptical to a more spherical configuration (final frame), is driven by neurohumoral activation and increased systolic wall stress resulting in diffuse myocyte hypertrophy associated with increased apoptosis (not shown) and increases in interstitial collagen.[10] *Source:* Adapted with permission from Konstam et al., *JACC: Cardiovasc Imaging.* 2011;4(1):98-108.

## LOADING CONDITIONS AND MYOCYTE PHENOTYPE

In 1975, Grossman and coworkers proposed the hypothesis that increased wall stress in either systole or diastole initiates either concentric or eccentric (dilated) hypertrophy (Figure 4.5).[12] Since then, the molecular mechanisms for components of this control circuit have been identified. One mechanism involves a deformable sarcomere protein that undergoes differential phosphorylation based on the direction of stress and strain.[13] Other molecular signals for the development of hypertrophy include stretch of the sarcomere-spanning protein titin and release of locally acting growth factors.[14]

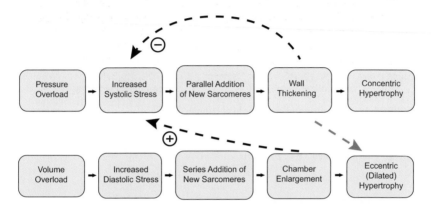

FIGURE 4.5    **Loading conditions and sarcomere growth patterns.** Hypothesized mechanism by which increased wall stress initiates concentric versus eccentric (dilated) hypertrophy. This hypothesis requires that the heart can "detect" systolic and diastolic wall stress occurring with pressure and volume overload, respectively, resulting in the selective addition of new sarcomeres in either a parallel or series position to return wall stress toward normal. If pressure overload is sustained, it can eventually also lead to eccentric hypertrophy **(red arrow)**.[12] *Source:* Adapted with permission from Grossman W et al., *J Clin Invest.* 1975;56(1):56-64.

## EXTRACELLULAR ENVIRONMENT

The extracellular environment provides scaffolding for and participates in differentiation of cardiac muscle and nonmuscle cells.[15] In parallel with changes of intracellular components, extracellular matrix modifications[16] also participate in ventricular remodeling (Figure 4.6). Following ischemic or nonischemic insults, increased deposition of fibrous proteins, including collagen[17] and fibronectin,[18] further modulate the mechanical properties of the remodeled left ventricle.

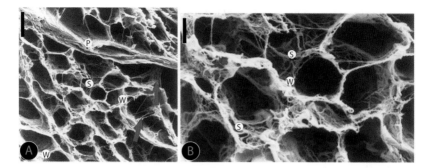

**FIGURE 4.6   Connective tissue skeleton of human heart with an organization similar to a honeycomb.** The perimysium (P) envelops groups of myocytes. The endomysial weave (W), as final arborization of the perimysium, supports and connects individual cells and is connected to adjacent myocytes by lateral struts (S). Collagen struts also connect myocytes to interstitial microvessels **(lower arrow)** or perimysium **(upper arrow)**. **Panel A:** Low magnification ×1415, scale bar = 20 μm; **Panel B:** High magnification × 2830, scale bar = 10 μm.[19] *Source:* Adapted with permission from Rossi MA et al., *Circulation.* 1998;97(9):934-935.

# Neurohumoral Circulatory Responses

Complex neurohumoral responses amplify maladaptive remodeling and circulatory changes initiated by any insult to the heart.

### ACUTE VERSUS CHRONIC NEUROHUMORAL RESPONSES

Regulatory mechanisms of sodium retention and vasoconstriction are appropriate to maintain homeostasis in response to acute hypoperfusion and hypotension following reductions in circulating blood volume such as hemorrhage (Table 4.1). These same responses, however, may be inappropriate if initiated in response to the development of chronic cardiac dysfunction and may contribute to further deterioration, thus becoming targets of therapy.[20]

**TABLE 4.1** **Neurohumoral responses to impaired cardiac performance and their effects on the circulation.**[20]

| RESPONSE | SHORT-TERM EFFECTS | LONG-TERM EFFECTS |
|---|---|---|
| SALT AND WATER RETENTION | Augments preload | Pulmonary congestion, edema/anasarca |
| VASOCONSTRICTION | Maintains blood pressure for perfusion of vital organs (brain, heart) | Exacerbates pump dysfunction (excessive afterload, increases cardiac energy expenditure) |
| SYMPATHETIC STIMULATION | Increases heart rate and contractility | Increases energy expenditure |

## NEUROHUMORAL MEDIATORS OF ADVERSE CARDIAC REMODELING

Following a primary myocardial injury, such as acute myocardial infarction or viral myocarditis, the onset of symptoms of pump failure may occur immediately, follow days of fluid retention, or follow months to years of maladaptive ventricular remodeling. The same neurohumoral mediators that act as vasoconstrictors or mediators of sodium and water retention can also act as growth factors that promote the progression of adverse ventricular hypertrophy, if sustained (Figure 4.7).

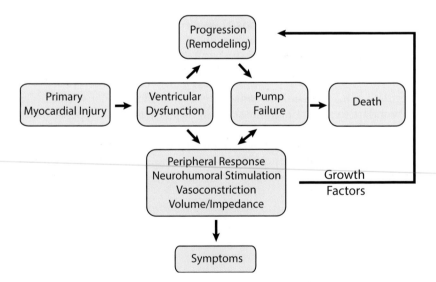

**FIGURE 4.7** **The Adverse Cardiac Remodeling Cascade.** Effects of neurohormones and cytokine stimulation on the heart and the systemic vasculature in heart failure.[11] *Source:* Adapted with permission from Jaski BE, *Basics of Heart Failure.* Springer Science + Business Media B.V.; 2000: 45.

## PLASMA NOREPINEPHRINE PREDICTS PROGNOSIS

Neurohumoral activation implies a poor prognosis for the patient with heart failure. The circulating level of the primary sympathetic nervous system neurotransmitter, norepinephrine, was the single most significant measured predictor of survival in chronic congestive heart failure patients in the VA Heart Failure Trial (Figure 4.8).[21]

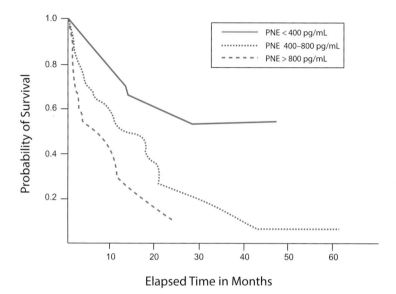

Elapsed Time in Months

**FIGURE 4.8  Plasma norepinephrine levels (PNE) and heart failure survival.** Increases in baseline PNE levels predicted a progressively worse prognosis in patients from the first VA Heart Failure Trial (*n* = 106). The three Kaplan-Meier survival curves (shown above) showed statistically significant differences.[21] *Source:* Adapted with permission from Cohn et al., *N Engl J Med.* 1984;311(13):819-823.

Multiple neurohumoral mechanisms may be activated with impaired heart function. Cournot et al. found that predischarge BNP levels ≥ 360 pg/mL and a decrease of < 50% between admission and discharge levels were associated with higher postdischarge event rates (Figure 4.9).[22] Just as activation of neurohumoral systems implies a worse prognosis, blockade of neurohormonal mediators can improve prognosis.[23,24]

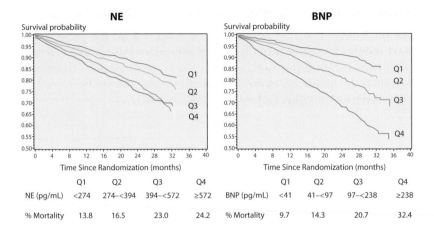

| | Q1 | Q2 | Q3 | Q4 | | Q1 | Q2 | Q3 | Q4 |
|---|---|---|---|---|---|---|---|---|---|
| NE (pg/mL) | <274 | 274–<394 | 394–<572 | ≥572 | BNP (pg/mL) | <41 | 41–<97 | 97–<238 | ≥238 |
| % Mortality | 13.8 | 16.5 | 23.0 | 24.2 | % Mortality | 9.7 | 14.3 | 20.7 | 32.4 |

**FIGURE 4.9    Neurohormonal levels and HF mortality.** Comparison between in-hospital BNP and norepinephrine (NE) levels in relation to predicting mortality in patients with heart failure. BNP exhibited a stronger association with mortality and morbidity than NE (*P* < 0.0001). In these patients, BNP may be a biomarker for general neurohumoral activation.[25] *Source:* Adapted with permission from Anand et al., *Circulation.* 2003;107(9):1278-1283.

## THE EXAMPLE OF ALDOSTERONE

Aldosterone receptors, in addition to mediating sodium reuptake from the distal tubule of the kidney, are also present on cardiac fibroblasts and can contribute to increases in myocardial fibrosis.[26] Aldosterone is also involved in the depressed responsiveness of carotid baroreceptor activity observed in heart failure.[27] Beneficial effects of aldosterone blockade may be more marked in patients with higher levels of the circulating biomarker of myocyte wall stress named ST2 (see Chapter 2, Figure 2.17).[28] Improvements in heart failure patient survival with pharmacologic blockade of aldosterone receptors with spironolactone or eplerenone may reflect blunting a combination of all aldosterone effects (see Chapter 8).[29–31]

# Intracellular Mechanisms of Progression

Progression of heart failure is also determined by intracellular mechanisms involving calcium uptake and release by the sarco(endo)plasmic reticulum, and by the mitochondrial response to the chemical byproducts of myocardial stress.

## SARCO(ENDO)PLASMIC RETICULUM AND CA²⁺ ION EXCHANGE

One of the abnormalities in both human and experimental models of heart failure is a defect in sarcoplasmic reticulum (SR) function, which in turn causes abnormal intracellular calcium ion handling.[32] Sarco(endo) plasmic reticulum calcium ATPase 2a (SERCA2a) is the major enzyme responsible for reuptake of calcium in the SR from the cytoplasm (Figure 4.10).

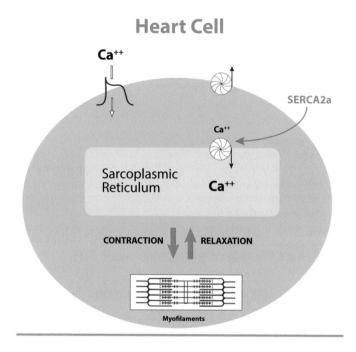

FIGURE 4.10    Diagram of heart cell emphasizing role of SERCA2a.[11] *Source:* Adapted with permission from Jaski BE, *Basics of Heart Failure.* Springer Science + Business Media B.V.; 2000: 73.

SERCA2a expression declines in heart failure of any etiology (Figure 4.11).[33] A further decrease in activity is mediated by a decrease in phosphorylation of the SERCA2a activator protein phospholamban.[34] This impaired intracellular calcium pump action results in abnormally high levels of cytoplasmic calcium in diastole and low levels in systole. Because calcium concentration determines actin and myosin force generation throughout the cardiac cycle, these defects contribute to both impaired cardiac relaxation and contraction (Figure 4.11).[34]

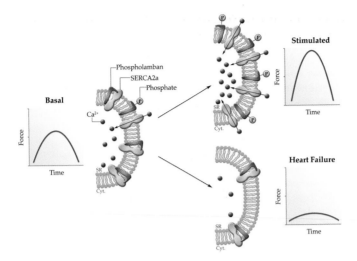

FIGURE 4.11    **Phospholamban phosphorylation and myocardial force.** Under *basal conditions,* unphosphorylated phospholamban binds to and inhibits sarco(endo)plasmic reticulum calcium ATPase 2a (SERCA2a). During cardiac stimulation (**upper right diagram**) phosphorylated phospholamban dissociates from SERCA2a and increases SERCA2a mediated $Ca^{2+}$ ion movement into the sarcoplasmic reticulum. Regardless of the etiology, as heart failure progresses (**lower right diagram**), both SERCA2a expression and phospholamban phosphorylation are reduced, resulting in less SERCA2a $Ca^{2+}$ transport activity. Abbreviations: SR, sarcoplasmic reticulum; Cyt, cytoplasm.[34] *Source:* Adapted with permission from MacLennan & Kranias, *Nat Rev Molec Cell Biol.* 2003;4(7):566-577.

## CATECHOLAMINE-RELATED PROTEIN MEDIATORS

Multiple cellular systems can contribute to adverse myocardial remodeling as the heart failure syndrome progresses.[35] These include dysregulation of multiple components of the catecholamine myocardial signaling cascade, such as the beta-adrenergic receptor, beta-adrenergic receptor kinase (BARK), and phosphokinase A (PKA). Current agents target extracellular norepinephrine binding to membrane receptors. Future therapies may target more specific intracellular pathways of this and other neurohumoral systems to optimize net reverse remodeling effects.[36]

## MITOCHONDRIAL PROCESSES INFLUENCE HEART MUSCLE CELL SURVIVAL

In response to varying levels of stress (hypoxia, inflammation, mechanical overload), myocardial cells can manifest different degrees of autophagy, apoptosis, and necrosis (Figure 4.12).[37-41] Each process serves a unique function in the balance between cell survival and death, and provides a contribution to cardiac remodeling. Molecular events at the subcellular level of the mitochondrion, such as opening of permeability transition pores (mPTPs), effect the initiation of all three. Whereas apoptosis and necrosis result in irreversible cell loss, autophagy, at least initially, may act as a protective cell-survival mechanism.

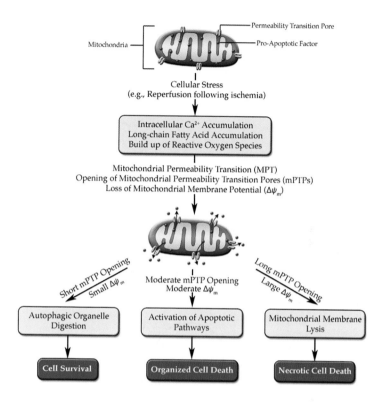

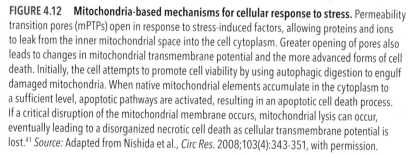

**FIGURE 4.12** **Mitochondria-based mechanisms for cellular response to stress.** Permeability transition pores (mPTPs) open in response to stress-induced factors, allowing proteins and ions to leak from the inner mitochondrial space into the cell cytoplasm. Greater opening of pores also leads to changes in mitochondrial transmembrane potential and the more advanced forms of cell death. Initially, the cell attempts to promote cell viability by using autophagic digestion to engulf damaged mitochondria. When native mitochondrial elements accumulate in the cytoplasm to a sufficient level, apoptotic pathways are activated, resulting in an apoptotic cell death process. If a critical disruption of the mitochondrial membrane occurs, mitochondrial lysis can occur, eventually leading to a disorganized necrotic cell death as cellular transmembrane potential is lost.[41] *Source:* Adapted from Nishida et al., *Circ Res.* 2008;103(4):343-351, with permission.

## Autophagy

During ischemic stress, autophagy (derived from the Greek words "auto" meaning "self" and "phagein" meaning "to eat")[42] attempts to maintain homeostasis by sequestering intracellular components. Recycling denatured proteins and damaged organelles can provide amino acids for new protein synthesis and reduce stress from oxygen-derived radicals

(Figure 4.13).[43] Although potentially allowing a myocardial cell to deflect a serious injury such as myocardial ischemia,[44] continuous and prolonged activation of the autophagic pathway can result in cell death from excessive accumulation of autophagosomes (Figure 4.14).[43]

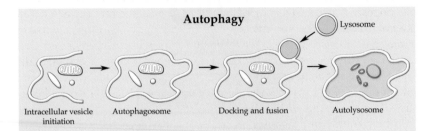

**FIGURE 4.13   Autophagy mechanism.** Autophagy begins with the formation of an isolation membrane within the cell cytoplasm. This vesicle then undergoes elongation, engulfing and sequestering cytoplasmic constituents such as proteins and organelles, as it forms the autophagosome. Autophagosomes dock and fuse with lysosomes to form autolysosomes, where engulfed entities are degraded for use within the cell.[41] *Source:* Adapted with permission from Nishida et al., *Circ Res.* 2008;103(4):343-351.

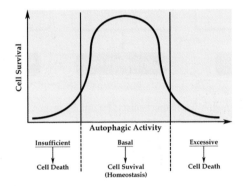

**FIGURE 4.14   Autophagic activity and cell survival.** A basal level of autophagic activity promotes cell viability, while insufficient or excessive amounts of autophagy can result in cell death.[41] *Source:* Adapted with permission from Nishida et al., *Circ Res.* 2008;103(4):343-351.

### Apoptosis and Necrosis

Derived from the Greek word meaning "dropping off" or "falling off," apoptosis is a highly regulated, organized process of programmed cell death.[42,45] In response to moderate levels of cellular stress, myocardial cells may undergo apoptotic cell death, characterized by cell shrinkage and organized chromosomal DNA fragmentation (Figure 4.15). Cellular components and DNA fragments are packaged into membrane-bound apoptotic bodies that are subsequently phagocytosed by surrounding macrophages and neutrophils.

Apoptosis is associated with a minimum of inflammation in the surrounding tissues.[46,47] Cardiac apoptosis can contribute to the development of congestive heart failure by reducing the contractile mass of myocytes, loss of nonmyocytes, and maladaptive remodeling.[48] Through the use of transgenic mouse models, Wencker and colleagues demonstrated that even slight increases in the incidence of myocyte apoptosis can be sufficient to lead to the development of cardiac myopathy, and that inhibition of apoptosis could prevent the development of cardiac dilation and contractile dysfunction within these models.[46]

In contrast to apoptosis, necrosis is a disorganized cellular death process accompanied by inflammation resulting from high levels of stress, such as that seen in myocardial infarction. Ischemia-induced factors (such as increases in intracellular calcium, long-chain fatty acids and reactive oxygen species) can induce a transition in mitochondrial membrane permeability that triggers either apoptotic or necrotic cell death (Figure 4.15). The actual process depends on the level of mitochondrial dysfunction caused by the loss of mitochondrial membrane potential, intra-mitochondrial components, and other factors.[38]

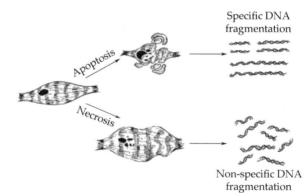

**FIGURE 4.15    Comparison of cellular changes in necrosis and apoptosis.** Apoptotic cell death is characterized by cell shrinkage, organized chromosomal DNA fragmentation, and packaging of cellular components into vesicles, which bud off the cell in a process called "blebbing." In contrast, necrotic cell death is characterized by cell swelling and lysis due to loss of plasma membrane integrity; cellular components are not fragmented or vesicularized, and this evokes an inflammatory response in surrounding tissue.[45] *Source:* Adapted with permission from Khoynezhad et al., *Tex Heart Inst J.* 2007;34(3):352-359.

# Gene Mutations in Heart Failure

Several types of heart failure are known to have a genetic basis (Figure 4.16). Nevertheless, the impact of genetic factors on cardiac structure and function can be complex (Figure 4.17). Diverse nucleotide substitutions within a single gene may lead to similar or variable clinical phenotypes.[49,50] For example, of nine genes associated with hypertrophic cardiomyopathy (HCM), more than 400 different mutations have been discovered.[51] The relationship between genotype and phenotype can be further modulated by other genetic, epigenetic, and environmental factors, leading to variable penetrance of a known gene mutation. Thus, family members with the same nucleotide gene mutation may present with different clinical sequelae. Because of these factors, patient care cannot be directed simply by identifying the gene associated with a specific disease state. However, once an abnormal gene is identified in an affected family, it may serve as a useful construct to identify additional phenotypic features in affected family members.

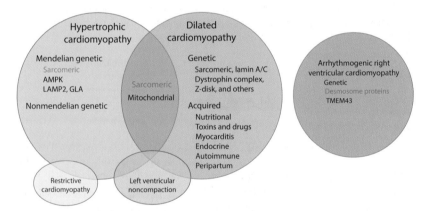

FIGURE 4.16   **Inherited cardiomyopathies and their genetic basis.** Classes of genes highlighted in red denote the most common locations of mutations. Abbreviations: AMPK, AMP-activated protein kinase; GLA, α-galactosidase A; LAMP2, lysosomal-associated membrane protein 2; TMEM43, transmembrane protein 43.[51] *Source:* Adapted with permission from Watkins et al., *N Engl J Med.* 2011;364(17):1643-1656.

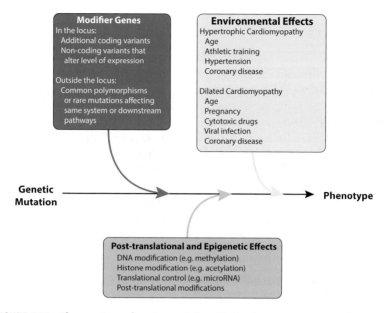

**FIGURE 4.17** **The genotype-phenotype relationship involves many compounding factors which include: genetic mutation, molecular responses, and environmental effects.**[51] *Source:* Adapted with permission from Watkins H et al., *N Engl J Med.* 2011;364(17):1643-1656.

## HYPERTROPHIC CARDIOMYOPATHY

Termed a "disease of the sarcomere," hypertrophic cardiomyopathy (HCM) most commonly stems from mutations of specific sarcomeric genes that can lead to increased energy utilization (Figure 4.18).[51] Patients with HCM can present with regional (especially septal) or global left ventricular hypertrophy (see Chapter 7). Less commonly mitochondrial defects and mutations in the cardiac energy-sensing apparatus can lead to similar morphologic changes of the left ventricle. Sarcomeric mutations are transmitted in an autosomal dominant pattern with a high penetrance, conveying a greater than 95% lifetime risk of detectable HCM.[52]

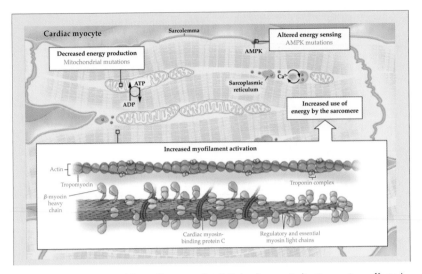

**FIGURE 4.18** **Hypertrophic cardiomyopathy.** Cellular diagram indicating regions affected by genetic abnormalities associated with hypertrophic cardiomyopathy.[51] *Source:* Adapted with permission from Watkins et al., *N Engl J Med.* 2011;364(17):1643-1656.

## FAMILIAL DILATED CARDIOMYOPATHY

The geneses of familial nonischemic dilated cardiomyopathies, characterized by left ventricular enlargement and systolic dysfunction, include mutations to sarcomeric and nonsarcomeric genes (Figure 4.19). In this case, the sarcomeric mechanisms are different from those of HCM and involve decreased myofilament activation.[53] Nonsarcomeric mutations have varied molecular mechanisms, including loss of cell structural integrity that can lead to myocyte cell damage. When multiple cases of cardiomyopathy are recognized within a family, the pattern of affected members can suggest the mode of inheritance: autosomal dominant or recessive, X or Y-linked, or mitochondrial (Figure 4.20).

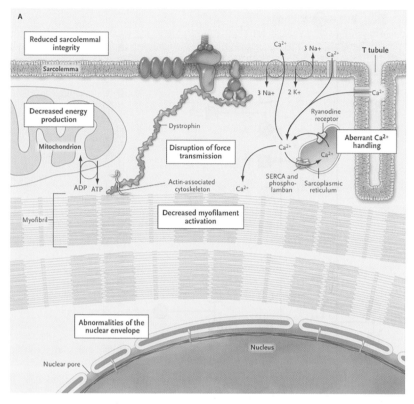

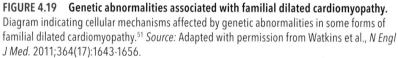

**FIGURE 4.19    Genetic abnormalities associated with familial dilated cardiomyopathy.** Diagram indicating cellular mechanisms affected by genetic abnormalities in some forms of familial dilated cardiomyopathy.[51] *Source:* Adapted with permission from Watkins et al., *N Engl J Med.* 2011;364(17):1643-1656.

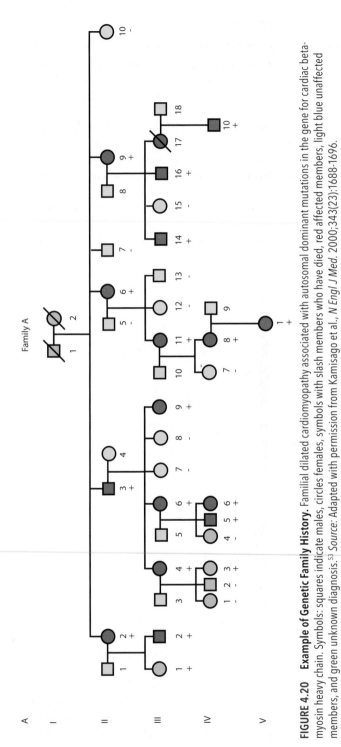

**FIGURE 4.20   Example of Genetic Family History.** Familial dilated cardiomyopathy associated with autosomal dominant mutations in the gene for cardiac beta-myosin heavy chain. Symbols: squares indicate males, circles females, symbols with slash members who have died, red affected members, light blue unaffected members, and green unknown diagnosis.[53] *Source:* Adapted with permission from Kamisago et al., *N Engl J Med.* 2000;343(23):1688-1696.

## OTHER GENETIC CARDIOMYOPATHIES

Restrictive cardiomyopathy (RCM) is the least common form of familial cardiomyopathy. RCM is characterized by diastolic dysfunction with normal ventricular chamber size and systolic function, and dilated atria. Wall thickness is frequently mildly increased overlapping the phenotype of hypertrophic cardiomyopathy.

Left ventricular noncompaction cardiomyopathy, also called spongiform cardiomyopathy, results from a genetic defect for transformation of myocardial trabeculations into compact ventricular muscle during cardiac development.[54] Noncompaction is diagnosed when endocardial trabeculations (imaged by echocardiogram or cardiac magnetic resonance imaging [MRI]) are more than twice the thickness of the compact associated epicardial ventricular wall (Figure 4.21). Patients are frequently asymptomatic, but can develop heart failure, arrhythmias, thromboembolic events, and sudden cardiac death.[55] This cardiomyopathy may present with either HF-pEF or HF-rEF.

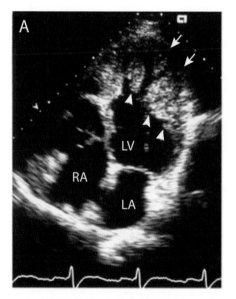

**FIGURE 4.21  Noncompaction cardiomyopathy.** Echocardiogram showing prominent apical trabeculations and recesses **(arrowheads)**. Note thin epicardial layer **(thin arrows)**.[55] *Source:* Adapted with permission from Oechslin et al., *J Am Coll Cardiol.* 2000;36(2):493-500.

Arrhythmogenic right ventricular cardiomyopathy is a distinct category associated with ventricular tachycardia, left ventricular dysfunction, and at times, marked right ventricular dilation. Recognition of this condition may trigger an evaluation for an implanted cardioverter-defibrillator (ICD) device.[51] In patients without a pacemaker or ICD, MRI is appropriate to detect the morphological and tissue characteristic changes of this disorder. Echocardiography is also useful in detection and monitoring of this cardiomyopathy. Rarely, severe right heart failure can necessitate heart transplantation.

## EPIGENETICS

Epigenetic effects include potentially heritable biochemical modifications of DNA, RNA, or associated protein histones that do not involve changes in a nucleotide sequence. These chemical changes such as locus-specific DNA methylation and histone acetylation may result in differential gene expression (Figure 4.22). These modifications in gene expression may result from changes in environmental factors, including diet,[56] and are considered to persist longer than the ordinary binding process of transcription factors, but shorter than mutation changes in the nucleotide sequence. As an example of such a process, regions of the human myocyte genome in normal versus end-stage cardiomyopathic tissue display different methylation profiles that correlate with specific sites of increased or decreased transcription.[57]

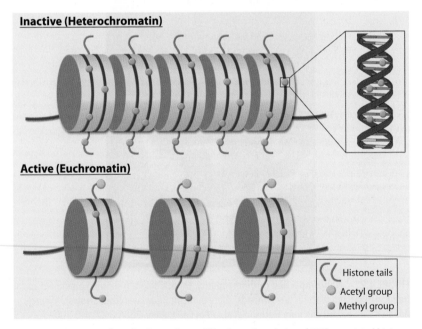

FIGURE 4.22   Examples of epigenetic modifications. Acetylation of DNA-associated histone proteins or DNA methylation of DNA cytosine residues can affect DNA to RNA transcription.

# References

1. Dawkins R. *River Out of Eden: A Darwinian View of Life.* Science masters series. New York, NY: Basic Books; 1995: 172.

2. Leri A, Kajstura J, Anversa P. Role of cardiac stem cells in cardiac pathophysiology: a paradigm shift in human myocardial biology. *Circ Res.* 2011;109(8):941-961.

3. Mohammed SF, et al. Comorbidity and ventricular and vascular structure and function in heart failure with preserved ejection fraction: a community-based study. *Circ Heart Fail.* 2012;5(6):710-719.

4. Popescu BA, et al. Left ventricular remodelling and torsional dynamics in dilated cardiomyopathy: reversed apical rotation as a marker of disease severity. *Eur J Heart Fail.* 2009;11(10):945-951.

5. Konstam MA. "Systolic and diastolic dysfunction" in heart failure? Time for a new paradigm. *J Card Fail.* 2003;9(1):1-3.

6. Willis MS, et al. Build it up-tear it down: protein quality control in the cardiac sarcomere. *Cardiovasc Res.* 2009;81(3):439-448.

7. Lionetti V, et al. Control of autocrine and paracrine myocardial signals: an emerging therapeutic strategy in heart failure. *Heart Fail Rev.* 2010;15(6):531-542.

8. Mann DL,Bristow MR. Mechanisms and models in heart failure: the biomechanical model and beyond. *Circulation.* 2005;111(21):2837-2849.

9. Jaski BE, Serruys PW. Epicardial wall motion and left ventricular function during coronary graft angioplasty in humans. *J Am Coll Cardiol.* 1985;6(3):695-700.

10. Konstam MA, et al. Left ventricular remodeling in heart failure: current concepts in clinical significance and assessment. *JACC Cardiovasc Imaging.* 2011;4(1):98-108.

11. Jaski BE. *Basics of Heart Failure: A Problem Solving Approach.* Boston: Kluwer Academic Publishers; 2000.

12. Grossman W, Jones D, McLaurin LP. Wall stress and patterns of hypertrophy in the human left ventricle. *J Clin Invest.* 1975;56(1):56-64.

13. Russell B, et al. Mechanical stress-induced sarcomere assembly for cardiac muscle growth in length and width. *J Molec Cell Cardiol.* 2010;48(5):817-823.

14. Linke WA. Sense and stretchability: the role of titin and titin-associated proteins in myocardial stress-sensing and mechanical dysfunction. *Cardiovasc Res.* 2008;77(4): 637-648.

15. Deschamps AM, Spinale FG. Disruptions and detours in the myocardial matrix highway and heart failure. *Curr Heart Fail Rep.* 2005;2(1):10-17.

16. Weber KT. Extracellular matrix remodeling in heart failure: a role for de novo angiotensin II generation. *Circulation.* 1997;96(11):4065-4082.

17. Jugdutt BI. Ventricular remodeling after infarction and the extracellular collagen matrix: when is enough enough? *Circulation.* 2003;108(11):1395-1403.

18. Borer JS, et al. Myocardial fibrosis in chronic aortic regurgitation: molecular and cellular responses to volume overload. *Circulation.* 2002;105(15):1837-1842.

19. Rossi MA, Abreu MA, Santoro LB. Images in cardiovascular medicine. Connective tissue skeleton of the human heart: a demonstration by cell-maceration scanning electron microscope method. *Circulation.*1998;97(9):934-935.

20. Katz AM. *Heart Failure. Pathophysiology, Molecular Biology, and Clinical Management.* 2000, Philadelphia: Lippincott Williams & Wilkins. 109-110; 319-324.

21. Cohn JN, et al. Plasma norepinephrine as a guide to prognosis in patients with chronic congestive heart failure. *N Engl J Med.* 1984;311(13):819-823.

22. Cournot M, et al. Optimization of the use of B-type natriuretic peptide levels for risk stratification at discharge in elderly patients with decompensated heart failure. *Am Heart J.* 2008;155(6):986-991.

23. Effect of enalapril on survival in patients with reduced left ventricular ejection fractions and congestive heart failure. The SOLVD Investigators. *N Engl J Med.* 1991;325(5):293-302.

24. Packer M, et al. The effect of carvedilol on morbidity and mortality in patients with chronic heart failure. U.S. Carvedilol Heart Failure Study Group. *N Engl J Med.* 1996;334(21):1349-1355.

25. Anand IS, et al. Changes in brain natriuretic peptide and norepinephrine over time and mortality and morbidity in the Valsartan Heart Failure Trial (Val-HeFT). *Circulation.* 2003;107(9):1278-1283.

26. MacFadyen RJ, Barr CS, Struthers AD. Aldosterone blockade reduces vascular collagen turnover, improves heart rate variability and reduces early morning rise in heart rate in heart failure patients. *Cardiovasc Res.* 1997;35(1):30-34.

27. Wang W, McClain JM, Zucker IH. Aldosterone reduces baroreceptor discharge in the dog. *Hypertension.* 1992;19(3):270-277.

28. Weir RA, et al. Serum soluble ST2: a potential novel mediator in left ventricular and infarct remodeling after acute myocardial infarction. *J Am Coll Cardiol.* 2010;55(3): 243-250.

29. Pitt B, et al. The effect of spironolactone on morbidity and mortality in patients with severe heart failure. Randomized Aldactone Evaluation Study Investigators. *N Engl J Med.* 1999;341(10):709-717.

30. Pitt B, et al. The EPHESUS trial: eplerenone in patients with heart failure due to systolic dysfunction complicating acute myocardial infarction. Eplerenone Post-AMI Heart Failure Efficacy and Survival Study. *Cardiovasc Drugs Ther.* 2001;15(1):79-87.

31. Zannad F, et al. Eplerenone in patients with systolic heart failure and mild symptoms. *N Engl J Med.* 2011;364(1):11-21.

32. Kranias EG, Hajjar RJ. Modulation of cardiac contractility by the phospholamban/SERCA2a regulatome. *Circ Res.* 2012;110(12):1646-1660.

33. Periasamy M, Bhupathy P, Babu GJ. Regulation of sarcoplasmic reticulum Ca2+ ATPase pump expression and its relevance to cardiac muscle physiology and pathology. *Cardiovasc Res.* 2008;77(2):265-273.

34. MacLennan DH, Kranias EG. Phospholamban: a crucial regulator of cardiac contractility. *Nat Rev Mol Cell Biol.* 2003;4(7):566-577.

35. Mann DL. Mechanisms and models in heart failure: A combinatorial approach. *Circulation.* 1999;100(9):999-1008.

36. Rengo G. Lymperopoulos A, Koch WJ. Future g protein-coupled receptor targets for treatment of heart failure. *Curr Treat Options Cardiovasc Med.* 2009;11(4):328-338.

37. Weiss JN, et al. Role of the mitochondrial permeability transition in myocardial disease. *Circ Res.* 2003;93(4):292-301.

38. Nakayama H, et al. Ca2+- and mitochondrial-dependent cardiomyocyte necrosis as a primary mediator of heart failure. *J Clin Invest.* 2007;117(9):2431-2444.

39. Di F, et al. Mitochondria and cardioprotection. *Heart Fail Rev.* 2007;12(3-4):249-260.

40. Lodish H, et al. in *Molecular Cell Biology.* 2007, W. H. Freeman.

41. Nishida K, Yamaguchi O, Otsu K. Crosstalk between autophagy and apoptosis in heart disease. *Circ Res.* 2008;103(4):343-351.

42. Depre C, Vatner SF. Cardioprotection in stunned and hibernating myocardium. *Heart Fail Rev.* 2007;12(3-4):307-317.

43. Nishida K, Otsu K. Cell death in heart failure. *Circ J.* 2008;72 (suppl A):A17-A21.

44. Cao DJ, Gillette TG, Hill JA. Cardiomyocyte autophagy: remodeling, repairing, and reconstructing the heart. *Curr Hypertens Rep.* 2009;11(6):406-411.

45. Khoynezhad A, Jalali Z, Tortolani AJ. A synopsis of research in cardiac apoptosis and its application to congestive heart failure. *Tex Heart Inst J.* 2007;34(3):352-359.

46. Wencker D, et al. A mechanistic role for cardiac myocyte apoptosis in heart failure. *J Clin Invest.* 2003;111(10):1497-1504.

47. Nakagawa T, et al. Cyclophilin D-dependent mitochondrial permeability transition regulates some necrotic but not apoptotic cell death. *Nature.* 2005;434(7033): 652-658.

48. van Empel VP, et al. Myocyte apoptosis in heart failure. *Cardiovasc Res.* 2005;67(1): 21-29.

49. Jacoby D, McKenna WJ. Genetics of inherited cardiomyopathy. *Eur Heart J.* 2012. 33(3):296-304.

50. Creemers EE,Wilde AA, Pinto YM. Heart failure: advances through genomics. *Nat Rev Genet.* 2011;12(5):357-362.

51. Watkins H, Ashrafian H, Redwood C. Inherited cardiomyopathies. *N Engl J Med.* 2011;364(17):1643-1656.

52. American College of Cardiology Foundation/American Heart Association Task Force on, et al. 2011 ACCF/AHA guideline for the diagnosis and treatment of hypertrophic cardiomyopathy: a report of the American College of Cardiology Foundation/ American Heart Association Task Force on Practice Guidelines. *J Thorac Cardiovasc Surg.* 2011;142(6):e153-203.

53. Kamisago M, et al. Mutations in sarcomere protein genes as a cause of dilated cardiomyopathy. *N Engl J Med.* 2000;343(23):1688-1696.

54. Klaassen S, et al. Mutations in sarcomere protein genes in left ventricular noncompaction. *Circulation.* 2008;117(22):2893-2901.

55. Oechslin EN, et al. Long-term follow-up of 34 adults with isolated left ventricular noncompaction: a distinct cardiomyopathy with poor prognosis. *J Am Coll Cardiol.* 2000;36(2):493-500.

56. Cooney CA, Dave AA, Wolff GL. Maternal methyl supplements in mice affect epigenetic variation and DNA methylation of offspring. *J Nutr.* 2002;132(8 Suppl): 2393S-2400S.

57. Movassagh M, et al. Distinct epigenomic features in end-stage failing human hearts. *Circulation.* 2011;124(22):2411-2422.

# CHAPTER 5

# Stage B: Asymptomatic Structural Heart Disease

## FAST FACTS

- Stage B includes those with a history of myocardial infarction without heart failure symptoms.

- Stage B may also manifest as asymptomatic left ventricular hypertrophy, systolic dysfunction, or diastolic dysfunction detected by Doppler echocardiography.

- Medication treatment for hypertension can result in regression of increased left ventricular wall thickness.

- Comorbidities of renal insufficiency, anemia, and chronic obstructive lung disease increase the likelihood that Stage B patients will progress to symptomatic Stage C heart failure.

- Screening for Stage B patients at a population level is not widely implemented at present because of limited cost effectiveness.

- When cancer treatment affects myocardial function, chemotherapy more commonly leads to systolic dysfunction, whereas radiation leads to diastolic dysfunction.

- Patients with Stage B asymptomatic systolic dysfunction can be treated with beta-blockers, ACE inhibitors, angiotensin receptor blockers, or implantable cardioverter-defibrillators as indicated.

*"Before heart failure occurs, hypertrophy has generally become well developed and moreover it appears to have developed in a pattern unique to the inciting stress."*

—William Grossman, 1975[1]

# Who Is the Stage B Pre-Heart Failure Patient?

Stage B is composed of patients who have structural heart disease associated with risk of subsequent heart failure. By definition, the advancement from Stage A to Stage B heart failure can occur without recognition by patients especially if noncardiac factors limit physical activity. Thus, the clinical definition of the Stage B patient is often somewhat difficult to pinpoint. For example, the Mayo Clinic criteria include an assessment of physical activity (see complete criteria below).

## STAGE B CLINICAL DEFINITIONS

**AHA/ACC Guidelines[2]**
Patients with structural heart disease that is strongly associated with the development of heart failure (HF) but without HF signs or symptoms.

**Mayo Clinic[3]**
Previous myocardial infarction; left ventricular hypertrophy by echocardiogram or ECG; left ventricular dilatation or hypocontractility; moderate to severe valvular heart disease.

Asymptomatic physical capacity of > 7 mets.*

* > 7 mets activity e.g., carrying 24 lbs. up a flight of 8 steps
(1 met = oxygen consumption at rest = 3.5 mL O2/kg/min)

## STAGE B SYSTOLIC DYSFUNCTION

Stage B outcomes depend on the population studied and the criteria used to define structural heart disease. In patients with left ventricular systolic dysfunction (LVSD), it is estimated that there are four times as many asymptomatic (Stage B) as symptomatic Stage C and D patients combined.[4]

The Framingham Study assessed 4257 asymptomatic participants (age ≥ 40 years) and found an ejection fraction (EF) < 50% to be present in 6.0% of men and in 0.8% of women. As systolic function worsened, prognosis approached that of symptomatic systolic dysfunction (Figure 5.1).[5]

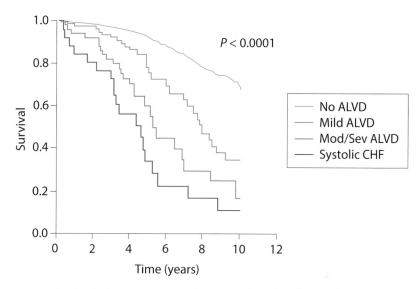

**FIGURE 5.1** **Survival curves in relationship to systolic dysfunction.** Kaplan-Meier curves for survival (n = 4257). In the key, ALVD stands for asymptomatic left ventricular (systolic) dysfunction. No ALVD consists of subjects with normal left ventricular systolic function (EF > 50%) and no history of congestive heart failure (CHF). Mild ALVD indicates an EF of 40% to 50%. Mod/Sev ALVD indicates EF < 40%. Systolic CHF indicates symptomatic patients with systolic dysfunction.[4] *Source:* Adapted with permission from Goldberg & Jessup, *Circulation.* 2006;113(24):2851-2860.

Subsequently, an analysis by Lam et al. in an elderly subset of the Framingham study population (mean age, 76 ± 5 years) assessed both LV systolic and diastolic dysfunction. Systolic dysfunction was defined as echocardiographic EF ≤45%, and diastolic dysfunction was defined by abnormal Doppler mitral inflow patterns showing abnormal relaxation, pseudonormal, or restrictive filling (see Chapter 7). Using these definitions, they found a prevalence of asymptomatic systolic dysfunction of 5% and diastolic dysfunction of 36%.[6]

## STAGE B SYSTOLIC AND DIASTOLIC DYSFUNCTION

The Mayo Clinic sampled a cross-section of 2029 Olmsted County, Minnesota residents aged ≥45 years. When using clinical criteria including post-MI, systolic dysfunction, valvular heart disease, and left ventricular hypertrophy (LVH) either by ECG or on echocardiogram, they found a Stage B prevalence of 23%. When Doppler diastolic dysfunction (see Table 5.1) was included, the prevalence increased to 34% (Figure 5.2).[3]

**TABLE 5.1    Mayo Clinic Definition Stage B Abnormal Echocardiogram.**
Echocardiographic findings can be abnormal based on systolic or diastolic dysfunction. E/A ratio refers to transmitral Doppler velocity in early diastole (E) or during atrial inflow (A)[3] (see also Chapter 7, Figure 7.2).

| SYSTOLIC DYSFUNCTION: EF < 50% | |
| --- | --- |
| DIASTOLIC DYSFUNCTION | E/A RATIO |
| Normal | Normal E/A ratio |
| Mild diastolic dysfunction | Decreased E/A ratio < 0.75 |
| Moderate/"pseudonormal" diastolic dysfunction with other Doppler indices of elevated left ventricular end-diastolic filling pressure | E/A ratio 0.75 to 1.5 |
| Severe diastolic dysfunction | Increased E/A ratio of > 1.5, deceleration time < 140 ms, Doppler indices of elevated left ventricular end-diastolic filling pressure |

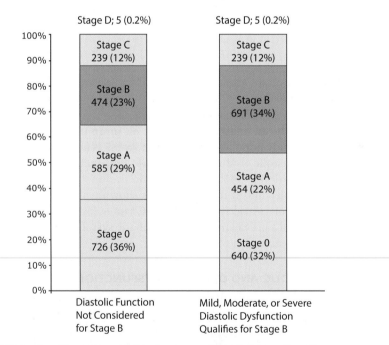

**FIGURE 5.2    Prevalence of heart failure by stages with and without diastolic dysfunction as criteria for Stage B.** All individuals were ≥ 45 years old. Stage 0 refers to the absence of any Stage A risk factors. Using the Mayo Clinic's criteria, the inclusion of diastolic ventricular dysfunction (Table 5.1) as a qualifying abnormality for Stage B heart failure increases the prevalence of Stage B heart failure.[3] *Source:* Adapted with permission from Ammar et al., *Circulation.* 2007;115(12):1563-1570.

# Neurohumoral Continuum from Stage B to Stage C Systolic Dysfunction

The patient with structural heart disease can manifest a progressive increase in virtually all neurohumoral mediators.[7] These activated systems can have acute circulatory and long-term gene expression effects in myocardial and vascular cells. High baseline levels of mediators can also blunt compensatory reserve for acute adjustments to circulatory stress.

### NEUROHUMORAL ACTIVATION CAN PRECEDE SYMPTOMATIC HF-rEF

The Studies of Left Ventricular Dysfunction (SOLVD) trials evaluated normal subjects without heart disease (control group), patients with a left ventricular EF less than 35% prior to the development of heart failure symptoms (Stage B prevention group), and patients with recent development of heart failure symptoms (Stage C treatment group).[8] Increasing levels of norepinephrine, plasma renin activity, and vasopressin were observed with increases in disease severity.

*Norepinephrine*

Plasma norepinephrine levels in Stage B patients with systolic dysfunction are elevated compared to normal controls but not as high as in patients with Stage C heart failure (Figure 5.3).

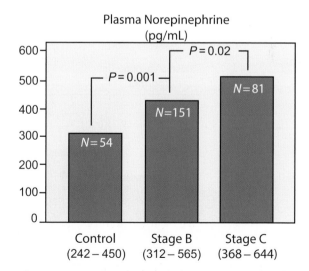

FIGURE 5.3   **Plasma norepinephrine activity in SOLVD patient groups.**[7] *Source:* Adapted with permission from Francis et al., *Circulation.* 1990;82(5):1724-1729.

*Plasma Renin Activity*

Plasma renin activity, a mediator of angiotensin II formation, also increased within the three SOLVD groups (Figure 5.4).

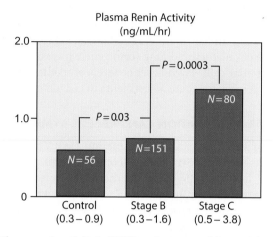

**FIGURE 5.4   Plasma renin activity in SOLVD patient groups.**[7] *Source:* Adapted with permission from Francis et al., *Circulation.* 1990;82(5):1724-1729.

*Vasopressin/Antidiuretic Hormone*

Although pituitary vasopressin release is primarily stimulated by increases in plasma osmolality, it can also be triggered by baroreceptor activation with low cardiac output states and by angiotensin II (Figure 5.5). In advanced Stage C and Stage D patients, high levels of vasopressin can lead to hyponatremia (see Chapter 10).

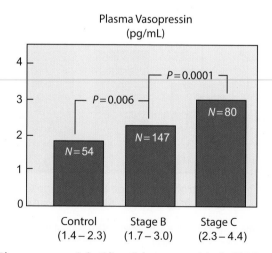

**FIGURE 5.5   Plasma vasopressin/antidiuretic hormone activity in SOLVD patient groups.**[7]
*Source:* Adapted with permission from Francis et al., *Circulation.* 1990;82(5):1724-1729.

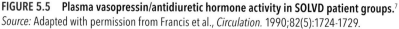

# The Continuum from Hypertension to HF-pEF

Similar to the pattern of neurohormonal activation, a continuum of diastolic dysfunction-associated abnormalities is seen when Doppler echocardiography assessments are made in a normal control group, in hypertensives with LVH identified by echocardiography but without heart failure symptoms, and in Stage C hypertensives with HF-pEF (Figure 5.6).

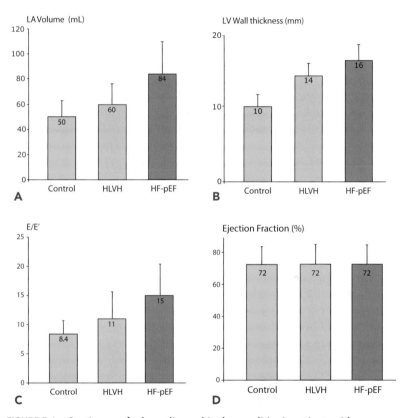

**FIGURE 5.6   Continuum of echocardiographic abnormalities in patients with progressive stages of heart failure.** Data were obtained in a cross-sectional study comparing normotensive control subjects without LVH (*n* = 56), hypertensive left ventricular hypertrophy (HLVH) subjects without heart failure (*n* = 40), and HF-pEF patients (*n* = 37). Diastolic dysfunction parameters in **Panels A, B,** and **C** are left atrial (LA) volume, left ventricular wall thickness, and E/E% respectively (see Chapter 7). **Panel D** shows EF% in the same study population. Overall EF% does not change even when diastolic dysfunction worsens.[9] *Source:* Adapted with permission from Melenovsky et al., *J Am Coll Cardiol.* 2007;49(2):198-207.

## HYPERTENSIVE LEFT VENTRICULAR HYPERTROPHY AS TARGET FOR THERAPY

Most classes of medications that lower high blood pressure are associated with regression of LVH by echocardiography that can be detected as early as 3 months after initiation of therapy.[10] Whether left ventricular wall thickness or mass per se is justified as a target of antihypertensive therapy is uncertain.[11] At present, blood pressure goals alone are most strongly correlated with improved patient outcomes, and the goal of regression of hypertrophy is not incorporated into therapeutic guidelines. Although hypertension is the most common cause of increased left ventricular wall thickness, many other causes exist (Tables 5.2, 5.3, and 5.4)

TABLE 5.2   Common causes of left ventricular hypertrophy.

| CONDITION: CLINICAL PEARLS AND FEATURES | DIAGNOSTIC POINTERS |
|---|---|
| **Hypertension:**<br>5%–10% due to secondary causes in adults | **ECG:** presence of LVH (prevalence ~30%) can predict prognosis<br>**Echo:** concentric LVH<br>**MRI:** may help identify aortic coarctation |
| **Aortic stenosis:**<br>• Ejection systolic murmur may be absent in low cardiac output state<br>• Distinguish from dynamic LV outflow tract obstruction | **ECG:** LVH<br>**Echo:** Low valve gradient and reduced valve area in patients with low ejection fraction |
| **Obesity:**<br>• BMI > 30 kg/m²<br>• Increased waist circumference | **ECG:** Attenuated ECG LVH due to body habitus (prevalence ~10%) |
| **Physiological LVH**<br>**Athletic heart:**<br>• High-level endurance training<br>• Resting bradycardia<br>• LVH regression with deconditioning | **ECG:** LVH<br>**Echo:**<br>• Mild concentric LVH (rarely > 13 mm)<br>• Volume-loaded (dilated) LV cavity<br>• Preserved diastolic and long-axis function<br>**MRI:** No late gadolinium enhancement |

*Abbreviations:* BMI, body mass index; ECG, electrocardiogram; Echo, echocardiogram; LV, left ventricle; LVH, left ventricular hypertrophy; MRI, magnetic resonance imaging.[12] *Source:* Adapted from Yousef et al., *Eur Heart J.* 2013;34(11):802-808.

**TABLE 5.3    Less common causes of left ventricular hypertrophy.**

| CONDITION: CLINICAL PEARLS AND FEATURES | DIAGNOSTIC POINTERS |
|---|---|
| **Sarcomere protein disease/hypertrophic cardiomyopathy:**<br>• Family history (population prevalence 1:500)<br>• Leading cause of sudden death in young athletes<br>• Risk stratification for sudden cardiac death | **ECG:** If LVH with anterior T-wave inversion, consider apical LVH<br>**Echo:**<br>• Asymmetrical septal hypertrophy common (but also can present with concentric or apical LVH, and right ventricular involvement)<br>• Normal LV dimensions in early stages of disease<br>• Systolic anterior motion of mitral valve, dilated left atrium, diastolic dysfunction, and dynamic LV outflow tract obstruction<br>**MRI:** Intramyocardial late gadolinium enhancement<br>**Genetics:** Autosomal dominant |
| **Amyloidosis:**<br>• Senile amyloid relatively common (20% in population over 80 years old)<br>• Multisystem involvement with variable signs including: proteinuria, petechiae, peripheral and autonomic neuropathy, hepatosplenomegaly, macroglossia | **ECG:** Low voltage QRS, heart block, atrial fibrillation<br>**Echo:**<br>• LVH with preserved LV size and bi-atrial dilatation<br>• Speckled LV septum<br>• Restrictive physiology<br>• Thickened interatrial septum and valve leaflets<br>**MRI:** Subendocardial late gadolinium enhancement<br>**Other:** Congo red staining of target organ biopsies |
| **Hemochromatosis:**<br>• Late presentation in females<br>• Transfusion overload<br>• Clinical constellation includes: bronze skin, arthritis, diabetes (and other endocrine abnormalities), and liver cirrhosis | **ECG:** LVH<br>**Echo:** LVH with bi-ventricular and bi-atrial dilatation. Restrictive physiology<br>**MRI:** Rapid signal decay (< 20 ms) on T2* imaging may suggest indication for venesection and/or iron chelation therapy<br>**Genetics:** Human hemochromatosis protein (HFE) gene testing (autosomal recessive) |
| **Left ventricular noncompaction:**<br>• May have preserved or reduced ejection fraction<br>• Warfarin may be useful for prevention of systemic embolism | **Echo:** Ratio of non-compacted to compacted myocardium > 2:1. Color flow Doppler demonstrates blood flow in deep inter-trabecular sinuses<br>**MRI:** Tendency to over diagnose condition<br>**Genetics:** Autosomal dominant in familial cases |

*Abbreviations:* ECG, electrocardiogram; Echo, echocardiogram; LV, left ventricle; LVH, left ventricular hypertrophy; MRI, magnetic resonance imaging.[12] *Source:* Adapted with permission from Yousef et al., *Eur Heart J.* 2013;34(11):802-808.

**TABLE 5.4    Uncommon genetic causes of left ventricular hypertrophy.**

| CONDITION: CLINICAL PEARLS AND FEATURES | DIAGNOSTIC POINTERS |
|---|---|
| **Fabry disease:**<br>• Deficiency of $\alpha$-galactosidase A<br>• Enzyme replacement therapy available | **ECG:** LVH, short P–R interval, heart block<br>**Laboratory:** Proteinuria<br>**Genetics:** Absence of male–male transmission due to X-linked inheritance. Female presentation later in life. |
| **Pompe disease:**<br>• Acid maltase deficiency<br>• Limb-girdle and respiratory muscle weakness | **ECG:** LVH, short P–R interval, accessory pathways<br>**Laboratory:** Serum CK elevated, no fasting hypoglycemia<br>**Echo:** Concentric LVH with restrictive physiology<br>**Genetics:** Autosomal recessive |
| **Danon disease:**<br>• Lysosomal-associated membrane protein 2 (LAMP2) deficiency<br>• Skeletal muscle weakness, and mental retardation | **ECG:** LVH, short P–R interval, accessory pathways<br>**Laboratory:** Reduced LAMP2 activity (a membrane protein assay)<br>**Echo:** Concentric LVH with restrictive physiology<br>**Genetics:** Autosomal recessive |
| **PRKAG2 cardiomyopathy:**<br>• Mutation of AMP-activated protein kinase $\gamma 2$ gene | **ECG:** LVH, short P–R interval, accessory pathways<br>**Echo:** Concentric LVH with restrictive physiology<br>**Genetics:** Autosomal dominant |
| **Primary carnitine deficiency:**<br>• Functional carnitine transporter deficiency<br>• Skeletal muscle weakness, hepatomegaly, abnormal fatty acid metabolism | **ECG:** LVH<br>**Echo:** Concentric LVH with restrictive physiology<br>**Laboratory:** Hypoglycemia, hyperammonemia, low plasma carnitine level<br>**Genetics:** Autosomal recessive |
| **Mitochondrial:**<br>• Skeletal muscle weakness<br>• Neurologic abnormalities | **ECG:** LVH<br>**Laboratory:** Serum CK and glucose normal or elevated<br>**Echo:** Concentric LVH with restrictive physiology<br>**Muscle biopsy:** typical ragged red fibers<br>**Genetics:** Mitochondrial DNA mutation analysis |

*Source:* Adapted with permission from Yousef et al., *Eur Heart J.* 2013;34(11):802-808.[12]

# Cardiac and Noncardiac Interactions

Lam and coworkers evaluated the Framingham database for the interaction of cardiac and noncardiac organ dysfunction leading to the syndrome of heart failure. The coexistence of Stage B heart failure (either systolic or diastolic dysfunction) and anemia, renal, or pulmonary dysfunction favored the subsequent development of Stage C heart failure (Figure 5.7). In contrast, impaired liver function and white blood cell count did not affect the risk of subsequent heart failure.

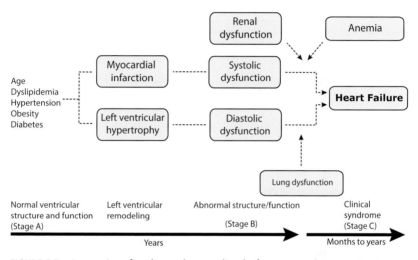

**FIGURE 5.7   Interaction of cardiac and noncardiac dysfunctions and progression to heart failure.**[13] *Source:* Adapted with permission from Klein, *Circulation.* 2011;124(1):4-6.

In a multivariate analysis, Stage C heart failure classification was separated into HF-rEF and HF-pEF and the antecedent factors determined. HF-rEF was associated with antecedent left ventricular systolic dysfunction, greater serum creatinine, and lower hemoglobin concentration; HF-pEF was associated with antecedent left ventricular diastolic dysfunction and lower ratio of forced expiratory volume in 1 second to forced expiratory volume ($FEV_1$ : FVC) on pulmonary function testing.[6] The combined impact of these indicators of noncardiac organ system dysfunction on the cumulative incidence of heart failure is shown in Figure 5.8.

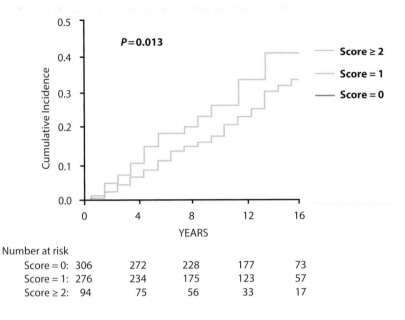

Number at risk

|  | | | | |
|---|---|---|---|---|
| Score = 0: | 306 | 272 | 228 | 177 | 73 |
| Score = 1: | 276 | 234 | 175 | 123 | 57 |
| Score ≥ 2: | 94 | 75 | 56 | 33 | 17 |

**FIGURE 5.8  Noncardiac Risk Score based on noncardiac major organ system dysfunction and cumulative incidence of symptomatic heart failure.** Risk score ranges from 0 to 3. One point each was awarded for the presence of the following three parameters: serum creatinine > 1.05 mg/dL (92.8 µmol/L), $FEV_1$ : FVC < 91% predicted, and hemoglobin concentration < 13 g/dL.[6] *Source:* Adapted with permission from Lam et al., *Circulation.* 2011; 124(1):24-30.

The presence of any 1 of the 3 significant noncardiac organ dysfunctions conferred a 30% increase in risk of subsequent development of symptomatic heart failure. When more than 1 dysfunction was present, risks were additive (Table 5.5 and Figure 5.8).[6] Thus, the syndrome of heart failure represents more than the end result of all direct insults to the heart accumulated over time. It also reflects the contributions of vital noncardiac organs to circulatory homeostasis. Although more complex, this paradigm expands the scope of interventions beyond cardiovascular alone to include other organ systems that may potentially influence the development of heart failure in individuals at risk.

**TABLE 5.5   Association of cardiac and noncardiac dysfunction with symptomatic heart failure.**[6] *Left ventricular systolic dysfunction defined as an EF < 50%. **Left ventricular diastolic dysfunction defined as heart failure and EF > 50%. † Noncardiac Risk Score (range 0–3). One point each for: serum creatinine > 1.05 mg/dL (92.8 μmol/L), $FEV_1$ : FVC < 91% predicted, and hemoglobin concentration < 13 g/dL. CI = confidence interval.

| CHARACTERISTICS | HAZARD RATIO 95% CI | P |
|---|---|---|
| ALL HEART FAILURE (HF-rEF + HF-pEF) | | |
| LV systolic dysfunction* | 1.97 (1.05–3.68) | 0.034 |
| LV diastolic dysfunction** | 1.40 (1.02–1.93) | 0.039 |
| Noncardiac Risk Score† (incremental risk/1-unit increase) | 1.30 (1.06–1.60) | 0.013 |
| HF-rEF | | |
| LV systolic dysfunction* | 3.93 (1.86–8.30) | <0.01 |
| Serum creatinine > 1.05 mg/dL | 1.32 (1.04–1.69) | 0.025 |
| Hemoglobin concentration/1-unit decrease | 1.31 (1.10–1.55) | 0.002 |
| HF-pEF | | |
| LV diastolic dysfunction** | 1.88 (1.13–3.13) | 0.016 |
| $FEV_1$ : FVC ratio < 91% predicted | 1.38 (1.04–1.83) | 0.024 |

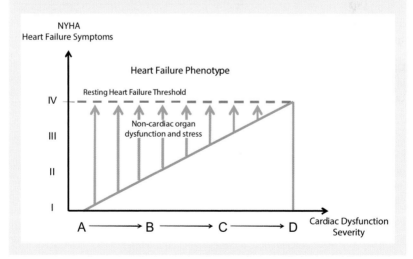

**Significant noncardiac organ dysfunction (in purple) can induce NYHA symptoms (class II and higher) even in the Stage A or B patient.**

# Screening Tests for Stage B Heart Failure

Because Stage B patients are (by definition) still asymptomatic, the issue of appropriate screening tests is paramount. Two candidates are BNP and echocardiogram testing.

## BNP FOR STAGE B SCREENING

Redfield and coworkers used a single BNP determination to predict the presence of asymptomatic Doppler echocardiogram abnormalities. A trend for higher BNP levels with worsening systolic or diastolic dysfunction was not statistically different between normal, mildly impaired, and severely impaired groups. They concluded that cost-effectiveness of screening with BNP would not be optimal (Figure 5.9).[14]

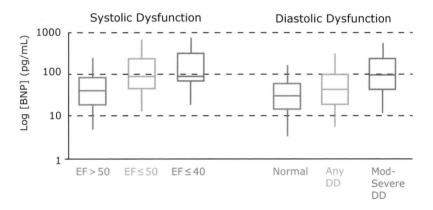

**FIGURE 5.9   Distribution of BNP according to ventricular systolic or diastolic function in Stage B individuals without heart failure and in normal controls (EF > 50 or no DD).** **Left panel:** BNP according to ejection fraction. **Right panel:** BNP according to Doppler diastolic function (see Table 5.1). $N = 817$, subjects $\geq 65$ years old. Overlap of BNP values between individuals with Stage B preclinical heart failure (**orange or red box plots**) and normal controls (**shown in green box plots**) implies poor discriminatory utility of an isolated BNP measurement for population screening. Box plot display of the log BNP: Vertical line extends to 5th and 95th percentile, boxes show the quartiles: horizontal lines for 25th, 50th (**middle line**), and 75th percentile values.[14] *Source:* Adapted from Redfield et al., *Circulation.* 2004;109(25):3176-3181, with permission.

## DOPPLER ECHOCARDIOGRAM FOR STAGE B SCREENING

If Stage B patients are identified by Doppler echocardiographic abnormalities, the predictive value of progression to symptomatic Stage C is also relatively low and thus not suitable for screening. Aurigemma and coworkers evaluated systolic and diastolic function parameters by Doppler echocardiogram to detect the subsequent development of heart failure in the Cardiovascular Health Study.[15] Participants were free of known coronary heart disease, heart failure, or atrial fibrillation at the time of their initial echocardiogram. After a mean follow-up of 5.2 years, only 6.4% developed heart failure—and 57% of those patients who did had HF-pEF. Although multivariate modeling identified variables associated with subsequent heart failure, the low incidence of clinical heart failure progression led to low positive predictive values (Table 5.6).

TABLE 5.6    Predictive value for development of symptomatic heart failure based on echocardiographic parameters. Numbers given are percent. Left ventricular hypertrophy (LVH) is defined as a left ventricle mass index exceeding 95% of the healthy reference population. LV fractional shortening is defined as left ventricular internal dimension fractional shortening with systole. Depressed shortening is that which falls below 5th percentile of the healthy reference population. E/A is the ratio of early to late Doppler mitral inflow velocity.[15]

| ECHO PARAMETERS | SENSITIVITY | SPECIFICITY | + PREDICTIVE VALUE | − PREDICTIVE VALUE |
|---|---|---|---|---|
| LVH | 24 | 92 | 18 | 95 |
| Depressed LV fractional shortening | 13 | 95 | 15 | 94 |
| E/A > 1.5 or < 0.7 | 40 | 83 | 14 | 95 |

## COMBINATIONS OF SCREENING TESTS

Cohn and coworkers have proposed a battery of 10 tests to assess cardiovascular risk that can be performed within one hour at their cardiovascular center. The cost effectiveness of this combination of tests to predict risk in a population setting is uncertain.[16]

## STAGE B HEART FAILURE IN CANCER PATIENTS AND SURVIVORS

Chemotherapy and radiation treatments have increased the survival of cancer patients. Some treatments, however, may cause reversible or irreversible structural heart disease. Cardiotoxicity can affect any heart component including the valves, myocardium, cardiac conduction system, coronary arteries, or pericardium. Combined chemotherapy and radiation therapy may have cumulative toxicity. Although cardiac impairment may occur acutely during cancer treatment,[17] cardiac manifestations may first become detected only years or decades later. This has led to the emergence of the field known as cardio-oncology.[18]

During treatment with known cardiotoxic chemotherapy (e.g., anthracyclines, trastuzumab), patients should be monitored for systolic dysfunction usually by echocardiography. Asymptomatic cancer survivors previously treated with these medications should subsequently be considered as Stage B patients at indefinite risk for future Stage C heart failure.[19] Ultimately, some patients may develop Stage D heart failure and be candidates for a left ventricular assist device and/or cardiac transplant (see Chapter 11). At any stage, if left ventricular systolic dysfunction is identified, patients should be treated (see below).

Survivors of left-sided breast cancer or Hodgkin's or non-Hodgkin's lymphoma treated with chest irradiation (despite cardiac shielding) are at increased risk for developing heart failure.[20] Initial treatment of coronary artery or valvular disease may unmask a radiation related underlying restrictive myopathy with diastolic dysfunction. Careful assessment of all contributors to HF-pEF (see Chapter 7) may be important prior to cardiac intervention in these cases. This includes the possibilities of associated pulmonary, renal, or gastrointestinal radiation-induced toxicities as contributors to a patient's symptoms.

## Management of Stage B Patients

At present, when diastolic dysfunction is recognized, guidelines support using primary prevention measures described under Stage A recommendations. However, when asymptomatic systolic dysfunction is recognized, evidence-based guidelines are emerging for pharmacotherapy and even prophylactic defibrillator resynchronization therapy, when indicated (Figure 5.10).

## Stage B

| Goals | Drugs | In selected patients |
|---|---|---|
| • Prevent HF symptoms<br>• Prevent further cardiac remodeling | • ACEI or ARB as appropriate<br>• Beta Blockers as appropriate | • ICD<br>• Revascularization or valvular surgery as appropriate |

FIGURE 5.10  **Goals and therapies in Stage B patients.**[4] *Source:* Adapted with permission from Goldberg & Jessup, *Circulation.* 2006;113(24):2851-2860.

## JAY COHN
### (1930–PRESENT)

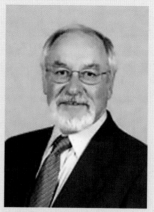

Understanding of structural heart disease leading to heart failure and associated therapies has been heavily influenced by the contributions of Dr. Jay Cohn. His laboratory and clinical research supported that left ventricular structural remodeling is the basis for progressive heart failure, and he was among the first to evaluate neurohumoral activation as a key contributor to this progression.

Beyond his work as a scientist, Dr. Cohn has shaped the structure and organization of heart failure research and practice in the United States and internationally. He organized and chaired the V-HeFT (Vasodilator Heart Failure Trial) series of studies and subsequently helped develop the Val-HeFT (Valsartan Heart Failure Trial) and A-HeFT (African-American Heart Failure Trial) studies. Dr. Cohn founded the Heart Failure Society of America and became the organization's first president including serving as the editor-in-chief of the society's *Journal of Cardiac Failure*.

*Source:* Image adapted from www.med.umn.edu

## References

1. Grossman, W, Jones D, McLaurin LP. Wall stress and patterns of hypertrophy in the human left ventricle. *J Clin Invest*. 1975;56(1):56-64.

2. Hunt SA, Abraham WT, Chin MH, et al. ACC/AHA 2005 Guideline Update for the Diagnosis and Management of Chronic Heart Failure in the Adult: a report of the American College of Cardiology/American Heart Association Task Force on Practice Guidelines (Writing Committee to Update the 2001 Guidelines for the Evaluation and Management of Heart Failure): developed in collaboration with the American College of Chest Physicians and the International Society for Heart and Lung Transplantation: endorsed by the Heart Rhythm Society. *Circulation*. 2005;112(12):e154-e235.

3. Ammar KA, Jacobsen SJ, Mahoney DW. Prevalence and prognostic significance of heart failure stages: application of the American College of Cardiology/American Heart Association heart failure staging criteria in the community. *Circulation*. 2007;115(12):1563-1570.

4. Goldberg LR, Jessup M. Stage B heart failure: management of asymptomatic left ventricular systolic dysfunction. *Circulation*. 2006;113(24):2851-2860.

5. Wang TJ, Evans JC, Benjamin EJ, Levy D, LeRoy EC, Vasan RS. Natural history of asymptomatic left ventricular systolic dysfunction in the community. *Circulation*. 2003;108(8):977-982.

6. Lam CS, Lyass A, Kraigher-Krainer E, et al. Cardiac dysfunction and noncardiac dysfunction as precursors of heart failure with reduced and preserved ejection fraction in the community. *Circulation*. 2011;124(1):24-30.

7. Francis GS, Benedict C, Johnstone DE, et al. Comparison of neuroendocrine activation in patients with left ventricular dysfunction with and without congestive heart failure. A substudy of the Studies of Left Ventricular Dysfunction (SOLVD). *Circulation.* 1990;82(5):1724-1729.

8. Effect of enalapril on survival in patients with reduced left ventricular ejection fractions and congestive heart failure. The SOLVD Investigators. *N Engl J Med.* 1991;325(5):293-302.

9. Melenovsky V, Borlaug BA, Rosen B, et al. Cardiovascular features of heart failure with preserved ejection fraction versus nonfailing hypertensive left ventricular hypertrophy in the urban Baltimore community: the role of atrial remodeling/dysfunction. *J Am Coll Cardiol.* 2007;49(2):198-207.

10. Liebson PR, Grandits GA, Dianzumba S, Prineas RJ, Grimm RH Jr, Neaton JD, Stamler J. Comparison of five antihypertensive monotherapies and placebo for change in left ventricular mass in patients receiving nutritional-hygienic therapy in the Treatment of Mild Hypertension Study (TOMHS). *Circulation.* 1995;91(3):698-706.

11. James PA, Oparil S, Carter BA, et al. 2014 Evidence-Based guideline for the management of high blood pressure in adults: Report from the panel members appointed to the Eighth Joint National Committee (JNC 8). *JAMA.* 2014;311(5):507-520.

12. Yousef Z, Elliot PM, Cecchi F, et al. Left ventricular hypertrophy in Fabry disease: a practical approach to diagnosis. *Eur Heart J.* 2013;34(11):802-808.

13. Klein L. Omnes viae Romam ducunt: Asymptomatic cardiac and noncardiac organ system dysfunction leads to heart failure. *Circulation.* 2011;124(1):4-6.

14. Redfield MM, Rodeheffer RJ, Jacobsen SJ, et al. Plasma brain natriuretic peptide to detect preclinical ventricular systolic or diastolic dysfunction: a community-based study. *Circulation.* 2004;109(25):3176-3181.

15. Aurigemma GP, Gottdiener JS, Shemanski L, Gardin J, Kitzman D. Predictive value of systolic and diastolic function for incident congestive heart failure in the elderly: the cardiovascular health study. *J Am Coll Cardiol.* 2001;37(4):1042-1048.

16. Cohn JN, Francis GS. Stage B, a pre-cursor of heart failure. *Heart Fail Clin.* 2012;8(1): xvii-xviii.

17. Chaudary S, Song SY, Jaski BE. Profound, yet reversible, heart failure secondary to 5-fluorouracil. *Am J Med.* 1988;85(3):454-456.

18. Ky B, Vejpongsa P, Yeh ET, Force T, Moslehi JJ. Emerging paradigms in cardiomyopathies associated with cancer therapies. *Circ Res.* 2013;113(6):754-764.

19. Yeh ET, Bickford CL. Cardiovascular complications of cancer therapy: Incidence, pathogenesis, diagnosis, and management. *J Am Coll Cardiol.* 2009;53(24):2231-2247.

20. Groarke JD, Nguyen PL, Nohria A, et al. Cardiovascular complications of radiation therapy for thoracic malignancies: the role for non-invasive imaging for detection of cardiovascular disease. *Eur Heart J.* 2014;35(10):612-623.

# CHAPTER 6

# Assessment of Stage C Patients with HF-rEF

## FAST FACTS

- The "3 Fs" of Heart Failure Assessment:
  - Fit: Does presentation fit the diagnosis of heart failure?
  - Function: Is systolic or diastolic ventricular function abnormal?
  - Factors: Are there treatable causes of heart failure present?
- Echo-Doppler is the single most important test to assess severity and etiology of heart failure.
- Frequent causes of HF-rEF with systolic dysfunction include:
  - Coronary artery disease (CAD)
  - Chronic pressure or volume overload
  - Dilated cardiomyopathy (Idiopathic/Other)
- Cardiac MRI can assess myocardial viability, inflammation, and fibrosis via gadolinium enhanced imaging.

*"It is a capital mistake to theorize before one has data."*

—Sherlock Holmes (Sir Arthur Conan Doyle)[1]

## The "3 Fs" of Ongoing Heart Failure Assessment

Care of a patient with Stage C heart failure requires repetition of a clinical cycle that includes assessment, initiation of a plan, and reassessment. New symptoms may fit the previous diagnosis of heart failure or herald new causes of heart failure or other disorders.

# Fit: Do Findings Fit the Diagnosis of Heart Failure?

**THREE-STEP ASSESSMENT OF HEART FAILURE (THE "3 Fs")**
1. Does presentation **fit** the diagnosis of heart failure?
2. Is systolic or diastolic left ventricular **function** abnormal?
3. Are there **factors** pointing to treatable causes of heart failure present?

Even an experienced clinician can miss the diagnosis of heart failure. Preexisting chronic obstructive lung disease or renal insufficiency can obscure the cardiac etiology of shortness of breath or fatigue. In a young person, shortness of breath due to either cardiomyopathy or myocarditis is often attributed to asthma or pneumonitis. Conversely, recurrent symptoms may be attributed entirely to a previous heart failure diagnosis rather than an alternative new diagnosis.

Few patients have symptoms due to heart failure with a normal BNP, ECG, and chest x-ray. A chest x-ray may show cardiomegaly or bilateral pulmonary infiltrates consistent with edema (see Chapter 2).

## ASSESSING THE HISTORY AND SYMPTOMS

**BASIC DATA FOR HEART FAILURE ASSESSMENT**
• History and physical exam
• Lab: Comprehensive metabolic panel, CBC, BNP, urinalysis
• Electrocardiogram (ECG)
• Chest x-ray (CXR)

The assessment of heart failure includes information from the standard components of medical diagnosis such as: cardinal symptoms, history, physical findings, and past medical history.

*Cardinal Symptoms*

The cardinal symptoms of heart failure are shortness of breath, fatigue, edema, or chest pain; although any of these may also be due to alternative etiologies. For each of these symptoms some common alternative etiologies also need to be considered (List 6.1).

**FOUR CARDINAL SYMPTOMS IN HISTORY FOR POSSIBLE HEART FAILURE**
• Shortness of breath (Pulmonary congestion)
• Fatigue (Inadequate cardiac output)
• Edema (Systemic congestion)
• Chest pain (Myocardial ischemia)

LIST 6.1    Alternate Etiologies of Cardinal Heart Failure Symptoms[2]

| Shortness of Breath | Fatigue |
|---|---|
| • Pulmonary | • Anemia |
| • Anemia | • Musculoskeletal |
| • Musculoskeletal | • Metabolic |
| • Functional | • Functional |
| Edema | Chest Pain |
| • Renal | • Gastrointestinal |
| • Hepatic | • Pulmonary |
| • Nutritional | • Musculoskeletal |
| • Venous insufficiency | • Functional |
| • Obstruction of venous return | |

In addition to the cardinal symptoms of heart failure, the clinician should be alert to less specific symptoms, especially in the elderly (List 6.2).

LIST 6.2    Less Specific Symptoms of Heart Failure

- Early satiety, nausea and vomiting, abdominal discomfort
- Wheezing or cough
- Unexplained fatigue
- Confusion/delirium
- Depression/weakness (especially in the elderly)

## PAST MEDICAL HISTORY

Details of the past medical, family, and social history can be important in assessing heart failure. Key questions regarding the patient's own medical history include:

1. Does the patient have previously known medical problems that could contribute to heart failure (List 6.3)?

2. Does the patient have risk factors for coronary artery disease, including hypertension, hyperlipidemia, smoking, and diabetes mellitus?

**LIST 6.3   Pertinent Past Medical History for Heart Failure**

- Myocardial infarction
- Cardiotoxic cancer therapy
- Coronary artery disease
- Autoimmune disease
- Hypertension
- Severe viral illness
- Diabetes mellitus
- Rheumatic fever as a child
- Thyroid disease

## FAMILY HISTORY

Key questions regarding the patient's family history include:

1. Is there a family history of heart failure or coronary artery disease?

2. Is there a family history of early unexplained or sudden death?

## SOCIAL HISTORY

Key questions regarding the patient's family history include:

1. Is there a history of noncompliance with medications or diet?

2. Is alcohol use excessive?

3. Is there a history of illicit drug use?

4. Is there an adequate family or social support structure?

5. Has there been any unusual travel and/or exposure (e.g., toxins)?

## PHYSICAL EXAM

Most individuals with ventricular dysfunction will appear completely comfortable at rest and with simple ambulation. Only with physical exertion or decompensated heart failure do patients appear overtly short of breath or fatigued.

Proper evaluation of vital signs is fundamental for assessment of heart failure syndromes. Each of the basic vital signs can have more than one etiology and the proper interpretation may guide a specific approach to heart failure. Tachycardia can represent compromised cardiac reserve at rest or arrhythmia mediating a cardiomyopathy; bradycardia can indicate medication effect, sinoatrial dysfunction, or AV node block. Hypertension may be the etiology of heart failure or identify a target for therapy; hypotension can imply intravascular depletion, pharmacologic effects, or profoundly low cardiac reserve. Tachypnea is consistent with pulmonary congestion, concomitant pulmonary disorders, or anemia. Fever may signal associated infection or active inflammatory myocarditis.

Beyond basic vital signs, the physical exam helps determine if a heart failure patient is "wet" (volume overloaded) or "dry" (intravascularly depleted). Criteria for "wet" include jugular venous neck distention, pulmonary rales, $S_3$ gallop, abdominojugular reflux (AJR), hepatomegaly, and peripheral edema (Figure 6.1). Any of these findings can indicate elevated ventricular filling pressures, suggesting that the patient is "wet." Physical exam findings that indicate intravascular depletion, suggesting that a patient is "dry," include hypotension, an orthostatic decrease in blood pressure, or decreased skin turgor. More commonly, decreased intravascular volume is suggested by the findings of weight loss, a history of a gastrointestinal syndrome, or laboratory evidence of an increased ratio of blood urea nitrogen (BUN) to creatinine (Cr). Some clinicians supplement the cardiovascular physical exam with a bedside focused cardiac ultrasound.[3]

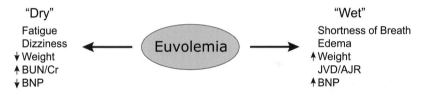

FIGURE 6.1   Assessing whether patients are "wet" or "dry".

The volume status of a patient contributes to important cardiac abnormalities and specific physical exam findings are associated with each abnormality (List 6.4).

**LIST 6.4    Cardiac Abnormalities and Associated Physical Exam Findings**

| Cardiac Abnormality | Physical Exam Sign |
|---|---|
| Elevated cardiac filling pressures and fluid overload | • Elevated jugular venous pressure<br>• $S_3$ gallop<br>• Rales<br>• Abdominojugular reflux<br>• Ascites<br>• Edema |
| Cardiac enlargement | • Laterally displaced or prominent apical impulse<br>• Murmurs suggesting valvular dysfunction |
| Reduced cardiac output | • Hypotension<br>• Narrow pulse pressure<br>• Cool extremities<br>• Tachycardia with pulsus alternans |
| Arrhythmia | • Irregular or rapid pulse suggestive of atrial fibrillation or frequent ectopy |

## CLINICAL ESTIMATION OF HEMODYNAMICS IN HEART FAILURE

Stevenson and Perloff evaluated clinical factors to determine which might be useful to predict pulmonary capillary wedge pressure (PCWP) and cardiac output measured by right heart catheterization.[4] Subjects were 50 patients with known HF-rEF who were being evaluated for heart transplant or adequacy of medical regimens. Orthopnea (a recent history of shortness of breath while patients were supine, requiring extra pillows) had a 91% sensitivity for being PCWP being ≥ 22 mm Hg (Figure 6.2). Physical exam findings of congestion were relatively insensitive to detect an elevated PCWP. Peripheral edema, neck vein distention, or rales were present in only 50% of patients with high wedge pressure. However, when any of these findings were present on physical exam, it was highly specific for a PCWP of ≥ 22 mm Hg.

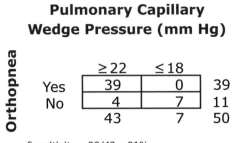

## Pulmonary Capillary Wedge Pressure (mm Hg)

|  | ≥ 22 | ≤ 18 |  |
|---|---|---|---|
| Yes | 39 | 0 | 39 |
| No | 4 | 7 | 11 |
|  | 43 | 7 | 50 |

Sensitivity = 39/43 = 91%
Specificity = 7/7 = 100%
Positive Predictive Value = 39/39 = 100%
Negative Predictive Value = 7/11 = 64%

**FIGURE 6.2    Orthopnea as a clinical indicator of PCWP.** Orthopnea was a sensitive specific predictor of a high PCWP in patients with known advanced heart failure.[4]

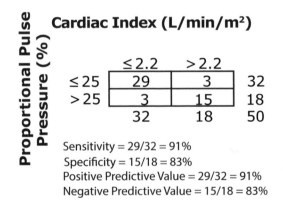

## Cardiac Index (L/min/m²)

|  | ≤ 2.2 | > 2.2 |  |
|---|---|---|---|
| ≤ 25 | 29 | 3 | 32 |
| > 25 | 3 | 15 | 18 |
|  | 32 | 18 | 50 |

Sensitivity = 29/32 = 91%
Specificity = 15/18 = 83%
Positive Predictive Value = 29/32 = 91%
Negative Predictive Value = 15/18 = 83%

**FIGURE 6.3    Proportional pulse pressure as a clinical indicator of low cardiac index.** Proportional pulse pressure ([Systolic–Diastolic] / Systolic) less than or equal to 25% has an overall predictive accuracy of 88%.[4]

Stevenson and Perloff also found that the best discriminator for predicting a low cardiac index ($\leq 2.2$ L/min/m²) was a proportional pulse pressure (pulse pressure divided by the systolic pressure) less than or equal to 25% (Figure 6.3). Proportional pulse pressure and cardiac index also correlated in a linear relationship over a range of values.

## LABORATORY TESTS

Laboratory tests are part of the standard evaluation for heart failure and often have a particular relationship of abnormal findings to cardiac pathology (List 6.5).

LIST 6.5   Laboratory Tests in Heart Failure

## CHEMISTRY

BUN : Cr:

Increased BUN and Cr are consistent with inadequate renal perfusion, often present with heart failure, or intrinsic renal disease. An increased ratio of BUN to Cr can imply renal hypoperfusion or neurohumoral activation.

Liver function tests:

Liver function tests include: bilirubin, albumin, AST, ALT, GGT, and alkaline phosphatase. Abnormalities in these tests may indicate passive congestion with right heart failure, primary hepatic dysfunction, or both.

Sodium (Na$^+$):

Low serum Na$^+$ concentration is associated with neurohormonal activation, including high arginine vasopressin (ADH) (see Chapter 10).

Potassium (K$^+$):

Serum potassium often decreases with diuretics, but increases with ACE inhibitors, mineralocorticoid receptor antagonists, and renal insufficiency.

Magnesium (Mg$^{2+}$):

Magnesium levels are potentially decreased with diuretics, which can contribute to arrhythmias.

## BIOMARKERS FOR SPECIFIC ETIOLOGIES

Troponin (I or T):

Troponin I and troponin T are sensitive and specific indicators of myocardial necrosis in acute coronary syndromes.

Thyroid stimulating hormone:

Thyroid stimulating hormone (TSH) is used to identify a hypo- or hyperthyroid state. Low TSH indicates high levels of circulating thyroid hormones (hyperthyroidism) while high TSH indicates low levels of circulating thyroid hormones (hypothyroidism).

Ferritin, iron/iron binding capacity:

A serum ferritin level < 100 mg/dL or < 300 mg/dL in combination with iron/iron binding capacity < 20% indicate iron deficiency. High levels may indicate primary or secondary hemochromatosis.

BNP/NT-proBNP:

BNP/NT-proBNP often differentiates clinical heart failure from other causes of dyspnea (see Chapter 2).

## COMPLETE BLOOD COUNT (CBC)

**Anemia:**

Anemia, regardless of underlying cause, contributes to heart failure decompensation or high output heart failure if sustained.

## URINALYSIS

**Proteinuria:**

Proteinuria implies intrinsic renal disease. Low serum protein can contribute to edema due to inadequate oncotic pressure.

## ECG

Abnormalities are often present on resting ECG in patients with heart failure (Table 6.1).

**TABLE 6.1   Corresponding ECG findings and suspected diagnoses.[2]**

| FINDINGS | SUSPECTED DIAGNOSIS |
| --- | --- |
| Acute ST-T changes | Myocardial ischemia |
| Atrial fibrillation, other tachyarrhythmia | Thyroid disease or heart failure due to rapid ventricular rate |
| Bradyarrhythmias | Heart failure due to low heart rate/heart block |
| Previous MI (e.g., Q waves) | Heart failure due to reduced left ventricular performance |
| Low voltage | Pericardial effusion, amyloidosis |
| Left ventricular hypertrophy | Diastolic dysfunction, hypertrophic cardiomyopathy |

## CHEST X-RAY (CXR)

A chest x-ray provides information on 2 important questions that may support a diagnosis of heart failure depending on results of further investigation:

1. Are pulmonary infiltrates present?
   - Edema?
   - Other causes of dyspnea (i.e., fibrosis, pneumonia, inflammation)?

2. Is the cardiac silhouette enlarged? (Figure 6.4)
   - Left ventricular dilation?
   - Left ventricular hypertrophy?
   - Right ventricular enlargement (may be present on lateral film only)?
   - Pericardial effusion?

An important caveat is that in the patient with chronic heart failure, a physical exam and chest x-ray can be free of findings of lung congestion despite a markedly elevated pulmonary capillary wedge pressure, as in Figure 6.4. This may relate to chronic enlargement of lung lymph vessels compensating for increased left heart filling pressures with increased return of interstitial edema to the venous system. Clear lung fields are also seen in isolated right heart failure.

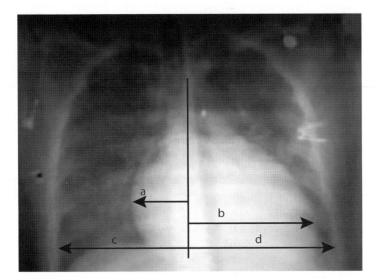

**FIGURE 6.4    Chest x-ray demonstrating enlarged cardiac silhouette.** Cardiac enlargement defined as (a + b/c + d > 0.5).[5] *Source:* Adapted with permission from Jaski BE, *Basics of Heart Failure.* Springer Science + Business Media B.V.; 2000: 108.

**CHEST X-RAY FINDINGS OF INCREASED HEART FILLING PRESSURE**

- Pulmonary venous redistribution
- Kerley B lines (horizontal interstitial lines in lateral lower lung bases)
- Peripheral infiltrates
- Pleural effusions
- Diffuse infiltrates
- Prominent azygos vein

*Additional Testing Requirements*

Because chest x-ray findings can be nonspecific, additional testing is often needed such as BNP, echocardiography, or (less often) right heart catheterization. BNP is usually elevated with ventricular dysfunction even in the absence of exam or chest x-ray abnormalities. If an empiric trial of diuretics leads to improvement, pulmonary congestion due to heart failure is the likely diagnosis, especially if abnormalities are present on the echocardiogram (see discussion of the second "F" for Function). Alternatively, when nonspecific interstitial infiltrates are present on chest x-ray, symptomatic patients may require either Doppler echocardiogram estimation or catheter measurement of pulmonary capillary wedge pressure to distinguish heart failure from pulmonary infection, inflammation, or fibrosis.

## Function: Is Left Ventricular Systolic Function Abnormal by Echocardiography?

For some patients, when standard echocardiogram imaging is inadequate, alternative tests for measurement of left ventricular ejection fraction (EF) are available, such as contrast echocardiography, radionuclide ventriculography, cardiac magnetic resonance imaging (MRI), catheterization ventriculography, or cardiac computed tomography (CT). Echocardiography is the primary diagnostic test for determining systolic function (Figure 6.5).

A left ventricular EF ≤ 40% is consistent with HF-rEF and systolic dysfunction as the etiology of heart failure. Although an EF between 40% and 55% is also below normal, in the absence of associated diastolic dysfunction or comorbidities, it is uncommon for this degree of systolic dysfunction alone to result in the clinical findings of heart failure (Figure 6.6).

Patients with an EF > 40% may still have symptomatic heart failure with a preserved ejection fraction, HF-pEF, especially if associated with other conditions (see Chapter 7).

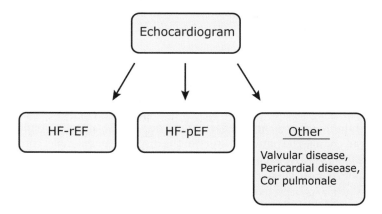

FIGURE 6.5  Echocardiography triage for cardiac function when heart failure is clinically suggested.

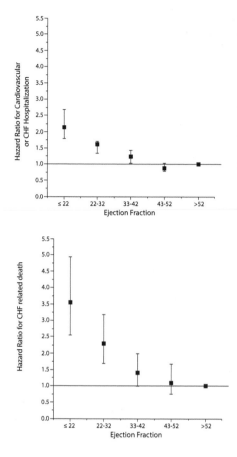

**FIGURE 6.6    Clinical Findings of Heart Failure and EF.** CHF hospitalizations or death increase in patients with heart failure at EF ≤ 42%. Hazard ratio based on left ventricular EF for heart failure–related death **(bottom)**, and cardiovascular death or hospitalization for heart failure **(top)** in the CHARM Trial of heart failure patients with spectrum of ejection fractions (EF range 5%–80%, N = 7599). CHF indicates chronic heart failure.[6]

# Factors: What Are the Etiologies of Heart Failure?

Determining the etiology of heart failure may reveal treatable conditions that can change the natural history of the disease. For example, coronary artery disease (CAD) is a common cause of heart failure and is potentially treatable by revascularization.

When a patient has systolic dysfunction, look for the presence or absence of regional wall motion abnormalities (Figure 6.7). Typically with ischemic or cardiomyopathy, the contraction of the base of the heart is preserved compared to impaired function more distant from the origin of the coronary arteries at the apex. Regional wall motion abnormalities that do not fit a simple vascular distribution can be found in patients with nonischemic systolic dysfunction, including Takotsubo cardiomyopathy (see p. 124). In the absence of regional wall motion abnormalities, however, dilated cardiomyopathy or chronic pressure or volume overload is more likely.[7]

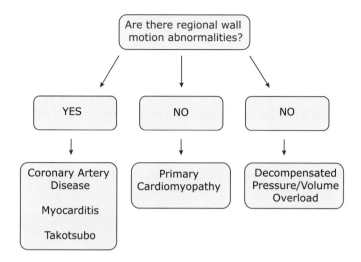

**FIGURE 6.7    Regional wall motion abnormalities in heart failure suggest CAD as the etiology.** An atypical distribution of regional wall motion abnormalities that does not correspond to a coronary artery distribution may suggest myocarditis or Takotsubo cardiomyopathy (**see text**).

## CORONARY ARTERY DISEASE (CAD)

A history of angina, myocardial infarction (MI), or regional wall motion abnormalities on echocardiography helps identify the patient with CAD. When initial screening suggests myocardial ischemia as an etiology of heart failure, coronary angiography should be considered. Percutaneous or surgical revascularization may lead to benefit in the presence of angina or findings of ischemia on noninvasive testing.

### Noninvasive Imaging Techniques for CAD

Noninvasive imaging techniques for assessment of CAD in the stable patient with heart failure include stress myocardial perfusion scintigraphy or echocardiography, cardiac CT, cardiac MRI, and positron-emission tomography (PET). Exercise electrocardiography alone, without imaging, is usually not specific enough to assess CAD as an etiology of heart failure.

### Cardiac CT and MRI for Detection of CAD

Cardiac CT can directly image coronary anatomy and is useful to exclude CAD in a patient with diffuse hypokinesis with a low pretest probability of an ischemic etiology. At present, most patients require beta blockade to slow resting heart rate and allow adequate spatial resolution to evaluate CAD by CT. Cardiac CT with intravenous contrast has a sensitivity of 95% for the visualization of significant morphological coronary stenosis. In addition, the negative predictive value has been observed to be as high as 99%–100%, making CT useful in ruling out CAD.[8] Another advantage of CT is the simultaneous detection and characterization of coronary atherosclerotic plaques within the artery wall (Figure 6.8). Although MRI does not directly image coronary anatomy, it is not dependent on heart rate and is useful for looking for regional left ventricular wall fibrosis associated with previous myocardial infarction and assessment of myocardial viability.

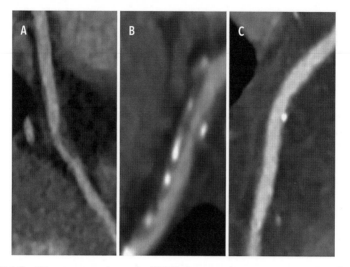

**FIGURE 6.8    CT coronary angiography (CTCA).** Coronary plaque composition: **(Panel A)** a noncalcified, **(Panel B)** a mixed, and **(Panel C)** a calcified coronary arterial plaque.[8] *Source:* Adapted with permission from Nikolaou et al., *Insights Imaging.* 2011;2(1):9-24.

## DILATED CARDIOMYOPATHY (IDIOPATHIC/OTHER)

The presence of diffuse hypokinesis without obvious causes of pressure or volume overload usually implies the presence of cardiomyopathy. Although nonischemic cardiomyopathies are often idiopathic (no identifiable cause), a variety of identifiable and treatable causes exist.

### Causes of Primary Dilated Cardiomyopathy

Cardiomyopathy refers to primary disorders of the heart muscle. If a definite etiology can be identified (Table 6.2), then a specific treatment often improves outcome.[9] Familial dilated cardiomyopathy implies a genetic etiology of ventricular dysfunction and accounts for up to 35% of patients with "idiopathic" dilated cardiomyopathy.[10] To date, only a small number of specific genetic causes of familial dilated cardiomyopathy have been identified (see Chapter 4).[11–13] Many more are likely to be found in the future.

**TABLE 6.2 Etiologies of dilated cardiomyopathy.** Relatively common causes are indicated by the symbol ++.[9] *Source:* Adapted with permission from Hosenpud JD. The cardiomyopathies. In: *Congestive Heart Failure: Pathophysiology, Diagnosis, and Comprehensive Approach to Management.* New York: Springer-Verlag, 1994.

IDIOPATHIC++
  Peripartum++

METABOLIC/ENDOCRINE
  Acromegaly
  Hypo- or hyperthyroidism++
  Pheochromocytoma
  Diabetes++
  Beriberi
  Selenium deficiency
  Kwashiorkor
  Hemochromatosis++

GENETIC (SEE CHAPTER 4)
  Familial++
  X-linked
  Dystrophin-associated glycoprotein
  Metavinculin deficiency

COLLAGEN VASCULAR DISEASE
  Lupus erythematosus
  Dermatomyositis
  Polyarteritis nodosa
  Scleroderma

INFECTIOUS

*VIRAL++*
  Coxsackievirus
  Echovirus
  Adenovirus
  Arbovirus

*BACTERIAL*
  Diphtheria
  Tuberculosis
  Leptospirosis
  Rickettsia
  Typhus
  Q fever

NEUROMUSCULAR DISEASE
  Duchenne's
  Becker's
  Friedreich's ataxia
  Limb-girdle muscular dystrophy
  Neurofibromatosis
  Myasthenia gravis

*PROTOZOAL*
  Chagasic
  Malarial
  Leishmaniasis

GRANULOMATOUS DISEASE
  Idiopathic
  Sarcoidosis++
  Giant cell++
  Wegener's

TOXINS
  Alcohol++
  Arsenic
  Cobalt
  Lead
  Carbon tetrachloride
  Carbon monoxide
  Catecholamines++
  Amphetamines++
  Cocaine++
  Adriamycin++
  Cyclophosphamide
  5-Fluorouracil

## Lab Testing in Dilated Cardiomyopathy

Laboratory testing in patients with dilated cardiomyopathy can be used to identify certain etiologies that have specific treatments such as thyroid disease, iron overload, autoimmune disease, and some infectious etiologies.

**Thyroid disease:** Either hyper- or hypothyroidism, if sustained, may lead to heart failure. Hyperthyroidism can present as high-output heart failure with or without atrial fibrillation; both should respond to treatment of hyperthyroidism with beta-blockers, propylthiouracil, or radioactive iodine. Hypothyroidism can produce dilated cardiomyopathy. This may relate to changes in myosin gene expression mediated by the level of thyroid hormone and should respond to thyroid hormone replacement (e.g., levothyroxine sodium).

**Iron overload:** Iron studies provide an index for cardiomyopathy related to iron overload; either primary hemochromatosis or secondary iron overload due to multiple transfusions (e.g., associated with β-thalassemia major) or ineffective bone marrow erythropoiesis. An elevated iron–iron binding capacity ratio of > 50% in men and > 45% in women and a ferritin level > 1000 µg/L are consistent with this diagnosis. In menstruating women with iron-overload cardiomyopathy, these levels may be lower. Patient diagnosis is ultimately dependent on finding increased tissue stores of iron (see below).[14]

The etiology of hereditary hemochromatosis has been related to mutations of genes that regulate iron absorption. The most common is the *HFE* gene on chrome 6 with a recessive pattern of inheritance.[15] Affected individuals have increased gastrointestinal absorption of iron with a normal diet. This gene occurs in as many as 10% of subjects of European origin who are clinically unaffected heterozygotes and may be tested for as a confirmatory or screening test in patients with family history of hemochromatosis. Three to 5 per 1000 people of European descent are homozygotes with potential for progressive iron overload involving the heart, liver, pancreas, joints, and endocrine glands. A negative test for *HFE* gene does not rule out other genetic or secondary causes of iron overload, however.

Iron-overload cardiomyopathy may present as either a dilated or restrictive pattern by echocardiography. The dilated cardiomyopathy may be a more advanced stage of the disorder. In either case, confirmation of the diagnosis can be made by a characteristically reduced signal by MRI or by endomyocardial biopsy showing increased iron stores within myocytes (Figure 6.9). Electron microscopy will show marked electron-dense bodies within myocytes. Phlebotomy or chelation therapy (e.g., intravenous deferoxamine) may lead to improvement of iron overload and reversal of heart failure findings, especially if begun early in the course of structural heart disease.[16]

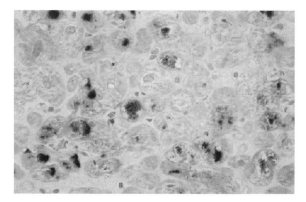

**FIGURE 6.9   Endomyocardial biopsy showing hemochromatosis.** Slide prepared with Prussian blue stain shows increased blue iron deposits within the myocytes of a patient with hemochromatosis.[5] *Source:* Adapted with permission from Jaski BE, *Basics of Heart Failure.* Springer Science + Business Media B.V.; 2000: 119.

**Other lab tests:** Erythrocyte sedimentation rate (ESR) in heart failure is usually low in the absence of inflammation. An elevated ESR is a nonspecific finding in inflammatory conditions including viral or idiopathic myocarditis. Elevated troponins most often indicate myocardial ischemia; however, in the absence of acute coronary syndrome, they are consistent with myocardial inflammation. Acute viral serologies are neither specific nor sensitive for an early diagnosis of viral myocarditis, but may be compared to subsequent convalescent titers to support this etiology during later follow-up. Antinuclear antibodies screen for autoimmune conditions, including systemic lupus erythematosus.

Chagas disease due to previous infection with *Trypanosoma cruzi*, a protozoan parasite, is characterized by heart failure, ventricular arrhythmias, heart blocks, thromboembolic phenomena, and sudden death.[17] Serologic blood testing for chronic Chagas disease may be indicated in patients with dilated cardiomyopathy who have a history of residing in rural Central or South America, which are known endemic regions of this disease. Although endomyocardial biopsy in affected patients often shows evidence of inflammation, it does not usually contribute to clinical assessment.

## MYOCARDITIS

Myocarditis is usually a clinical diagnosis suggested by a patient presenting with acute nonischemic HF-rEF possibly preceded by a viral prodrome. A variety of specific etiologies, including viral infection, autoimmune, or drug hypersensitivity can be considered. Cardiac biopsy can confirm the presence of inflammatory infiltrates.

In general, there is no specific treatment for adults with myocarditis. In a randomized trial in patients with a cardiac biopsy diagnosis of subacute or chronic myocarditis and a left ventricular EF < 45% who received conventional therapy alone or combined with a 24-week regimen of immunosuppressive therapy, no difference was seen in the primary endpoint of improvement of EF at 28 weeks. Overall, patients had a high mortality of 56% at mean 4.3 years of follow-up.[18]

Giant cell myocarditis is one exception where immunosuppressive treatment may lead to clinical improvement.[19] This etiology is suggested clinically by rapid progression of heart failure or marked ventricular arrhythmias. Cardiac biopsy is necessary to demonstrate characteristic giant cells (Figure 6.10). Thus, when myocarditis is being considered, a reason to perform a diagnostic endomyocardial biopsy is to evaluate for giant cell myocarditis, as this will lead to a change in therapy.

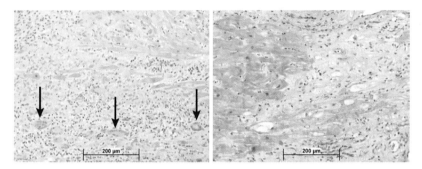

**FIGURE 6.10    Giant cell myocarditis. Left panel:** Cardiac biopsy showing characteristic multinucleated giant cells (arrows) in a patient with giant cell myocarditis. **Right panel:** Cardiac biopsy showing replacement fibrosis after 30 days of therapy.[19] *Source:* Adapted with permission from Cooper et al., *Am J Cardiol.* 2008;102(11):1535-1539.

When a myocarditis syndrome with severe hemodynamic compromise is present, a diagnosis of fulminant myocarditis can be made and temporary inotropic or mechanical circulatory support may be required (see Chapter 9). In these cases, even severe myocardial dysfunction can improve, if not complicated by multisystem organ failure.[20]

## PERIPARTUM CARDIOMYOPATHY

Peripartum cardiomyopathy is a type of idiopathic dilated cardiomyopathy with clinical onset between the last month of pregnancy and the first 5 months postpartum. The incidence in a large series was 28 of 67,369 deliveries (about 1/2500).[21] It is unknown if this presentation is due to a specific etiology related to pregnancy or due to an unmasking of left ventricular dysfunction from a preexisting cause.[21] Although the findings of heart failure may regress within 6 months of symptom onset, peripartum cardiomyopathy may also lead to either death or need for heart transplant. In peripartum women, history or physical exam findings should lead to an echocardiogram for diagnosis of systolic dysfunction.

## TACHYCARDIA-MEDIATED CARDIOMYOPATHY

Dilated cardiomyopathy may develop secondary to a sustained supraventricular tachycardia. Abnormal rhythms associated with tachycardia-mediated cardiomyopathy include reentrant or ectopic atrial tachycardias, uncontrolled atrial fibrillation, or atrial flutter. Very frequent premature ventricular complexes, such as sustained ventricular bigeminy, may also lead to impaired ventricular function.[22] Ablation or rate control of the arrhythmia in any of these cases may lead to total resolution of the ventricular dysfunction (Figure 6.11).[23]

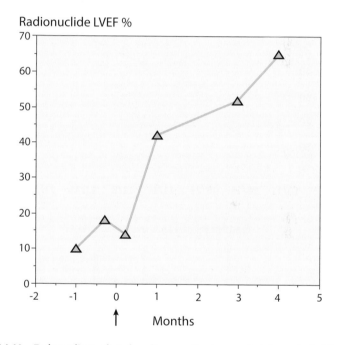

FIGURE 6.11  **Tachycardia-mediated cardiomyopathy.** Increase in left ventricular EF versus time following ablation of an ectopic atrial tachycardia in a patient with nonischemic cardiomyopathy. Arrow at time 0 indicates arrhythmia treatment by catheter ablation.[23]
*Sources:* Reprinted with permission from Rabbani et al., *Am Heart J.* 1991;121(3 Pt 1):816-819.

## PHEOCHROMOCYTOMA

Pheochromocytoma is an uncommon neuroendocrine tumor that secretes high amounts of catecholamines, especially norepinephrine. These tumors are usually located in the adrenal gland or, less often, in ganglia of the sympathetic nervous system. These tumors can cause resistant or malignant hypertension with symptoms associated with surges in the release of norepinephrine that may be episodic.[24] Individuals can develop dilated cardiomyopathy that resolves with pharmacologic alpha and beta adrenergic receptor blockade and subsequent tumor removal (Figure 6.12). The occurrence of this reversible cardiomyopathy supports the neurohumoral hypothesis that adrenergic activation of any cause, if sustained, is deleterious and can promote the progression of heart failure.

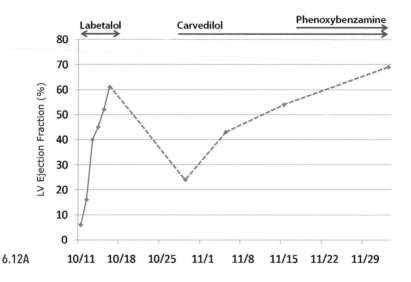

6.12A

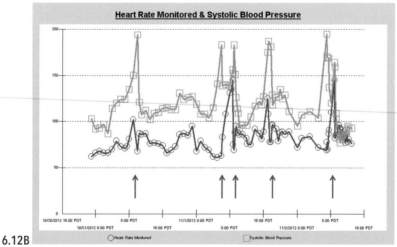

6.12B

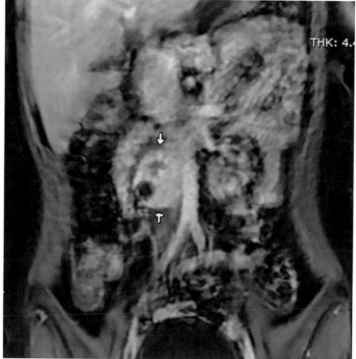

6.12C

**FIGURE 6.12** **Pheochromocytoma associated with highly symptomatic and recurrent heart failure.** A 27-year-old woman presented with hypertension, acute pulmonary edema, and cardio-embolic stroke. **Panel A:** By echocardiography, her EF improved from 6% on admission to 61% only 5 days later during treatment with the alpha- and beta-adrenergic blocker labetalol. Depressed EF recurred 13 days later after discontinuation of labetalol. Improved EF returned with reinstitution of adrenergic blockade. **Panel B:** Surges (**arrows**) in resting blood pressure (**green**) and heart rate (**blue**) were noted with recurrent left ventricular dysfunction. Plasma metanephrines and chromogranin A (CgA) were elevated threefold above upper limits. Her 24-hour urine normetanephrine level was 19,780 nmol/dL (normal < 3548 nmol/dL). **Panel C:** MRI revealed a 4.7 × 2.9 cm mass (**arrows**) in the right retroperitoneum compressing the inferior vena cava. Subsequent surgical specimen histology obtained after tumor removal confirmed tumor cells with diffuse, strong positive staining for multiple neuroendocrine markers CgA, synaptophysin, and CD56, consistent with pheochromocytoma. Subsequent to tumor removal, cardiac medication was discontinued with normal blood pressure and cardiovascular status.

## EXAMPLES OF TRANSIENT SYSTOLIC DYSFUNCTION WITH POTENTIAL FOR RECOVERY

There are at least 3 important syndromes where systolic dysfunction may be transient. Recognizing these conditions and providing appropriate intervention in a timely manner may lead to remarkable recovery of systolic function.

### Myocardial Stunning

Acute CAD syndromes associated with delayed heart contractile recovery after revascularization illustrates the phenomenon of myocardial stunning. Whereas myocardial hibernation is associated with chronic ischemia (as seen in heart failure associated with long-standing occlusive CAD), myocardial stunning is associated with acute ischemia (especially ST elevation myocardial infarction) and may present as heart failure even after intervention and reperfusion. By definition, both hibernating and stunned myocardium are associated with the potential for gradual myocyte contractile recovery following reperfusion that may take days or weeks. Prior to reperfusion, both activate autophagic pathways—adaptively adjusting gene and protein expression to promote cell survival, and inhibiting death pathways thus delaying the permanent loss of myocardial function (see Chapter 4).[25]

### Takotsubo Cardiomyopathy

Takotsubo (or stress-related) cardiomyopathy represents a transient, but profound, myocardial dysfunction not due to CAD, but associated with severe emotional distress, stroke, or seizure. The left ventricle typically displays marked apical dyskinesis, presenting a morphology similar to a type of Japanese pot (used for catching octopus) called *takotsubo*, which is the origin of the disorder's name (Figure 6.13).[26] The presentation can mimic acute myocardial infarction; however, the coronary arteries are not obstructed. Although the exact mechanism is uncertain, excessive myocardial catecholamine release may contribute to an autophagic mechanism to account for this transient dysfunction.[27] Although the syndrome can initially be life threatening, ventricular dysfunction usually recovers spontaneously over a period of days with temporary hemodynamic support, if needed.

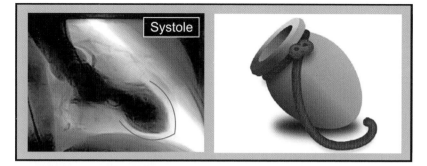

**FIGURE 6.13    Takotsubo cardiomyopathy.** Left ventriculogram of a patient presenting with Takotsubo cardiomyopathy showing characteristic apical dyskinesis (**red outline**) despite normal coronary arteries by angiogram. Note the morphologic similarity to the Japanese *takotsubo* octopus-catching pot.[26] *Source:* Adapted with permission from Koulouris et al., *Hellenic J Cardiol.* 2010;51(5):451-457.

### Systemic Inflammatory Response Syndrome (SIRS)

Transient global cardiac dysfunction may also be seen in patients presenting with severe systemic infections or other inflammatory states with a diffuse reduced ventricular EF.[28] The etiology of this disorder may relate to the production and systemic release of cytokines, such as tumor necrosis factor-α and interleukin-1β, which act to depress myocardial function and increase heart rate without any direct myocardial involvement.29,30 Inflammation-associated intravascular volume depletion coupled with venous dilation can exacerbate an inadequate cardiac output by under-filling the heart.[29]

Postmortem studies in patients with SIRS show only minimal myocardial cell death[29,31–34] correlating with the observed eventual reversibility of cardiac dysfunction following resolution of septic or inflammatory conditions in most patients (Figure 6.14). This reversible myocardial depression could be a protective mechanism of the heart during sepsis, analogous to ischemia-induced hibernation.[29] Similar to hibernation, patients with sepsis have been found to have up-regulated autophagy in myocardial cells.[35] Because of their potential for complete recovery, these patients warrant aggressive circulatory support during the acute phase of their illness.

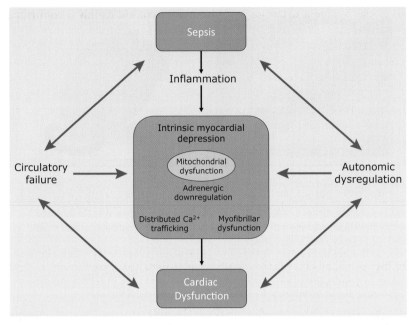

**FIGURE 6.14    Sepsis-induced cardiac dysfunction.** Elements involved in systemic inflammatory response syndrome (SIRS) include sepsis-induced cardiac dysfunction.[29] *Source:* Adapted with permission from Rudiger A & Singer M, *Crit Care Med.* 2007;35(6):1599-1608.

## Important Diagnostic Techniques for Heart Failure

The different presentations of heart failure require astute clinical observations and assessment. In addition, there are several important diagnostic tests or procedures that can be essential for accurate diagnosis and treatment decisions.

### TRANSVENOUS CARDIAC BIOPSY

Percutaneous transvenous endomyocardial biopsy (EMB) is typically performed from the right internal jugular vein with sampling of the right ventricular interventricular septum although left ventricular sampling can also be performed.[36] Indications include assessment for possible cardiac transplant rejection (see Chapter 11) and giant cell myocarditis (previously discussed in Figure 6.10).[37] In addition, EMB is useful for confirming the diagnosis of amyloidosis (see Figure 7.9), hemochromatosis (Figure 6.9), and inflammatory, infectious, or eosinophilic myocarditis (Figure 6.15). Cardiac involvement from sarcoidosis and doxorubicin (Adriamycin) cardiotoxicity can also be determined from EMB. Identifying any of these etiologies helps to guide treatment decisions and improve outcomes. An EMB-confirmed histologic diagnosis also has the potential to exclude constrictive pericarditis and thus avoid attempts at open-thoracotomy pericardial stripping. Less common findings after EMB include Loffler's endomyocardial fibrosis, Fabry disease, and the glycogen storage diseases.[38]

In 2007, guidelines for EMB[37] in otherwise unexplained heart failure included two class I ("procedure should be performed") indications with level of evidence B ("data derived from nonrandomized trials"):

1. New-onset heart failure of < 2 weeks duration and hemodynamic compromise.

2. Heart failure up to 3 months duration if associated with new ventricular arrhythmias, high-grade AV block, or failure to respond to usual care within 2 weeks.

These guidelines have not been universally endorsed in part because of the restricted options for specific treatments of myocarditis other than giant cell myocarditis.

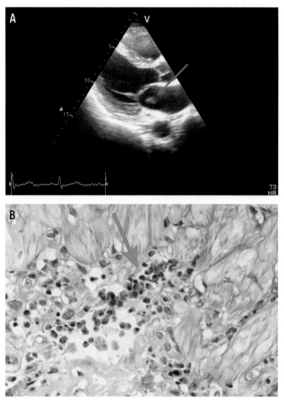

**FIGURE 6.15   Eosinophilic myocarditis.** Eosinophilic myocarditis was associated with Churg-Strauss syndrome and cardioembolic cerebrovascular accident in a 73-year-old male with a history of asthma, allergic rhinitis, and eosinophilia. **Panel A:** Echocardiogram showed EF 40% with left atrial thrombus (**arrow**). **Panel B:** Transvenous endomyocardial biopsy showing extensive infiltration with eosinophils (**arrow**), focal myocyte necrosis, and small-vessel vasculitis. Patient was treated with corticosteroids and anticoagulation with resolution of eosinophilia, neurologic symptoms, and the abnormal echocardiogram findings.

## CARDIAC MAGNETIC RESONANCE IMAGING (MRI)

Cardiac MRI can assess myocardial perfusion, function, and viability. Compared to CT imaging, MRI techniques avoid exposure to ionizing radiation, but cannot directly image coronary artery stenosis.[8] After intravenous administration of gadolinium contrast that remains confined to the extracellular space, delayed imaging with enhancement of the myocardial MRI signal correlates with the presence of interstitial fibrosis or inflammation.

Although echocardiographic imaging of the heart is sufficient for evaluating most patients with heart failure, MRI, including delayed-enhancement imaging, can help differentiate ischemic from nonischemic left ventricular dysfunction (Figure 6.16). Furthermore, morphologic patterns of hyperenhancement can suggest specific types of nonischemic cardiomyopathy.[39]

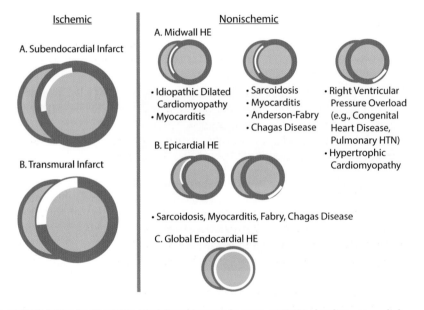

**FIGURE 6.16   Cardiac MRI with delayed hyperenhancement (HE) to localize myocardial fibrosis.** After intravenous gadolinium administration, HE (shown in white) may facilitate differentiation between ischemic and nonischemic left ventricular dysfunction.[39] *Source:* Adapted with permission from Shah DJ & Kim RJ. Magnetic resonance of myocardial viability. In: Edelman RR. *Clinical Magnetic Resonance Imaging,* 3d ed. New York: Elsevier; 2006.

While MRI provides an accurate assessment of morphologic and functional abnormalities associated with cardiomyopathy, there are restrictions in its use. Patients with pacemakers or implantable cardioverter-defibrillators (ICDs) cannot undergo routine magnetic resonance imaging, although investigational registries have reported safety with proper monitoring.[40] Coronary stents are not a contraindication.

Although renal insufficiency may contraindicate the use of contrast with either CT or MRI, gadolinium contrast with MRI is usually better tolerated than iodinated contrast with CT in the presence of mild to moderate renal insufficiency. Marked renal insufficiency (estimated glomerular filtration rate < 30 mL/min) may contraindicate use of intravenous gadolinium contrast due to a possible association with nephrogenic systemic fibrosis characterized by a severe skin and internal organ fibrotic reaction.[41]

## EVALUATION FOR MYOCARDIAL REVASCULARIZATION

In patients with heart failure, myocardial ischemia diagnostic testing and revascularization may be indicated for angina, recurrent pulmonary edema, or for identifying large areas of ischemia post-MI.

### Diagnostic Coronary Angiography

Patients with active angina or recurrent acute pulmonary edema should be considered for diagnostic angiography without preliminary stress testing. This applies to heart failure patients without contraindications to revascularization who have exercise-limiting angina, angina at rest, or recurrent episodes of acute pulmonary edema. Younger patients or patients being considered for aggressive treatments of Stage D heart failure (see Chapter 11) usually undergo early angiography to define what forms of revascularization could be alternative options.

### Stress Testing in Patients with MI but without Angina

If candidates for revascularization, most patients with heart failure and history of MI will benefit from an assessment for coronary revascularization with either initial stress testing with perfusion imaging or coronary angiography. Patients with large areas of ischemia may benefit from revascularization.[42] Because many patients with left ventricular dysfunction have a blunted exercise capacity, pharmacologic stress rather than exercise stress is more diagnostic. One common agent is the adenosine agonist regadenoson (Lexiscan®), which acts as a coronary arteriole vasodilator for nuclear perfusion imaging. Less commonly, dobutamine stress with assessment of wall motion by echocardiography may be used. Positron emission tomography is an alternative imaging modality for assessing myocardial ischemia and viability, but it is not as widely available.

## Revascularization with CABG: The STICH Trial

The randomized Surgical Treatment for Ischemic Heart Failure (STICH) trial provided cautious support for coronary artery bypass surgery (CABG) in heart failure patients with CAD and EF ≤35%.[43] An as-treated analysis of 620 patients with CABG versus 592 patients with medical therapy showed a mortality benefit for CABG revascularization (hazard ratio 0.70, $P < 0.001$) within the first year. However, based on an intention-to-treat analysis the primary end-point of all-cause mortality only showed a trend to improvement in the CABG group ($P = 0.12$). In a substudy of this trial, single photon–emission computed tomography (SPECT), dobutamine echocardiography, or both were used to assess myocardial viability. In both medical and CABG treated patients, the presence of hibernating myocardium was associated with improved long-term survival; however, the assessment of myocardial viability did not identify patients with a differential survival benefit from CABG, as compared with medical therapy alone.[44] It is unknown if newer methods including MRI with gadolinium contrast for defining myocardial viability, described below, would have influenced this result.

## Myocardial Viability Assessment with Cardiac MRI

Since the initiation of the STICH trial, other studies have found that MRI imaging with gadolinium contrast can detect viable versus nonviable myocardium, providing a basis for predicting recovery of myocardial function after revascularization procedures.[45]

Kim et al. (using gadolinium intravenous contrast MRI) analyzed myocardial segments with late hyperenhancement as a marker for fibrotic or nonviable myocardium (Figure 6.17). The study examined 50 patients with left ventricular dysfunction before undergoing revascularization. Left ventricular segments with contraction abnormalities were identified. In these abnormal segments, the likelihood of improvement after revascularization of these segments decreased as hyperenhancement (fibrosis) increased.[45] Furthermore, 78% of hypocontractile segments that did not show hyperenhancement had increased contractility after revascularization.

In the CE-MARC study, Greenwood et al. observed better sensitivity and predictive values with MRI compared to SPECT imaging for diagnosing coronary heart disease.[46] In an animal model of myocardial infarction comparing both techniques, SPECT and MRI detected transmural myocardial infarcts at similar rates; however, MRI detected subendocardial infarcts that were missed by SPECT (Figure 6.18).[47]

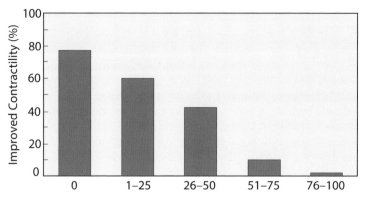

FIGURE 6.17  **Inverse relationship between improved contractility and transmural hyperenhancement.** Hyperenhancement as a marker of fibrosis before revascularization decreases the likelihood of increased contractility after revascularization. A greater amount of MRI-identified fibrosis corresponded to a lower likelihood of improved left ventricular segmental regional wall contractility.[45] *Source:* Adapted with permission from Kim et al., *N Engl J Med.* 2000;343(20):1445-1453.

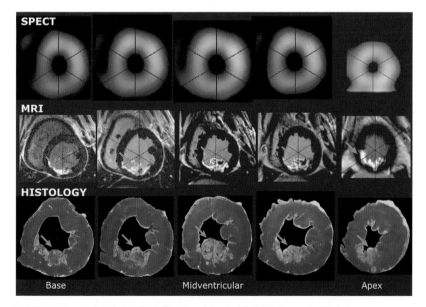

FIGURE 6.18  **Subendocardial infarction detected by MRI.** Example of inferior subendocardial infarcted myocardium in a canine model of myocardial infarction detected by MRI **(middle images, hyperenhancement indicated by green arrows)** apparent by Histology **(below)**, but not by SPECT imaging **(above)** techniques.[47] *Source:* Adapted with permission from Wagner et al., *Lancet.* 2003;361(9355):374-379.

# References

1. Doyle AC, Rathbone B, Sackler H. *The Stories of Sherlock Holmes.* New York: Caedmon; 1964.

2. Konstam MA, Dracup K, Baker DW. *Heart Failure: Evaluation and Care of Patients with Left Ventricular Systolic Dysfunction.* U.S. Department of Health and Human Services, 1994;1-11.

3. Spencer KT, Kimura BJ, Korcarz CE, et al. Focused cardiac ultrasound: recommendations from the American Society of Echocardiography. *J Am Soc Echocardiogr.* 2013;26(6):567-581.

4. Stevenson LW, Perloff JK. The limited reliability of physical signs for estimating hemodynamics in chronic heart failure. *JAMA.* 1989;261(6):884-888.

5. Jaski BE. *Basics of Heart Failure: A Problem Solving Approach.* Boston: Kluwer Academic Publishers; 2000.

6. Solomon SD, Anavekar N, Skali H. Influence of ejection fraction on cardiovascular outcomes in a broad spectrum of heart failure patients. *Circulation.* 2005;112(24):3738-3744.

7. Richardson P, McKenna W, Bristow M, et al. Report of the 1995 World Health Organization/International Society and Federation of Cardiology Task Force on the Definition and Classification of cardiomyopathies. *Circulation.* 1996;93(5):841-842.

8. Nikolaou K, Alkadhi H, Bamberg F, Leschka S, Wintersperger BJ. MRI and CT in the diagnosis of coronary artery disease: indications and applications. *Insights Imaging.* 2011;2(1):9-24.

9. Hosenpud JD. The cardiomyopathies. In: Hosenpud JD & Greenberg BH (eds.), *Congestive Heart Failure, Pathophysiology, Diagnosis and Comprehensive Approach to Management,* New York: Springer-Verlag, 1994;196-222.

10. Hershberger RE, et al, Genetic evaluation of cardiomyopathy—Heart Failure Society of America practice guideline. *J Card Fail.* 2009;15(2):83-97.

11. Hershberger RE, et al., Progress with genetic cardiomyopathies: screening, counseling, and testing in dilated, hypertrophic, and arrhythmogenic right ventricular dysplasia/cardiomyopathy. *Circ Heart Fail,* 2009;2(3):253-261.

12. Muntoni F, Cau M, Ganau A, et al. Brief report: deletion of the dystrophin muscle-promoter region associated with X-linked dilated cardiomyopathy. *N Engl J Med.* 1993;329(13):921-925.

13. Piran S, et al. Where genome meets phenome: rationale for integrating genetic and protein biomarkers in the diagnosis and management of dilated cardiomyopathy and heart failure. *J Am Coll Cardiol.* 2012;60(4):283-289.

14. Kremastinos DT, Farmakis D. Iron overload cardiomyopathy in clinical practice. *Circulation,* 2011;124(20):2253-2263.

15. Gulati V, et al. Cardiac involvement in hemochromatosis. *Cardiol Rev.* 2014;22(2): 56-68.

16. Gujja P, Rosing DR, Tripodi DJ, Shizukuda Y. Iron overload cardiomyopathy: better understanding of an increasing disorder. *J Am Coll Cardiol.* 2010;56(13):1001-1012.

17. Nunes MC, Dones W, Encina JJ, Ribeiro AL. Chagas disease: an overview of clinical and epidemiological aspects. *J Am Coll Cardiol.* 2013;62(9):767-776.

18. Mason JW, O'Connell JB, Herskowitz A, et al. A clinical trial of immunosuppressive therapy for myocarditis. The Myocarditis Treatment Trial Investigators. *N Engl J Med*. 1995;333(5):269-275.

19. Cooper LT, Jr, Hare JM, Tazelaar HD, et al. Usefulness of immunosuppression for giant cell myocarditis. *Am J Cardiol*. 2008;102(11):1535-1539.

20. Dembitsky WP, Moore CH, Holman WL, et al. Successful mechanical circulatory support for noncoronary shock. *J Heart Lung Transplant*. 1992;11(1 Pt 1):129-135.

21. Witlin AG, Mabie WC, Sibai BM. Peripartum cardiomyopathy: an ominous diagnosis. *Am J Obstet Gynecol*. 1997;176(1 Pt 1):182-188.

22. Ezzat VA, Liew R, Ward  DE, et al. Catheter ablation of premature ventricular contraction-induced cardiomyopathy. *Nat Clin Pract Cardiovasc Med*. 2008;5(5):289-293.

23. Rabbani LE, Wang PJ, Couper GL, Friedman PL. Time course of improvement in ventricular function after ablation of incessant automatic atrial tachycardia. *Am Heart J*. 1991;121(3 Pt 1):816-819.

24. Desai AS, et al., Clinical problem-solving. A crisis in late pregnancy. *N Engl J Med*. 2009;361(23):2271-2277.

25. Depre C, Vatner SF. Cardioprotection in stunned and hibernating myocardium. *Heart Fail Rev*. 2007;12(3-4):307-317.

26. Koulouris S, et al. Takotsubo cardiomyopathy: the "broken heart" syndrome. *Hellenic J Cardiol*. 2010;51(5):451-457.

27. Nef HM, Mollmann H, Elsasser A. Tako-tsubo cardiomyopathy (apical ballooning). *Heart*. 2007; 93(10):1309-1315.

28. Zanotti-Cavazzoni SL, Hollenberg SM. Cardiac dysfunction in severe sepsis and septic shock. *Curr Opin Crit Care*. 2009;15(5):392-397.

29. Rudiger A, Singer, M. Mechanisms of sepsis-induced cardiac dysfunction. *Crit Care Med*. 2007;35(6):1599-1608.

30. Werdan K, Schmidt H, Ebelt H, et al. Impaired regulation of cardiac function in sepsis, SIRS, and MODS. *Can J Physiol Pharmacol*. 2009;87(4):266-274.

31. ver Elst KM, Spapen HD, Nguyen DN, et al. Cardiac troponins I and T are biological markers of left ventricular dysfunction in septic shock. *Clin Chem*. 2000;46(5): 650-657.

32. Rossi MA, Celes MR, Prado CM, Saggioro FP. Myocardial structural changes in long-term human severe sepsis/septic shock may be responsible for cardiac dysfunction. *Shock*. 2007;27(1):10-18.

33. Soriano FG, Nogueira AC, Caldini EG, et al. Potential role of poly(adenosine 5'-diphosphate-ribose) polymerase activation in the pathogenesis of myocardial contractile dysfunction associated with human septic shock. *Crit Care Med*. 2006.;34(4): 1073-1079.

34. Fernandes Júnior CJ, Iervolino M, Neves RA, Sampaio EL, Knobel E. Interstitial myocarditis in sepsis. *Am J Cardiol*. 1994;74(9):958.

35. Ceylan-Isik AF, Zhao P, Zhang B, Xiao X, Su G, Ren J. Cardiac overexpression of metallothionein rescues cardiac contractile dysfunction and endoplasmic reticulum stress but not autophagy in sepsis. *J Mol Cell Cardiol*. 2010;48(2):367-378.

36. Chimenti C, Frustaci A. Contribution and risks of left ventricular endomyocardial biopsy in patients with cardiomyopathies: a retrospective study over a 28-year period. *Circulation*. 2013;128(14):1531-1541.

37. Cooper LT, Baughman KL, Feldman AM, et al. The role of endomyocardial biopsy in the management of cardiovascular disease: a scientific statement from the American

Heart Association, the American College of Cardiology, and the European Society of Cardiology. Endorsed by the Heart Failure Society of America and the Heart Failure Association of the European Society of Cardiology. *J Am Coll Cardiol.* 2007;50(19): 1914-1931.

38. Mason JW, O'Connell JB. Clinical merit of endomyocardial biopsy. *Circulation.* 1989;79(5):971-979.

39. Shah DJ, Kim RJ. Magnetic resonance of myocardial viability. In: Edelman RR. 2006, *Clinical Magnetic Resonance Imaging,* 3d ed. New York: Elsevier.

40. Russo RJ. Determining the risks of clinically indicated nonthoracic magnetic resonance imaging at 1.5 T for patients with pacemakers and implantable cardioverter-defibrillators: rationale and design of the MagnaSafe Registry. *Am Heart J.* 2013;165(3): 266-272.

41. Zou Z, Zhang HL, Roditi GH, Leiner T, Kucharczyk W, Prince MR. Nephrogenic systemic fibrosis: review of 370 biopsy-confirmed cases. *JACC Cardiovasc Imaging* 2011;4(11):1206-1216.

42. Coronary Revascularization Writing Group, Patel MR, Dehmer GJ, et al. ACCF/SCAI/STS/AATS/AHA/ASNC/HFSA/SCCT 2012 appropriate use criteria for coronary revascularization focused update: a report of the American College of Cardiology Foundation Appropriate Use Criteria Task Force, Society for Cardiovascular Angiography and Interventions, Society of Thoracic Surgeons, American Association for Thoracic Surgery, American Heart Association, American Society of Nuclear Cardiology, and the Society of Cardiovascular Computed Tomography. *J Thorac Cardiovasc Surg.* 2012;143(4):780-803.

43. Velazquez EJ, Lee KL, Deja MA, et al. Coronary-artery bypass surgery in patients with left ventricular dysfunction. *N Engl J Med.* 2011;364(17):1607-1616.

44. Bonow RO, Maurer G, Lee KL, et al. Myocardial viability and survival in ischemic left ventricular dysfunction. *N Engl J Med.* 2011;364(17):1617-1625.

45. Kim RJ, Wu E, Rafael A, et al. The use of contrast-enhanced magnetic resonance imaging to identify reversible myocardial dysfunction. *N Engl J Med.* 2000;343(20): 1445-1453.

46. Greenwood JP, Maredia N, Younger JF, et al. Cardiovascular magnetic resonance and single-photon emission computed tomography for diagnosis of coronary heart disease (CE-MARC): a prospective trial. *Lancet.* 2012;379(9814):453-460.

47. Wagner A, Mahrholdt H, Holly TA, et al. Contrast-enhanced MRI and routine single photon emission computed tomography (SPECT) perfusion imaging for detection of subendocardial myocardial infarcts: an imaging study. *Lancet.* 2003;361(9355): 374-379.

# CHAPTER 7

# Assessment of Stage C Patients with HF-pEF

## FAST FACTS

- HF-pEF is associated with conditions that cause diastolic dysfunction:
  - Hypertensive heart disease
  - Coronary artery disease
  - Hypertrophic cardiomyopathy (HCM)
  - Restrictive cardiomyopathy
- Doppler echocardiography assesses left ventricular diastolic function.
- In patients with HCM and a family history of HCM, 60%–70% will have an identifiable genetic mutation of the sarcomere.
- Amyloidosis is the most common identifiable cause of restrictive cardiomyopathy.
- Other causes of heart failure without left ventricular systolic dysfunction include valvular disease, pericardial disease, and cor pulmonale.
- Heart failure associated with obstructive or central sleep apnea may be improved by night-time use of continuous positive airway pressure (CPAP).

*"In the heart, the velocity and extent of relaxation, in other words, the ease with which the muscle stretches under the distending force of venous pressure is probably quite as important a factor in the heart's behavior as the force and rapidity of the systolic contraction."*

–Yandell Henderson, 1923[1]

*The 4 Stages of Heart Failure* © 2015 Brian E. Jaski. Cardiotext Publishing, ISBN: 978-1-935395-30-0.   135

# Diagnosis of HF-pEF

Heart failure with preserved ejection fraction (HF-pEF) can be diagnosed when clinical findings of congestion due to elevated pulmonary or systemic venous pressures present with no more than mild left ventricular systolic dysfunction (EF > 40%). Although HF-pEF is associated with echocardiography findings of left ventricular diastolic dysfunction, this is not always the case (see Chapter 2). Similarly, left ventricular hypertrophy by echocardiography is often present, but HF-pEF may still be present due to coronary artery disease or other conditions without increased left ventricular wall thickness (Figure 7.1). Beyond pathologic processes that directly affect myocardial structure, inflammation from noncardiac comorbidities and increased arterial stiffness can indirectly contribute to cardiomyocyte hypertrophy, interstitial fibrosis, and impaired left ventricular diastolic filling.[2]

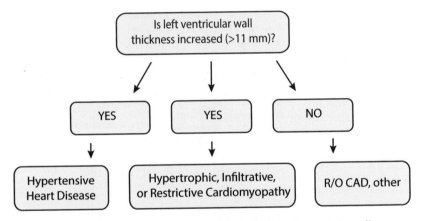

FIGURE 7.1    Causes of diastolic dysfunction and associated left ventricular wall thickness.

## DIFFERENTIAL DIAGNOSIS

Infiltrates on chest x-ray and preserved systolic function by echocardiogram can also be seen with interstitial lung disease or non-cardiogenic pulmonary edema. However, interstitial lung disease does not improve with diuretics. Non-cardiogenic pulmonary edema (also called adult respiratory distress syndrome) can occur in a patient with an acute severe noncardiac systemic illness. In this setting, lung edema develops due to a "capillary leak" despite normal left heart filling pressures. BNP may be normal or mildly elevated secondary to right ventricular strain.

In most patients, clinical findings and Doppler echocardiographic assessment (see List 7.1) are adequate to distinguish these conditions from HF-pEF. In some cases with indeterminate or overlapping findings, right heart catheterization should be performed; pulmonary capillary wedge pressure is high in HF-pEF and normal or low in primary pulmonary disorders.

**LIST 7.1    Echo-Doppler Findings in Diastolic Dysfunction**

- Left ventricular hypertrophy (wall thickness > 11 mm)
- Left atrial enlargement
- Mitral and pulmonary vein Doppler flow abnormalities
- Increased pulmonary artery systolic pressure estimated from velocity of tricuspid regurgitation
- Ratio of early diastolic mitral inflow to mitral annulus tissue velocities (E/e′) ≥ 10

## ECHOCARDIOGRAPHIC FINDINGS WITH DIASTOLIC DYSFUNCTION

Diastolic filling of the left ventricle can be assessed by Doppler echocardiography.[3] Left atrial enlargement can indicate the presence of longstanding structural heart disease.

Echocardiographic measurement of left atrial size by dimension or calculated volume has been called the "hemoglobin A1C" of left atrial pressure and, when increased, serve as an index of chronically elevated left-sided heart filling pressures.[4] In patients with symptomatic HF-pEF, progressive shortening of the transmitral deceleration time (DT) and increasing E/A ratio can be seen with decreasing ventricular compliance and increasing left atrial pressure (Figure 7.2).[5] Acute alterations in mitral inflow velocities may occur in response to patient treatment or other changes in hemodynamic status.

Tissue Doppler imaging (TDI) of mitral annulus motion can also assess myocardial relaxation. With systolic ejection of blood, there is contraction of the left ventricle in part achieved by mitral annular descent toward a relatively fixed apex. Following this, during ventricular filling, the annulus returns towards its initial position (Figure 7.3). Tissue Doppler imaging (TDI) displays the velocity profile of these movements. The velocity of the mitral annulus away from the left ventricular apex during early diastole (e′) reflects the rate of myocardial relaxation and may be less dependent on pressure gradients than transmitral blood flow velocity.[3]

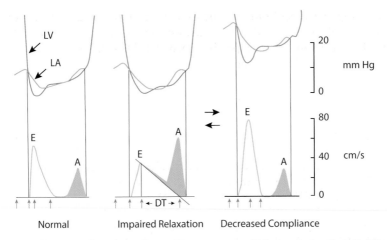

**FIGURE 7.2   Doppler echocardiographic assessment of left ventricular diastolic filling.** Changes in Doppler mitral velocities with correlation to left ventricle (**blue**) and left atrial (**orange**) pressures during diastole. Filling velocities and extrapolated deceleration times (**red arrows**) are in response to the transmitral pressure gradient. **Blue arrows** indicate interval of isovolumic relaxation time from aortic valve closure to mitral valve opening. Abbreviations: LV, left ventricle; LA, left atrium; E, early diastolic mitral inflow; A, diastolic filling during atrial systole; DT, deceleration time.[5] *Source:* Adapted with permission from Nagueh et al., *Eur J Echocardiogr.* 2009;10(2):165-193.

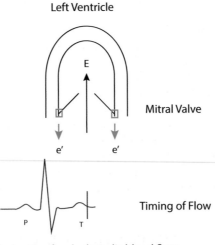

E/e′: A ratio of early diastolic blood flow
(E) versus tissue (e′) velocities that
correlates with left atrial pressure.

**FIGURE 7.3   Derivation of the E/e′ ratio.** Transmitral early diastolic blood flow (E) and mitral annulus tissue velocities (e′). High left atrial filling pressures with impaired diastolic filling are associated with increased blood flow E and decreased e′ tissue velocities.

In HF-pEF, the E/e′ ratio can be used as an initial measurement for an estimate of left ventricular filling pressures (Figure 7.4). Because of its utility, Doppler echocardiography has been called the "Rosetta Stone" for evaluation of diastolic function.[6]

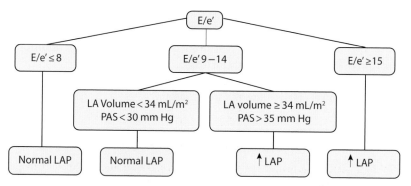

FIGURE 7.4    **Diagnostic algorithm for estimating left ventricular filling pressures based on Doppler echocardiographic findings in patients with HF-pEF.** Abbreviations: E, early diastolic transmitral blood flow; e′, mitral annulus tissue velocity; LA, left atrium; PAS, pulmonary artery systolic pressure; LAP, left atrial pressure.[5] *Source:* Adapted with permission from Nagueh et al., *Eur J Echocardiogr.* 2009;10(2):165-193.

## KEY DIAGNOSTIC FEATURES OF HYPERTENSIVE HEART DISEASE

When a patient with HF-pEF has a history of high blood pressure and uniform left ventricular hypertrophy by echocardiogram, the diagnosis of hypertensive heart disease is likely.

Echocardiographic findings of diastolic dysfunction support this diagnosis. Consider that patients with hypertensive heart disease may also have associated coronary artery disease (CAD). Ventricular hypertrophy in the absence of a history of high blood pressure or CAD may imply the presence of a secondary process due to hypertrophic, infiltrative, or restrictive cardiomyopathy (see descriptions below).

> Look for uniform hypertrophy of the left ventricle in hypertensive heart disease.

## KEY FEATURES OF HYPERTROPHIC CARDIOMYOPATHY

Hypertrophic cardiomyopathy (HCM) can be defined as left and/or right ventricular hypertrophy occurring usually in an asymmetric pattern and often involving the interventricular septum not secondary to systemic hypertension or other systemic disease.[7] Left ventricular chamber volume is normal or reduced. Microscopically, there is myocyte hypertrophy and disarray surrounding areas of increased loose connective tissue. When hypertrophic cardiomyopathy is associated with an obstructive gradient across the left ventricular outflow tract (LVOT), either at rest or after provocation, management directed toward improving this gradient may be important. End-stage hypertrophic cardiomyopathy may progress to systolic dysfunction. Although many terms have been used historically to describe HCM, including idiopathic hypertrophic subaortic stenosis (IHSS) and hypertrophic obstructive cardiomyopathy (HOCM), currently, using the term hypertrophic cardiomyopathy (HCM) and additional descriptive features is preferred (List 7.2).

**LIST 7.2   Phenotypes of Hypertrophic Cardiomyopathy**

- Asymmetric septal hypertrophy
- Symmetric hypertrophy (distinguish from hypertensive or athletic hypertrophy)
- Apical hypertrophy

Within the spectrum of patients with heart failure, patients with hypertrophic cardiomyopathy represent a distinct subset because treatment options differ. Hypertrophic cardiomyopathy typically arises from either an inherited or spontaneous point mutation in genes coding for proteins within the sarcomere including the heavy chain of myosin (see Chapter 4). The prevalence of all forms of hypertrophic cardiomyopathy may be as common as 1 in 500 in the United States population; however, many patients are asymptomatic.[8] The location of regional or global hypertrophy within the left (or right) ventricle between individuals can vary, even within a single family. Other functional features include diastolic dysfunction, mitral regurgitation, myocardial ischemia, and arrhythmias.

Echocardiography or cardiac magnetic resonance imaging (MRI) can be used to visualize the distribution of hypertrophy (Figure 7.5). The most common pattern is asymmetric septal hypertrophy with a ratio of septal to posterior wall thickness of 1.3 or greater. When there is dynamic outflow tract obstruction, a characteristic "spike and dome" morphology may be observed in the aortic pressure waveform or LVOT velocity. This pattern arises from an initial unobstructed ejection of blood from the left ventricle followed by progressive obstruction of outflow during the period of mid-to-late systolic ejection. An increase in systolic Doppler velocity across the LVOT narrowed by septal hypertrophy and systolic anterior motion (SAM) of the mitral valve (Figure 7.5) can be observed at rest or following physiologic provocation such as after premature ventricular contractions, post-exercise, or during the strain phase of the Valsalva maneuver (Figure 7.6). Approximately one-third of patients have nonobstructive HCM defined as resting or peak gradient after provocation of < 30 mm Hg. Patients with resting or provocable gradients ≥ 50 mm Hg and persistent symptoms may benefit from surgical or percutaneous intervention.[7]

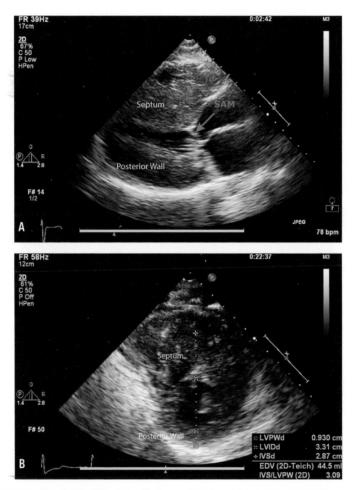

**FIGURE 7.5** **Imaging by 2D echocardiogram of cardiac abnormalities caused by hypertrophic cardiomyopathy.** Images show a 28-year-old female with HCM. Parasternal long axis (**Panel A**) reveals Systolic Anterior Motion (SAM) of the mitral valve leaflets. Echo parasternal short axis (**Panel B**) demonstrates asymmetric septal hypertrophy (left ventricle end-diastolic thickness: Septum measurement = 2.9 cm, Posterior wall = 0.9 cm).

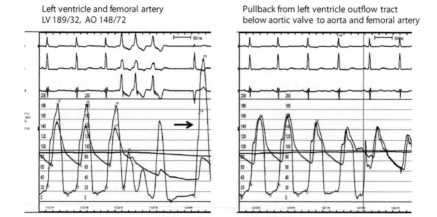

Left ventricle and femoral artery
LV 189/32, AO 148/72

Pullback from left ventricle outflow tract
below aortic valve to aorta and femoral artery

**FIGURE 7.6    Hemodynamics and provocation maneuvers in HCM with dynamic LVOT obstruction. Left panel:** Example of patient with a resting peak systolic left ventricular-aortic gradient of 41 mm Hg that increased to 192 mm Hg in a post-PVC beat (arrow). Despite the markedly increased left ventricular pressure of the post-PVC beat, arterial pulse pressure decreased (known as the Brockenbrough-Braunwald sign). Elevated left ventricular end-diastolic pressure of 32 mm Hg is consistent with diastolic dysfunction of the hypertrophic ventricle. Moderate to severe mitral regurgitation was also present. **Right panel:** No aortic valvular gradient was present during pullback from just below the aortic valve to the aorta, thus excluding aortic valve disease as contributing to the gradient. After surgical septal myectomy (data not shown), dynamic outflow tract gradient completely resolved.

Diffuse concentric hypertrophy of the left ventricle is another type of hypertrophic cardiomyopathy. However, this pattern of hypertrophy may also be seen with hypertensive, athletic, or infiltrative causes of hypertrophy. When global hypertrophy is detected and there is no history of hypertension or family history of HCM, additional diagnostic tests may be indicated. Cardiac MRI may identify delayed gadolinium hyperenhancement consistent with a HCM pattern of fibrosis (see Figure 6.16) or, endomyocardial biopsy may be needed when infiltrative causes are suspected.[9]

A less common manifestation of hypertrophic cardiomyopathy is hypertrophy confined to the apex of the left ventricle. This pattern often displays marked T-wave inversion across the precordial leads on a standard 12-lead electrocardiogram.

# Management of Hypertrophic Cardiomyopathy

Management of hypertrophic cardiomyopathy (HCM) includes three components: symptom management, risk stratification for sudden cardiac death (SCD), and counseling.[10]

## SYMPTOM MANAGEMENT

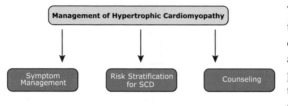

Two common symptoms of HCM are exertional dyspnea and chest pain. Chest pain often is not due to epicardial artery stenosis, but rather to functional ischemia due to increased myocardial oxygen demand from hypertrophy exceeding limited endocardial supply. Beta-blockers that decrease contractility and heart rate can lead to hemodynamic improvement in HCM by decreasing outflow tract obstruction and functional myocardial ischemia. The calcium channel blocker verapamil has negative inotropic and bradycardic effects that may also improve left ventricular outflow obstruction. However, it should be used cautiously, because its action as an arteriolar vasodilator may increase the dynamic outflow tract gradient. If these medications are poorly tolerated, the antiarrhythmic-negative inotropic agent disopyramide may be considered as an alternative.

In HCM with dynamic outflow tract obstruction, medications that increase myocardial contractility, such as digoxin or catecholamines, should be avoided. Also, vasodilators or diuretics should be used cautiously because they can reduce left ventricular size and worsen left ventricular outflow obstruction and gradient.

In patients with persistent, symptomatic HCM and obstructive physiology, invasive therapies may be appropriate, including surgical myectomy or septal ablation using percutaneous catheter infusion of alcohol.[11] Previously, dual-chamber (atrial-ventricular) pacing with right ventricular electrical activation was considered for palliation in patients who were high risk for surgery.[12] This has largely been superseded by septal alcohol ablation.

Paroxysmal, persistent, or permanent atrial fibrillation can exacerbate symptoms in HCM. Electrical cardioversion may be needed to rapidly restore sinus rhythm. To maintain sinus rhythm, disopyramide, sotalol, or amiodarone may be used. Catheter ablation or surgical Maze procedure for prevention of recurrent atrial fibrillation may be required in persistent cases.[13]

## SUDDEN CARDIAC DEATH IN HCM

Patients with HCM may have an increased risk for Sudden Cardiac Death (SCD) due to ventricular tachycardia or fibrillation. In high-risk individuals, implantable cardioverter-defibrillators (ICDs) can be more effective compared to drugs alone such as beta-blockers and amiodarone.[7] Identification of risk factors for SCD can help guide appropriate recommendations for ICD implant (List 7.3).

LIST 7.3    Risk Factors for SCD in HCM

One point for each factor:
- Family history of sudden death
- Unexplained syncope
- Nonsustained ventricular tachycardia on ambulatory monitoring (3 or more beats ≥ 120 bpm)
- Abnormal hypotensive blood pressure response (< 20 mm Hg increase or drop ≥ 20 mm Hg during exercise) to treadmill exercise testing (in patients < 50 years old)
- Severe left ventricular hypertrophy (> 30 mm)

| Risk Factors Score | Recommendation |
| --- | --- |
| • 0 | • Reassurance |
| • 1 | • Individualize |
| • 2+ | • Recommend ICD |
| • Prior SCD | • Recommend ICD |
| • Sustained VT | • Recommend ICD |

Cardiac MRI with late gadolinium enhancement can provide additional assessment of myocardial pathology. It has been proposed that visualization of myocardial scar in the area of left ventricular hypertrophy by this technique can be used to support decision making regarding recommendations for ICD implantation.[14] At present, the decision making for ICD implantation is based upon age, number and nature of risk factors, and clinical judgment.[10]

## GENETIC VARIANTS OF HCM

In individuals with HCM, genetic mutations associated with hypertrophic cardiomyopathy may be identified in approximately 60% to 70% of those with a positive family history, but only 10% to 50% of those without a family history (see Chapter 4).[7] Genetic testing from a blood sample may be considered when identification of a known mutation may help with screening family members. A negative genetic test does not exclude the potential to develop hypertrophic cardiomyopathy, unless screening fails to find a specifically identified mutation matched to an affected family member.

Approximately 5% of families with HCM will have 2 or more sarcomere mutations[15] that may be associated with a greater risk for sudden cardiac death.[16]

HCM with delayed penetrance and phenotypic expression may not be manifest until later in life. If an affected patient does not have a known mutation, then periodic imaging, usually by echocardiography, is used for phenotypic family screening of first-degree relatives.[17]

## COUNSELING

Counseling is important in caring for the patient with HCM for several reasons. Many types of HCM have a benign prognosis and it may be important to emphasize that the annual mortality in asymptomatic patients without high risk SCD or genetic findings may be less than 1%.[18] Asymptomatic individuals may prefer serial echo to gene testing to monitor risk for cardiomyopathy. Exercise guidelines are available, especially for individuals who are diagnosed with HCM at a young age.[19] In general, these guidelines have to be individualized to the severity of HCM and the type of exercise. Exercise treadmill testing can help assess the functional status of a patient with HCM for specific activities.

# Restrictive Cardiomyopathy Due to Amyloidosis

The most common identifiable cause of restrictive cardiomyopathy is amyloidosis. Four types of amyloidosis vary in prognosis and natural history (Table 7.1). One of the most severe is cardiac involvement from AL amyloidosis associated with immunoglobulin light chain deposition and plasma cell dyscrasia. Two different forms of amyloidosis may occur due to misfolding, aggregation, and deposition of transthyretin (a circulating protein produced by the liver that transports thyroxin and retinol). Familial amyloidosis (ATTR) is due to a mutation that increases this misfolding. Senile amyloidosis due to wild-type transthyretin protein can also lead to cardiac involvement, but is usually less aggressive and occurs late in life, predominantly in males. Amyloidosis secondary to chronic inflammation is not commonly associated with cardiac involvement.[20]

**TABLE 7.1  Types of amyloidosis.**[20]

| PHENOTYPE (NOMENCLATURE): AMYLOID FIBRIL PRECURSOR | ORGAN INVOLVEMENT | TREATMENT |
|---|---|---|
| LIGHT CHAIN (AL):<br>**Immunoglobulin light chain** | Heart<br>Other: kidney, liver, peripheral/autonomic nerves, soft tissue, gastrointestinal system | Chemotherapy |
| FAMILIAL (ATTR):<br>**Mutant transthyretin (TTR)** | Heart<br>Peripheral/autonomic nerves | • Liver transplantation<br>• New pharmacologic strategies to stabilize the TTR/tetramer (if cardiac involvement is present, cardiac amyloid may progress despite liver transplantation) |
| SENILE SYSTEMIC AMYLOID:<br>**Wild-type transthyretin** | Heart | Supportive |
| INFLAMMATORY (AA):<br>**Serum amyloid A** | Kidney<br>Heart (rarely) | Treat underlying inflammatory process |

Echocardiographic findings include hypertrophy of the left and right ventricles often with a "speckled" visual appearance within the thickened walls (Figure 7.7). ECG, however, shows a low QRS voltage. Systolic function is usually preserved until late in the disease, but not hyperdynamic as it may be with hypertensive or hypertrophic cardiomyopathy. When a biopsy confirms the diagnosis, immunochemical analysis can reveal the type of amyloid fibril and implied clinical features (Figures 7.8 and 7.9).

> Consider amyloidosis in patients with left ventricular hypertrophy by echocardiogram, but low voltage by electrocardiogram.

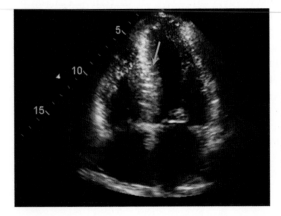

**FIGURE 7.7  Echo features of amyloidosis.** Echocardiogram in 4-chamber apical view shows left ventricular hypertrophy with linear "speckling" of septum (**arrow**), right ventricular free wall hypertrophy, and left atrial enlargement. Left ventricular ejection fraction was 63%.

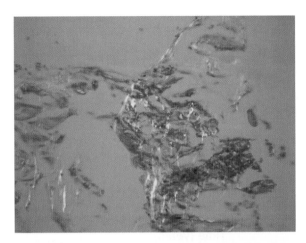

**FIGURE 7.8 Endomyocardial biopsy in amyloidosis.** Congo Red stain showing characteristic "apple green" birefringence under a polarizing microscope that often appears with yellow components. Vascular and interstitial depositions are also common.

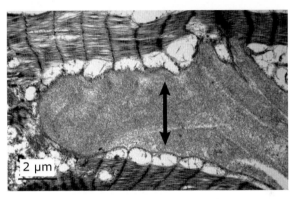

**FIGURE 7.9 Electron micrograph of endomyocardial biopsy in amyloidosis.** This specimen shows cotton-like fibrillar amyloid material (**arrows**) between myocytes from a patient with familial ATTR amyloid.

Diagnosis of AL amyloid is supported by findings of associated immunoglobulin on serum or urine protein electrophoresis with immunofixation or noncardiac organ amyloid involvement. It may be confirmed by endomyocardial biopsy showing interstitial myocardial deposits of amyloid protein. The poor prognosis of AL amyloid is associated with a low survival when awaiting transplant (Figure 7.10).[21] In AL amyloidosis, following cardiac transplantation, the amyloid deposits will recur in the transplanted heart unless the patient subsequently undergoes a bone marrow transplant.

**AMYLOIDOSIS CLASSIFICATION AND CLINICAL FEATURES**

**Light chain (AL):**
Plasma cell dyscrasia related to and occasionally associated with multiple myeloma. Heart disease occurs in one-third to half of AL patients; heart failure tends to progress rapidly and has a poor prognosis

**Familial (ATTR):**
Autosomal dominant transmission; amyloid derived from a mixture of mutant and wild-type transthyretin

**Senile systemic amyloid:**
Almost exclusively found in elderly men; slowly progressive symptoms

**Inflammatory (AA):**
Heart disease rare and, if present, rarely clinically significant

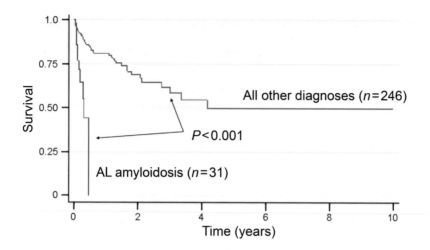

**FIGURE 7.10   Kaplan-Meier survival curves for patients awaiting heart transplant.**
Survival was lower for patients awaiting transplant with AL amyloidosis than for non-amyloid patients on the waiting list (P < 0.001).[21] *Source:* Adapted with permission from Gray Gilstrap et al., *J Heart Lung Transplant.* 2014;33(2):149-156.

MRI with late gadolinium enhancement may provide an index for the extent of amyloid protein in the myocardial interstitial space.[22] With the detection of such abnormalities, MRI can serve as a guide for treatment in this condition.

## Additional Causes of Restrictive Cardiomyopathy

Other causes of restrictive cardiomyopathy are numerous but uncommon (Table 7.2). It may require direct measurement of an elevated pulmonary capillary wedge pressure to make a diagnosis of restrictive cardiomyopathy. Unfortunately, specific treatment is unavailable for many restrictive cardiomyopathies. Although wall thickness is usually increased, it may also be normal (see Chapter 4). It is also important to exclude the potentially treatable diagnosis of constrictive pericarditis.

**TABLE 7.2  Classification of types of restrictive cardiomyopathy according to cause.**
Symbol ++ = relatively common.[23] *Source:* Reprinted with permission Kushwaha et al., *N Engl J Med.* 1997;336(4):267-276. Copyright ©1997 Massachusetts Medical Society. All rights reserved.

| MYOCARDIAL | ENDOMYOCARDIAL |
|---|---|
| INFILTRATIVE | Endomyocardial fibrosis |
|   Amyloidosis++ | Idiopathic fibrosis |
|   Sarcoidosis | Hypereosinophilic syndrome |
|   Gaucher's disease | Carcinoid heart disease |
|   Hurler's disease | Metastatic cancer |
|   Fatty infiltration | Radiation++ |
| NONINFILTRATIVE | Toxic effects of adriamycin |
|   Hypertrophic cardiomyopathy++ | Drugs causing fibrous endocarditis: |
|   Idiopathic cardiomyopathy |   • serotonin |
|   Familial cardiomyopathy |   • methysergide |
|   Scleroderma |   • ergotamine |
|   Pseudoxanthoma elasticum |   • mercurial agents |
|   Diabetic cardiomyopathy++ |   • busulfan |
| STORAGE DISEASES | |
|   Fabry disease | |
|   Glycogen storage disease | |
|   Hemochromatosis++ | |

# Other Important Causes of Heart Failure Syndrome

An echocardiogram can suggest three potentially treatable diagnoses other than HF-rEF or HF-pEF: valvular heart disease, pericardial disease, or cor pulmonale (Figure 7.11). These conditions require treatment distinct from the usual measures applied to left ventricular dysfunction. Any of these conditions may be a sole diagnosis or a new precipitant for deterioration in a patient with previously compensated heart failure.

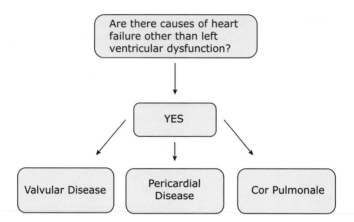

**FIGURE 7.11** Potentially treatable causes of heart failure other than left ventricular dysfunction.

## Valvular Heart Disease

Valvular heart disease represents an important treatable cause of heart failure. Valvular heart disease may be acquired or congenital. In the adult, the major types of valvular disease associated with heart failure are due to mechanical deformities of the aortic or mitral valve. The adult with congenital heart disease may also exhibit pressure or volume overload of either ventricle. When valvular disease is responsible for clinical heart failure, consider surgical or percutaneous correction.

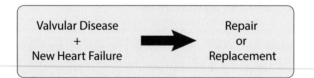

### AORTIC STENOSIS

The presence of aortic stenosis may be subtle in patients with heart failure. The typical systolic ejection murmur may be difficult to auscultate due to low cardiac output. In patients in cardiogenic shock, echocardiography may be the only way to identify aortic stenosis and even then aortic valve gradients are more difficult to interpret due to low cardiac output.

*Echocardiographic Findings*

By echocardiogram, the aortic valve appears calcified and restricted in motion. The peak pressure gradient across the valve can be estimated by the Bernoulli equation as $\Delta P = 4\,V_{AO}^2$. The valve area can be assessed by the continuity equation, as $Area_{AO} = (V_{LVOT}/V_{AO}) \times Area_{LVOT}$ (abbreviations below).

---

**Abbreviations for calculating aortic valve area**
$V_{AO}$ – peak velocity across valve by Doppler
LVOT – left ventricular outflow tract
$V_{LVOT}$ – Doppler velocity at LVOT
$Area_{LVOT}$ – cross-sectional area of LVOT by 2D echocardiography

---

A resting aortic peak velocity value of greater than 4.0 m/s, mean pressure gradient greater than or equal to 30 mm Hg, or valve area less than 1.0 cm$^2$ usually indicates hemodynamically significant aortic stenosis. Aortic valve replacement should be considered for patients with symptoms.[24] Treadmill testing may unmask symptoms when the clinical significance of aortic stenosis is uncertain, and hypotension (defined as a fall in systolic blood pressure of $\geq 20$ mm Hg from baseline) can imply a poor prognosis without valve replacement.[25]

When echocardiographic findings are equivocal or when coronary anatomy needs to be determined, cardiac catheterization can be used to directly measure the pressure gradient across the valve and determine cardiac output by thermodilution or Fick methods. A valve area can then be calculated from these direct measurements. A simplified formula estimate of aortic valve area (cm$^2$) is cardiac output (liters/minute) divided by the square root of the transvalvular peak pressure gradient (mm Hg).[26]

A patient with heart failure and aortic stenosis may have a significant stenosis with only a moderate pressure gradient. If aortic valve area is reduced, valve replacement may still be beneficial despite a low ejection fraction, especially if no other etiologies for heart failure are present.[27] Graded dobutamine infusion during echocardiogram evaluation can be used to help determine the significance of aortic stenosis versus myocardial dysfunction in low output states. Findings of an increase in valve gradient during dobutamine infusion and persistent low valve area suggest an expected clinical improvement with valve replacement.

*Transcatheter versus Surgical Aortic Valve Replacement*

Some patients with aortic stenosis may not be suitable for surgical valve replacement due to high risk secondary to advanced age, left ventricular dysfunction, or other coexisting conditions.[28] An alternate, less invasive, procedure for such patients is transcatheter aortic-valve replacement (TAVR), which functionally implants a stent-mounted bovine pericardial valve delivered via catheter (Figure 7.12).[28,29]

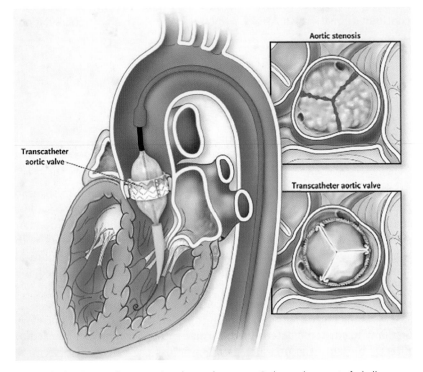

**FIGURE 7.12    Transcatheter aortic-valve replacement.** Catheter placement of a balloon expandable bovine pericardial valve.[29] *Source:* Adapted with permission from Smith et al., *N Engl J Med.* 2011;364(23):2187-2198.

In the PARTNER trial, patients deemed inoperable with severe aortic stenosis were randomly assigned to undergo transfemoral TAVR versus standard therapy, including balloon aortic valvuloplasty without valve replacement (Figure 7.13).[28] After a one-year follow up, the rate of death from any cause in the TAVR group was 30.7%, compared to a 50.7% death rate in patients who received standard therapy.

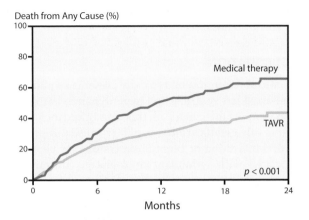

Death from Any Cause (%)

FIGURE 7.13    **Mortality rates after TAVR procedure.** In patients ($n = 179$) with comorbidities that contraindicated surgical aortic valve replacement, TAVR procedure reduced mortality compared to medical therapy for patients with severe aortic stenosis. (Hazard ratio 0.55)[28]
*Source:* Adapted with permission from Leon et al., *N Engl J Med.* 2010;363(17):1597-1607.

In patients with severe aortic stenosis at high risk for surgery who received either TAVR or surgical aortic valve replacement, all cause 1-year mortality was 24.2% in TAVR patients and 26.8% for those who received surgery ($P$ = NS).[29] Within 30 days, strokes were more common with TAVR, however, at 1 year this difference was no longer statistically significant.

## AORTIC REGURGITATION

Left ventricular volume overload due to aortic regurgitation can be acute or chronic.[30] Two important treatable causes of acute aortic regurgitation with a nondilated left ventricle are bacterial endocarditis of the aortic valve or aortic root dissection. Chronic aortic regurgitation with a dilated left ventricle may be due to aortic root dilatation or a congenitally deformed bicuspid aortic valve. Congenital conditions that affect connective tissue (e.g., Marfan's, Loey-Dietz syndrome), rheumatic heart disease, and rheumatoid arthritis are also associated with aortic regurgitation. Chronic severe aortic regurgitation can lead to dramatic physical exam findings including wide pulse pressure, visibly bounding pulse, double (or bisferiens) pulse, and marked cardiomegaly. When heart failure is present, aortic valve surgery should be considered. Prognosis for aortic valve replacement is related to the degree of left ventricle chamber enlargement. In the absence of symptoms, progressive or marked left ventricular enlargement should also suggest a need for aortic valve replacement since an end-systolic dimension greater than 5.5 cm by echocardiography is associated with a poorer survival after surgery.[30] Ascending aorta replacement may be required in patients with an excessively dilated ascending aorta. TAVR is currently not an option for patients with aortic regurgitation without aortic stenosis.

## MITRAL REGURGITATION

Acute severe mitral regurgitation typically presents as pulmonary edema with a normal-sized left ventricle and hyperdynamic left ventricular systolic function. Important causes of this condition include destructive bacterial mitral valve endocarditis, papillary muscle rupture associated with myocardial infarction or blunt chest trauma, or chordae tendineae rupture associated with redundant myxomatous mitral valve leaflets (Figure 7.14).

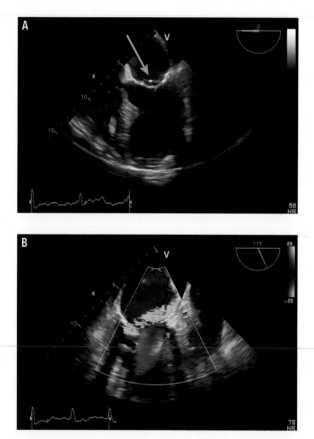

**FIGURE 7.14    Mitral regurgitation. Panel A:** Transesophageal echocardiogram showing a flail mitral leaflet from a ruptured chordae tendineae. **Panel B:** Color Doppler showing associated mitral regurgitation.

When chronic mitral regurgitation leads to heart failure, it is usually associated with eccentric (dilated) left ventricle chamber enlargement.

Ultimately myocardial dysfunction progresses due to excessive wall stress (pressure × radius/wall thickness) (see Chapter 4). In some cases, it can be a challenge to determine if mitral regurgitation has a primary valve cause or is secondary to ventricular enlargement and mitral annular dilation. Primary chronic mitral regurgitation can be the result of mitral valve prolapse, mitral annular calcification, or rheumatic heart disease. When mitral regurgitation is the cause for heart failure, either transthoracic or transesophageal echocardiography may identify mitral valve deformities suitable for mitral valve repair. If repair is not possible and the valve is replaced, preservation of the posterior valve apparatus can blunt subsequent ventricular enlargement. Left ventricular ejection fraction may initially decrease after correction of mitral regurgitation because of elimination of ventricular systolic ejection retrograde into the lower pressure left atrium.

Percutaneous options to repair primary or secondary mitral regurgitation are emerging. One example is the catheter placement of a clip that approximates the edges of the mitral leaflets. When compared to surgical repair at 12 months, the percutaneous approach was less effective at reducing mitral regurgitation, but associated with fewer adverse events and similar clinical outcomes.[31] Percutaneous mitral repair techniques are likely to increase in the future.

## MITRAL STENOSIS

Typically mitral stenosis develops decades after acute rheumatic fever. In the elderly, it can also occur with calcification of the mitral annulus without previous rheumatic fever.[32] Patients typically present with symptoms of shortness of breath due to pulmonary congestion. Because the left ventricle is "protected" by the narrowed mitral valve, catheter-based balloon valvuloplasty or surgical valve repair or replacement is usually associated with an excellent recovery of circulatory function.

Right ventricular failure manifested by symptoms of fatigue and a low cardiac output can predominate in patients with long-standing mitral stenosis who develop severe pulmonary hypertension. The increase in resistance to flow through the pulmonary arterial circulation is known as the "second stenosis" in patients with mitral stenosis.[33] High pulmonary vascular resistance associated with right ventricular failure can make operative risk higher and impair functional recovery in these patients. Once mitral stenosis is relieved, reversal of increased pulmonary vascular resistance usually occurs over a period of days to weeks.[34]

### Percutaneous Mitral Valvuloplasty

Percutaneous mitral valvuloplasty using a balloon catheter to dilate a stenotic mitral valve can be considered an alternative to open valve repair or replacement in appropriate patients. On average, the mean valve area doubles (from 1.0 to 2.0 cm$^2$), with a 50% to 60% reduction in trans-mitral gradient. [35] Complications include cardiac perforation, pericardial tamponade, severe mitral regurgitation, or cerebral vascular accident. Patients who have severely calcified valves often require open heart surgery to achieve a good result. [36] In patients with mitral stenosis but pliable valves, percutaneous mitral valvuloplasty may be preferable to surgical commissurotomy since it achieves similar results without the liabilities of thoracotomy and cardiopulmonary bypass. [37]

## TRANSESOPHAGEAL ECHOCARDIOGRAM FOR VALVE DISEASE

Performance of transesophageal echocardiogram (TEE) is not mandatory in the diagnosis of valvular diseases and heart failure. Nevertheless, a transesophageal echocardiogram can be useful when questions remain after transthoracic echocardiography. A flail mitral valve leaflet, either due to chordal rupture, papillary muscle tear, or endocarditis, often indicates a need for mitral valve surgery (Figure 7.14). TEE is also useful for better definition of possible valvular vegetations associated with endocarditis. TEE improves the assessment of prosthetic tissue or mechanical valves, especially in the mitral position, because echogenic struts limit visualization with transthoracic echocardiography. Generally, the mitral valve is better assessed than the aortic valve given the close anatomic location of the left atrium to the esophagus.

# Congenital Heart Disease

Diverse congenital heart lesions can occur in an adult: left-right shunts; right-left shunts (cyanotic heart disease); stenosis or hypoplasia of heart valves or ventricles; or great vessel abnormalities. If previously diagnosed during childhood, the abnormality may have been observed, palliated, or corrected. Echocardiography and transesophageal echocardiography can initially define the anatomic and functional significance of a suspected congenital lesion. Atrial or ventricular arrhythmias may occur associated with any significant congenital heart lesion even years after successful surgical correction. Collaboration with a cardiologist experienced in the management of congenital heart lesions can help in the management of these patients.[38]

# Pericardial Disease

Pericardial tamponade, pericardial constriction, and mixed effuso-constrictive disease can all be associated with heart failure findings.

Rapid accumulation of fluid within the pericardium can cause acute pericardial tamponade and circulatory collapse with as little as 100 mL of fluid. Examples include postoperative bleeding after open-heart surgery, catheter related coronary vessel or ventricular perforation, or ventricular rupture post-myocardial infarction. Tamponade is initially assessed by clinical findings and echocardiographic features (List 7.4).

Effuso-constrictive disease is a mixed diagnosis that is usually confirmed when a significant pericardial effusion is drained and a residual elevation of ventricular filling pressures remains consistent with pericardial constriction. Neoplastic involvement of the pericardium commonly results in this finding and may be initially associated with a liter or more of effusion.

**LIST 7.4   Features of Pericardial Disease**

Types of pericardial disease
- Pericardial tamponade
- Pericardial constriction
- Effuso-constrictive disease

Clinical findings of tamponade
- Pulsus paradoxus (> 10 mm Hg fall of blood pressure with inspiration)
- Hypotension
- Neck vein distention
- Electrical alternans on ECG
- Increase in size of cardiac silhouette on chest x-ray

Basic echocardiographic findings of tamponade
- Large pericardial effusion (anterior and posterior to heart)
- RV collapse with inspiration
- Atrial collapse with inspiration
- Exaggerated changes in respiratory pattern of transvalvular velocities

## CONSTRICTIVE VS. RESTRICTIVE CARDIOMYOPATHY

When a patient has heart failure and normal left ventricular size and systolic function, distinguishing HF-pEF due to restrictive cardiomyopathy from constrictive pericarditis can be important (Figure 7.15), as pericardial stripping can lead to marked clinical improvement in the case of constrictive pericarditis.[39] Echocardiography supplemented by CT or cardiac MRI can help to make a diagnosis of constrictive pericarditis if a thickened pericardium is identified.[40]

| | CP | RC |
|---|---|---|
| Thick or calcified pericardium by CXR, Echo, CT, or MRI | + | - |
| Respiratory variation in Doppler Exaggerated tricuspid inflow signal | + | - |
| LV and RV pressures track throughout diastole | + | - |
| Abnormal myocardial biopsy | - | + |

**FIGURE 7.15** Laboratory findings to help distinguish constrictive pericarditis (CP) from restrictive cardiomyopathy (RC).

A previous history of acute pericarditis, granulomatous disease (e.g., tuberculosis, histoplasmosis), and autoimmune diseases (e.g., rheumatoid arthritis), favors constrictive pericarditis. Conversely, a systemic illness, such as amyloidosis or history of chest radiation therapy, favors restrictive cardiomyopathy.

Physical exam and Doppler findings help distinguish the two conditions. A constricted pericardium is analogous to a rigid boot surrounding the heart that isolates the heart from respiratory changes in intrathoracic pressure and increases reciprocal changes in right and left ventricle inflow. With constriction, during inspiration (as venous thoracic flow increases), > 25% increases in tricuspid and decreases in mitral early diastolic transvalvular flows are seen by Doppler echocardiography.[39] Conversely, only small changes in inflow velocities with respiration are seen in restrictive cardiomyopathy.[41] In constrictive pericarditis, in contrast to restrictive cardiomyopathy, a paradoxical increase in central venous pressure occurs with respiration (positive Kussmaul's sign). Left and right heart cardiac catheterization demonstrates tracking of right and left ventricular diastolic pressure tracings prior to an "a" wave with constriction. Abnormal histology by endomyocardial biopsy favors restriction.

Occasionally, pericardial constriction can coexist with restrictive cardiomyopathy, following a previous episode of myopericarditis or radiation therapy for neoplasia.[42] Final validation of constrictive pericarditis is based on finding hemodynamic improvement following pericardial stripping.[39,43]

## Cor Pulmonale

Right heart failure (without left heart failure) due to a primary pulmonary reason with pulmonary hypertension, known as cor pulmonale, may occur for reasons such as acute or chronic pulmonary emboli, chronic obstructive lung disease, or obesity-related hypoventilation syndromes, including severe sleep apnea.[44] The diagnosis of primary pulmonary hypertension should be considered in the presence of a high pulmonary vascular resistance of unknown cause after thorough evaluation to exclude secondary causes of pulmonary hypertension, especially left heart failure or pulmonary emboli. Trials have shown benefit from treatment with oral and intravenous pulmonary vasodilators for patients with documented high pulmonary artery pressures and vascular resistance.[45]

Cor pulmonale can present with clinical findings from low cardiac output (fatigue or hypotension) and elevated right heart filling pressure (edema, ascites, and jugular venous distension). The echocardiogram in cor pulmonale reveals a large right ventricle, a small left ventricle, and a flattened interventricular septum. Together, this can give an appearance of a "D" sign on a short axis cross-section of the left ventricle as shown below (Figure 7.16).

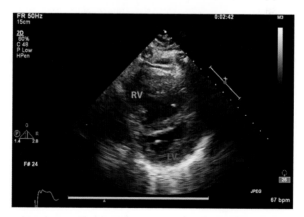

**FIGURE 7.16    Echocardiographic left ventricle "D" sign from right ventricular pressure overload.** This image came from a 46-year-old male with history of surgically corrected complex congenital heart disease with Eisenmenger's physiology (high pulmonary vascular resistance) and right heart failure. Pulmonary artery systolic pressure estimate was 85 mm Hg.

Marked right ventricular enlargement with dysfunction can simulate constrictive physiology, and even result in an elevated intrapericardial pressure.[45] This type of diastolic ventricular interaction is due to pericardial constraint, septal transmission of right ventricular chamber pressure, and the effect of circumferential myocardial fibers that encircle both ventricular chambers. It is important to differentiate this from constrictive pericarditis as a pericardial stripping procedure will not benefit the patient with right ventricular failure. Thickening of the pericardium by imaging is absent. Medical therapy that improves right heart failure, however, can decrease intrapericardial, left, and right heart filling pressures.[45]

## Sleep-Disordered Breathing in Heart Failure

Between 2006 and 2008, Bitter et al. found a 69% prevalence of sleep-disordered breathing (SDB) in patients with heart failure and ejection fraction > 55%. Forty percent had obstructive sleep apnea (OSA), and 30% had central sleep apnea (CSA).[46] As diastolic dysfunction became more severe, the incidence of SDB, especially CSA, increased (Figure 7.17). Cheyne-Stokes cyclic respiratory breathing is a hallmark of CSA.

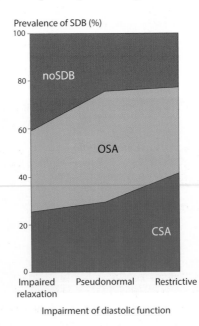

**FIGURE 7.17    Prevalence of obstructive sleep apnea (OSA) and central sleep apnea (CSA), in different stages of diastolic dysfunction.** Heart failure patients with normal left ventricular ejection fraction have increasing prevalence of OSA and CSA as diastolic dysfunction progresses.[46] *Source:* Adapted with permission from Bitter et al., *Eur J Heart Fail.* 2009;11(6):602-608.

## TREATMENT OF SLEEP APNEA IN HEART FAILURE

Nighttime continuous positive airway pressure (CPAP) is the most common management for sleep disordered breathing and heart failure with most trials done in patients with HF-rEF. In patients with OSA and HF-rEF, CPAP resulted in an improvement in left ventricular ejection fraction associated with reductions in left ventricular end-systolic dimensions (Figure 7.18).[47] In patients with HF-rEF and CSA, Bradley and coworkers found a decreased frequency of sleep apnea episodes and improved left ventricular ejection fraction at three months with the use of CPAP, but without change in patient survival or quality of life.[48]

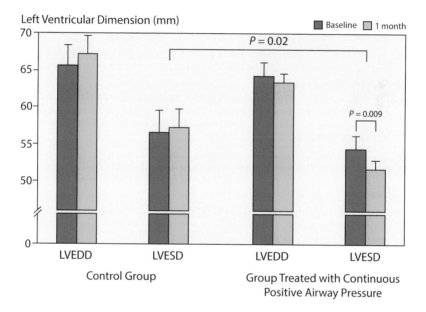

**FIGURE 7.18    CPAP improves left ventricle ejection fraction.** Patients with obstructive sleep apnea and systolic dysfunction treated with CPAP showed an improvement in left ventricular ejection fraction based on reduced left ventricular end-systolic dimension (LVESD) after one month of treatment.[47] *Source:* Adapted with permission from Kaneko et al., *N Engl J Med.* 2003;348(13):1233-1241.

Obesity-hypoventilation syndrome (previously known as Pickwickian syndrome) is a condition that can include components of sleep apnea.[49] In a patient with severe obesity, inadequate respiration leads to both hypoxia and hypercapnea. Secondary pulmonary hypertension can result with eventual right heart failure and cor pulmonale. Because obesity can also contribute to left sided HF-pEF, a combined biventricular heart failure picture can emerge.[50] If a patient cannot lose weight, CPAP or temporary more advanced respiratory support measures (BIPAP or mechanical ventilation) may help.

# References

1. Henderson Y. Volume changes of the heart. *Physiol Rev.* 1923;3(2):165-208.

2. Paulus WJ, Tschope C. A novel paradigm for heart failure with preserved ejection fraction: comorbidities drive myocardial dysfunction and remodeling through coronary microvascular endothelial inflammation. *J Am Coll Cardiol.* 2013;62(4):263-271.

3. Ommen SR, et al. Clinical utility of Doppler echocardiography and tissue Doppler imaging in the estimation of left ventricular filling pressures: a comparative simultaneous Doppler-catheterization study. *Circulation.* 2000;102(15):1788-1794.

4. Levine RA, Nattel S. Looking into the left atrial crystal ball: a ray of hope for patients with organic mitral regurgitation. *J Am Coll Cardiol.* 2010. 56(7):579-581.

5. Nagueh SF, et al. Recommendations for the evaluation of left ventricular diastolic function by echocardiography. *Eur J Echocardiogr.* 2009;10(2):165-193.

6. Nishimura RA, Tajik AJ. Evaluation of diastolic filling of left ventricle in health and disease: Doppler echocardiography is the clinician's Rosetta Stone. *J Am Coll Cardiol.* 1997;30(1):8-18.

7. Gersh BJ, et al. 2011 ACCF/AHA guideline for the diagnosis and treatment of hypertrophic cardiomyopathy: a report of the American College of Cardiology Foundation/American Heart Association Task Force on Practice Guidelines. *Circulation.* 2011;124(24):e783-831.

8. Maron BJ, et al. Prevalence of hypertrophic cardiomyopathy in a general population of young adults. Echocardiographic analysis of 4111 subjects in the CARDIA Study. Coronary Artery Risk Development in (Young) Adults. *Circulation.* 1995;92(4):785-789.

9. Petersen SE, et al. Differentiation of athlete's heart from pathological forms of cardiac hypertrophy by means of geometric indices derived from cardiovascular magnetic resonance. *J Cardiovasc Magn Reson.* 2005;7(3):551-558.

10. Ho CY. Hypertrophic cardiomyopathy in 2012. *Circulation.* 2012;125(11):1432-1438.

11. Firoozi S, et al. Septal myotomy-myectomy and transcoronary septal alcohol ablation in hypertrophic obstructive cardiomyopathy. A comparison of clinical, haemodynamic and exercise outcomes. *Eur Heart J.* 2002;23(20):1617-1624.

12. Nishimura RA, et al. Dual-chamber pacing for hypertrophic cardiomyopathy: a randomized, double-blind, crossover trial. *J Am Coll Cardiol.* 1997;29(2):435-441.

13. Darby AE, Dimarco JP. Management of atrial fibrillation in patients with structural heart disease. *Circulation.* 2012;125(7):945-957.

14. Bruder O, et al. Myocardial scar visualized by cardiovascular magnetic resonance imaging predicts major adverse events in patients with hypertrophic cardiomyopathy. *J Am Coll Cardiol.* 2010; 56(11):875-887.

15. Millat G, et al. Prevalence and spectrum of mutations in a cohort of 192 unrelated patients with hypertrophic cardiomyopathy. *Eur J Med Genet.* 2010;53(5):261-267.

16. Maron BJ, Maron MS, Semsarian C. Double or compound sarcomere mutations in hypertrophic cardiomyopathy: a potential link to sudden death in the absence of conventional risk factors. *Heart Rhythm.* 2012;9(1):57-63.

17. Lee DS, et al. Relation of disease pathogenesis and risk factors to heart failure with preserved or reduced ejection fraction: insights from the framingham heart study of the national heart, lung, and blood institute. *Circulation.* 2009;119(24):3070-3077.

18. Spirito P, et al. The management of hypertrophic cardiomyopathy. *N Engl J Med.* 1997;336(11):775-785.

19. Maron BJ, et al. Recommendations for physical activity and recreational sports participation for young patients with genetic cardiovascular diseases. *Circulation.* 2004;109(22):2807-2816.

20. Falk RH. Cardiac amyloidosis: a treatable disease, often overlooked. *Circulation.* 2011;124(9):1079-1085.

21. Gray Gilstrap L, et al. Predictors of survival to orthotopic heart transplant in patients with light chain amyloidosis. *J Heart Lung Transplant.* 2014;33(2):149-156.

22. Maceira AM, et al. Cardiovascular magnetic resonance in cardiac amyloidosis. *Circulation.* 2005;111(2):186-193.

23. Kushwaha SS, Fallon JT, Fuster V. Restrictive cardiomyopathy. *N Engl J Med.* 1997;336(4):267-276.

24. Grossman W, *Cardiac catheterization, angiography, and intervention.* 5 ed. 1996, Philadelphia: Lea & Febiger.

25. Das P, Rimington H, Chambers J. Exercise testing to stratify risk in aortic stenosis. *Eur Heart J.* 2005;26(13):1309-1313.

26. Hakki AH, et al. A simplified valve formula for the calculation of stenotic cardiac valve areas. *Circulation.* 1981;63(5):1050-1055.

27. Carabello BA, et al. Hemodynamic determinants of prognosis of aortic valve replacement in critical aortic stenosis and advanced congestive heart failure. *Circulation.* 1980;62(1):42-48.

28. Leon MB, et al. Transcatheter aortic-valve implantation for aortic stenosis in patients who cannot undergo surgery. *N Engl J Med.* 2010;363(17):1597-1607.

29. Smith CR, et al. Transcatheter versus surgical aortic-valve replacement in high-risk patients. *N Engl J Med.* 2011;364(23):2187-2198.

30. Bonow RO. Management of chronic aortic regurgitation. *N Engl J Med.* 1994;331(11): 736-737.

31. Feldman T, et al. Percutaneous repair or surgery for mitral regurgitation. *N Engl J Med.* 2011;364(15):1395-1406.

32. Carabello BA, Crawford FA Jr. Valvular heart disease. *N Engl J Med.* 1997; 337(1): 32-41.

33. Wood P. Pulmonary hypertension with special reference to the vasoconstrictive factor. *Br Heart J.* 1958;20(4):557-70.

34. Dalen JE, et al. Early reduction of pulmonary vascular resistance after mitral-valve replacement. *N Engl J Med.* 1967;277(8):387-394.

35. Bonow RO, et al. 2008 Focused update incorporated into the ACC/AHA 2006 guidelines for the management of patients with valvular heart disease: a report of the American College of Cardiology/American Heart Association Task Force on Practice Guidelines (Writing Committee to Revise the 1998 Guidelines for the Management of Patients With Valvular Heart Disease): endorsed by the Society of Cardiovascular Anesthesiologists, Society for Cardiovascular Angiography and Interventions, and Society of Thoracic Surgeons. *Circulation.* 2008;118(15): e523-661.

36. Abascal VM, et al. Prediction of successful outcome in 130 patients undergoing percutaneous balloon mitral valvotomy. *Circulation.* 1990;82(2):448-456.

37. Ben FM, et al. Percutaneous balloon versus surgical closed and open mitral commissurotomy: seven-year follow-up results of a randomized trial. *Circulation.* 1998;97(3): 245-250.

38. Warnes CA, et al. ACC/AHA 2008 Guidelines for the Management of Adults with Congenital Heart Disease: Executive Summary: a report of the American College of Cardiology/American Heart Association Task Force on Practice Guidelines (writing committee to develop guidelines for the management of adults with congenital heart disease). *Circulation.* 2008;118(23):2395-2451.

39. Vaitkus P T, Kussmaul WG. Constrictive pericarditis versus restrictive cardiomyopathy: a reappraisal and update of diagnostic criteria. *Am Heart J.* 1991;122(5): 1431-1441.

40. Verhaert D, et al. The role of multimodality imaging in the management of pericardial disease. *Circ Cardiovasc Imaging.* 2010;3(3):333-343.

41. Hatle LK, Appleton CP, Popp RL. Differentiation of constrictive pericarditis and restrictive cardiomyopathy by Doppler echocardiography. *Circulation.* 1989;79(2): 357-370.

42. Guntheroth WG. Constrictive pericarditis versus restrictive cardiomyopathy. *Circulation.* 1997;95(2):542-543.

43. Masui T, Finck S, Higgins CB. Constrictive pericarditis and restrictive cardiomyopathy: evaluation with MR imaging. *Radiology.* 1992;182(2):369-373.

44. Simonneau, G., et al., Clinical classification of pulmonary hypertension. *J Am Coll Cardiol.* 2004; 43(12 suppl S):5S-12S.

45. Jaber WA, et al. Differentiation of tricuspid regurgitation from constrictive pericarditis: novel criteria for diagnosis in the cardiac catheterisation laboratory. *Heart.* 2009;95(17):1449-1454.

46. Bitter T, et al. Sleep-disordered breathing in heart failure with normal left ventricular ejection fraction. *Eur J Heart Fail.* 2009;11(6):602-608.

47. Kaneko Y, et al. Cardiovascular effects of continuous positive airway pressure in patients with heart failure and obstructive sleep apnea. *N Engl J Med.* 2003;348(13): 1233-1241.

48. Bradley TD, et al. Continuous positive airway pressure for central sleep apnea and heart failure. *N Engl J Med.* 2005. 353(19):2025-2033.

49. Olson AL, Zwillich C. The obesity hypoventilation syndrome. *Am J Med.* 2005;118(9): 948-956.

50. Mathew B, et al. Obesity: effects on cardiovascular disease and its diagnosis. *J Am Board Fam Med.* 2008;21(6):562-568.

# CHAPTER 8

# Stage C: Improving Outcomes in Symptomatic Heart Failure

## FAST FACTS

- Oral loop diuretics differ in efficacy in part based on pharmacokinetic properties.

- Survival in patients with systolic dysfunction (HF-rEF) can be improved with angiotensin II inhibitors (ACEI/ARB), beta-blockers, and mineralocorticoid receptor antagonists.

- Adding isosorbide dinitrate and hydralazine benefits African Americans with persistent symptomatic HF-rEF.

- The incidence of sudden death in patients with persistent ejection fraction ≤ 35% is reduced with an implantable cardioverter-defibrillator (ICD).

- In appropriate patients with a prolonged QRS duration, cardiac resynchronization therapy reduces the risk of death or hospitalization, and in combination with an ICD, confers further survival benefit.

- With atrial fibrillation and heart failure, in addition to antithrombotic therapy, options are either restore and maintain sinus rhythm or lower resting heart rate to less than 100 bpm.

*"There are in fact, two things: science and opinion; the former begets knowledge, the latter ignorance."*

—Hippocrates

*The 4 Stages of Heart Failure* © 2015 Brian E. Jaski. Cardiotext Publishing, ISBN: 978-1-935395-30-0.   165

# Evidence-Based Therapies for Patients with HF-rEF

The basic algorithm for treating patients with HF-rEF is based on both the severity of symptoms and the degree of LV dysfunction (Figure 8.1). Pharmacologic therapies target different neurohormonal systems.

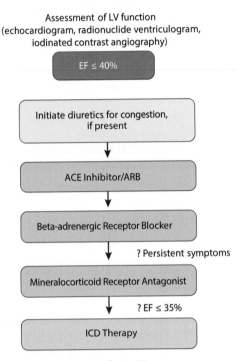

FIGURE 8.1    Steps in treating patients with HF-rEF.

## EVIDENCE-BASED THERAPIES REDUCE RISK

Optimal implementation of six evidence-based therapies improves survival in heart failure patients (Table 8.1, Appendix B). A proportion of patients, however, are currently undertreated (Table 8.2).[1] There may be several reasons for inconsistent application of evidence based guidelines, but hopefully, an explicit understanding of beneficial effects when consistently applying these recommended strategies, may lead to increased use in practice. Maximizing patient therapy could contribute to a decrease in heart failure symptoms and associated hospitalizations, and if mortality risk reductions of each modality are additive, then complete implementation of all 6 therapies has been estimated to save up to 67,996 deaths per year.[1] Commonly used doses of heart failure medications are listed at the end of this chapter (Table 8.4, p. 197).

TABLE 8.1    Mortality risk reduction for each component of heart failure therapy.[1]

| THERAPY | MORTALITY RELATIVE-RISK REDUCTION | CLINICAL TRIALS |
|---|---|---|
| ACEI/ARB | 17% | **The SOLVD Investigators** (Studies of Left Ventricular Dysfunction) |
| BETA-BLOCKER | 34% | **COPERNICUS** (Carvedilol Prospective Randomized Cumulative Survival Trial) |
| | | **MERIT-HF Investigators** (Metoprolol CR/XL Randomized Intervention Trial in Congestive Heart Failure) |
| ALDOSTERONE ANTAGONIST | 30% | **RALES** (Randomized Aldactone Evaluation Study Investigators) |
| | | **EPHESUS** (Eplerenone Post-Acute Myocardial Infarction Heart Failure Efficacy and Survival Study) |
| HYDRALAZINE/ NITRATE | 43% | **A-HeFT** (African-American Heart Failure Trial) |
| ICD | 23% | **SCD-HeFT** (Sudden Cardiac Death in Heart Failure Trial) |
| CRT | 36% | **COMPANION** (Comparison of Medical Therapy, Pacing, and Defibrillation in Heart Failure) |
| | | **CARE-HF Study Investigators** (Cardiac Resynchronization-Heart Failure) |

TABLE 8.2    Eligible heart failure patients not treated for guideline-recommended therapy.[1] (Not all patients with heart failure are eligible for every type of treatment.)

| THERAPY | TOTAL PATIENT POPULATION WITH HF ELIGIBLE FOR TREATMENT | ELIGIBLE HF POPULATION NOT TREATED | POTENTIAL ADDITIONAL LIVES SAVED PER YEAR IF TREATED |
|---|---|---|---|
| ACEI/ARB | 2,459,644 | 20.4% | 6,516 |
| BETA-BLOCKER | 2,512,560 | 14.4% | 12,922 |
| ALDOSTERONE ANTAGONIST | 603,014 | 63.9% | 21,407 |
| HYDRALAZINE/ NITRATE | 150,754 | 92.7% | 6,655 |
| ICD | 1,725,732 | 49.4% | 12,179 |
| CRT | 326,151 | 61.2% | 8,317 |

# Volume Management with Diuretics

Most patients with a history of pulmonary congestion require a loop diuretic such as furosemide. Some patients with mild volume overload can maintain euvolemia with sodium restriction alone or in conjunction with a thiazide diuretic.

## STRATEGIES FOR IMPROVING THE RESPONSE TO DIURESIS

If volume overload persists, changing a patient from furosemide to bumetanide or torsemide may enhance diuretic response (see below). In addition, intravenous administration avoids problems with bioavailability and improves efficacy. In other cases, as a "booster" for loop diuretics, oral metolazone 2.5–5 mg or hydrochlorothiazide 6.25–25 mg can be added every one to three days. An afternoon second dose of loop diuretic may be helpful.

| Generic Name | Brand Name | Equivalent IV Doses |
|---|---|---|
| • Furosemide | • Lasix® | • 40 mg |
| • Bumetanide | • Bumex® | • 1 mg |
| • Torsemide | • Demadex® | • 20 mg |
| • Ethacrynic acid | • Edecrin® | • 50 mg |

## LOOP DIURETICS: TORSEMIDE COMPARED TO FUROSEMIDE

The relative effectiveness of oral loop diuretics depends in part on differences in bioavailability and duration of action. Oral torsemide compared with furosemide has a greater bioavailability (80%–100% vs. 10%–90%), shorter onset of action ($T_{max}$ = 1.1 h vs. 2.4 h), and a longer duration of action (18–24 h vs. 4–6 h). Moreover, food intake can reduce furosemide's bioavailability, but does not affect torsemide.[2] Doses for effective diuresis vary among patients. One strategy is to titrate by doubling the dose of oral furosemide (up to 160 mg/day) or bumetanide (up to 4 mg/day), with a low threshold to change to torsemide (up to 200 mg/day) when a patient has persistent congestion. Fewer differences are seen among loop diuretics when administered intravenously.

# Angiotensin II Inhibition

At the systemic level, angiotensin converting enzyme (ACE) inhibitors and angiotensin II receptor blockers (ARBs) act as vasodilators by reducing the vasoconstricting effects of angiotensin II. Short-term, the arterial and venous vasodilation effects may contribute to improvements in symptoms of low cardiac output and congestion, respectively, unless offset by the effects of hypotension. Angiotensin II can also be generated from angiotensinogen locally in both the cardiac interstitium and intracellular compartments.[3] Long-term benefits of ACE inhibitors on heart failure outcomes may relate to reducing the local effects angiotensin II on organ function and structure as well as renal mechanisms.

## CONTRAINDICATIONS AND PRECAUTIONS FOR ACE INHIBITORS

Patients with heart failure due to left ventricular systolic dysfunction should be given a trial of ACE inhibitors, unless they have experienced life-threatening adverse reactions during previous medication exposure or if they are pregnant or plan to become pregnant. Other conditions that may be relative contraindications include low systemic blood pressure and renal dysfunction. Also consider alternatives to ACE inhibitors if a patient has a very low systemic blood pressure (systolic blood pressure < 80 mm Hg), markedly increased serum levels of creatinine (> 3 mg/dL), bilateral renal artery stenosis, or elevated levels of serum potassium (> 5.0 mEq/L). ACE inhibitors can be reconsidered when these parameters have improved. In the case of persistent renal insufficiency, half the usual dose can be considered. When treating a patient with ACE inhibitors, an increase in creatinine up to 0.5 mg/dL can be acceptable if blood pressure is maintained.

## SIDE EFFECTS

Although all ACE inhibitors lead to decreased production of angiotensin II, side effects may differ by specific agent. Any drug from this class can cause hypotension, cough, renal insufficiency, angioedema, and dysgeusia (change of taste). Agents with sulfhydryl groups, such as captopril, may also cause neutropenia, rash, and proteinuria.[4] ARBs have similar efficacy without the side effect of cough. Although angioedema can occur with ARBs, the incidence is much less than with ACE inhibitors.[5]

## CLINICAL TRIAL DATA FOR ACE INHIBITORS

### Studies of LV Dysfunction (SOLVD) Trial

The SOLVD Trial found that HF patients have improved survival beginning almost at the time of initiation of therapy with the ACE inhibitor enalapril (Figure 8.2). In this study, enalapril (target dose 10 mg twice daily) was compared to placebo in patients with heart failure symptoms and an EF ≤ 35%. The survival difference between patients receiving enalapril versus placebo increased over time.[6]

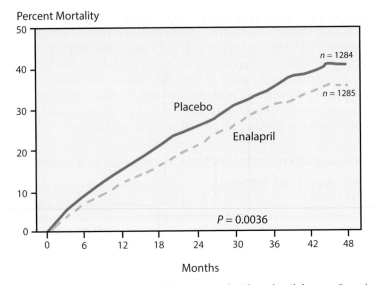

**FIGURE 8.2    The SOLVD trial and heart failure survival with enalapril therapy.** From the SOLVD Investigators, effect of enalapril on survival in patients with reduced left ventricular ejection fractions and congestive heart failure, further details in text.[6] *Source:* Reprinted with permission from *N Engl J Med.* 1991;325(5):293-302. Copyright © Massachusetts Medical Society. All rights reserved.

## Achieving Target Doses with ACE Inhibitors

Patient benefits improve when target doses of ACE inhibitor therapy are reached. The Assessment of Treatment with Lisinopril and Survival (ATLAS) trial found a dose-related response to ACE inhibition, achieving a better efficacy and cost-effectiveness with lisinopril goal of 32.5–35.0 mg per day compared to lower doses of 2.5–5.0 mg per day.[7] In most patients, a target of 20 mg per day of lisinopril or equivalent is desirable. If hypotension occurs during titration of ACE inhibitor dose, decreasing it may be necessary to decrease the diuretic dose.

## Captopril Blunts Post-MI Remodeling

In the Survival and Ventricular Enlargement (SAVE) trial,[8] patients who received the ACE inhibitor captopril had smaller increases in both left ventricular end-diastolic and end-systolic dimension at 1 year compared to placebo (Figure 8.3). During a mean follow-up of 3 years, captopril decreased adverse cardiovascular events (cardiovascular death, heart failure requiring hospitalization, or recurrent myocardial infarction). These findings demonstrate the mechanism of ACE inhibition: preventing adverse remodeling changes in left ventricular size and structure improves outcomes in heart failure post-MI.

# Effect of Captopril on Heart Size post-Myocardial Infarction

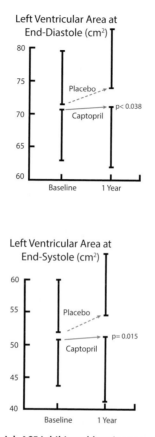

FIGURE 8.3    **The SAVE trial: ACE inhibitors blunt increases in heart size after myocardial infarction.** Left ventricular area measured by 2-dimensional echocardiography (Captopril, $n = 203$; Placebo, $n = 217$).[8] *Source:* Adapted with permission from St. John Sutton et al., *Circulation.* 1994;89(1):68-75.

## ACE INHIBITORS (ACEI) VERSUS ANGIOTENSIN II RECEPTOR BLOCKERS (ARBs)

Angiotensin II receptor blockers (ARBs) may be an alternative to ACE inhibitor therapy. Although use of either ACE inhibitors or ARBs will decrease the deleterious effects of angiotensin II, only ACE inhibitors will increase the level of the vasodilator bradykinin by blocking its degradation. Although bradykinin may have beneficial effects, including the release of nitric oxide and prostacyclin, it may also contribute to side effects such as angioedema and cough. Because ARBs do not affect bradykinin levels, these side effects are uncommon. Presently available ARBs block the angiotensin II type-1 receptor (responsible for the direct cardiovascular effects of angiotensin II) and not the type-2 receptor (possibly a desirable mediator for prevention of apoptosis).[5]

Thus, ARBs have related, but not equivalent, effects to ACE inhibitors. Nevertheless, clinical outcomes in heart failure with either agent have been similar. When the ARB candesartan was assessed in patients who were previously intolerant to ACE inhibitors, compared to placebo, candesartan significantly reduced cardiovascular death and hospital admission for heart failure by 30%, similar to the beneficial effects expected with ACE inhibitors (Figure 8.4).[9]

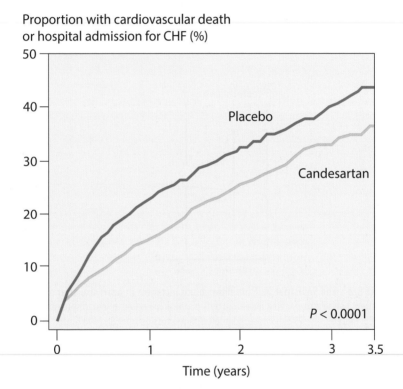

**FIGURE 8.4    CHARM trial: ARB therapy for HF-rEF.** The ARB candesartan, used in patients not on an ACE inhibitor, reduced cardiovascular death or hospital admission ($n$ = 2028; hazard ratio (HR), 0.77).[9] *Source:* Adapted with permission from Granger et al., *Lancet.* 2003;362(9386):772-776.

## INDICATIONS FOR ACE INHIBITORS AND ARBs

The indications for ACE inhibitors and ARBs have increased over time. Initially, ACE inhibitors were identified as treatment of symptomatic left ventricular systolic dysfunction. Subsequently, ACE inhibitors and ARBs were found to improve outcomes in three additional related categories of patients:

1. asymptomatic patients with ejection fractions ≤ 35% due to either ischemic or nonischemic cardiomyopathy[6,9]

2. patients 3–16 days following ST-elevation myocardial infarction (STEMI) with ejection fractions < 40%[10,11]

3. patients presenting within the first 24 hours after STEMI[12,13]

## NO BENEFIT TO COMBINATION THERAPY WITH ACE INHIBITOR AND ARB

Several large, multicenter trials (Val-HeFT: Valsartan Heart Failure Trial; CHARM: Candesartan in Heart Failure Assessment of Reduction in Morbidity and Mortality; and VALIANT: Valsartan in Acute Myocardial Infarction) have failed to find benefit of *adding* an ARB to patients on ACE inhibitor therapy. In the VALIANT trial,[11] valsartan, captopril, or both led to equivalent rates of death and other adverse cardiovascular outcomes in patients with myocardial infarction complicated by heart failure or left ventricular ejection fraction ≤ 35% (Figure 8.5). Thus, most patients with HF-rEF will benefit from either an ACE inhibitor or ARB, but not both.

However, addition of a mineralocorticoid receptor antagonist to either an ACE inhibitor or an ARB should be considered in patients with HF-rEF (see p. 181). Triple therapy with an ACE inhibitor, ARB, and mineralocorticoid receptor antagonist should be avoided because of no added benefit and increased risk of hyperkalemia and renal dysfunction.[14]

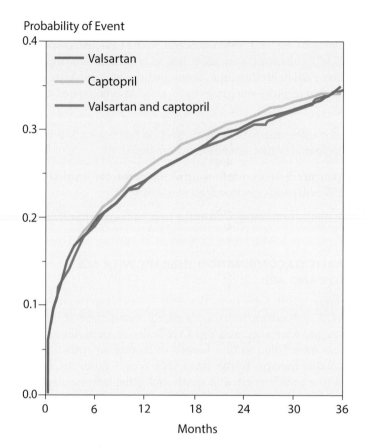

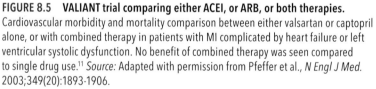

**FIGURE 8.5    VALIANT trial comparing either ACEI, or ARB, or both therapies.**
Cardiovascular morbidity and mortality comparison between either valsartan or captopril
alone, or with combined therapy in patients with MI complicated by heart failure or left
ventricular systolic dysfunction. No benefit of combined therapy was seen compared
to single drug use.[11] *Source:* Adapted with permission from Pfeffer et al., *N Engl J Med.*
2003;349(20):1893-1906.

## DIRECT INHIBITION OF RENIN

The direct renin inhibitor aliskiren (inhibits the enzyme renin, and cleavage of angiotensin I from angiotensinogen) has been approved for treatment of systemic hypertension. The possible use of aliskiren as an alternative or supplemental therapy to an ACE inhibitor or ARB for heart failure is uncertain at this time pending the results of randomized trials.[15]

# Beta Adrenoreceptor Blockade

Use of beta-blockers for the treatment of either ischemic or nonischemic cardiomyopathy has a history of initial skepticism followed by gradual acceptance for treatment of disease progression in patients with systolic dysfunction, regardless of symptom status.[14]

Beta-blockers can be classified as first, second, or third generation based on specific pharmacologic properties. First generation beta-blockers include propranolol with nonspecific blockade properties of both β1- and β2-catecholamine receptors. Second generation beta-blockers include metoprolol, bisoprolol, or atenolol, specific for the β1-receptor subtype. Third generation beta-blockers include carvedilol, nebivolol, and labetalol and have additional mechanisms of cardiovascular activity such as vasodilatation. The beta-blockers carvedilol, extended-release metoprolol, and bisoprolol improve survival in patients with symptomatic systolic dysfunction (HF-rEF). Of these, the data for survival benefit are strongest for carvedilol.

## THIRD GENERATION BETA-BLOCKERS: CARVEDILOL

Carvedilol is a nonspecific β1- and β2-receptor blocker with vasodilating α-receptor blocker properties and antioxidant effects.[16] The α-adrenergic receptor blockade could lead to hypotension and dizziness, but also preserves cardiac output via afterload reduction of the left ventricle.

In the U.S. Carvedilol Heart Failure study,[17] in patients with ejection fractions ≤ 35%, with a median duration of therapy of 6.5 months, there was a mortality of 7.8% in the placebo group and 3.2% in the carvedilol group—a 65% reduction in risk. The combined risk of death or cardiovascular hospitalization was reduced 38% (Figure 8.6).

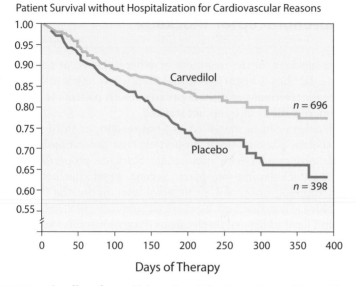

Patient Survival without Hospitalization for Cardiovascular Reasons

FIGURE 8.6   **The effect of carvedilol on rehospitalization and mortality in patients with chronic heart failure.** Patients in the carvedilol group had a 38% lower risk of death or hospitalization for cardiovascular disease than patients in the placebo group ($P < 0.001$).[17] *Source:* Adapted with permission from Packer et al., *N Engl J Med.* 1996;334(21):1349-1355.

### Carvedilol in Severe Heart Failure: COPERNICUS Trial.

In the COPERNICUS trial, 2289 patients with an ejection fraction of $< 25\%$ and severe heart failure symptoms (NYHA class IV) without congestion, were randomized to receive placebo or carvedilol. After an average of 10.4 months of follow-up, carvedilol reduced the risk of cardiovascular death or hospitalization by 27% ($P = 0.00002$), in addition to reducing patient days in the hospital for any cause by 27% ($P = 0.0005$).[18] Even in the highest-risk subset of patients, with recent or recurrent decompensation or an EF $\leq 15\%$, similar improvement was found (Figure 8.7).

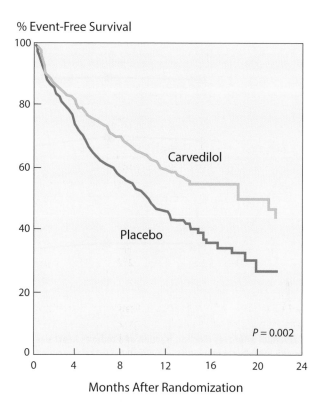

**% Event-Free Survival**

**Months After Randomization**

**FIGURE 8.7    Carvedilol for the highest-risk subgroup (*n* = 624) of patients with severe heart failure (COPERNICUS trial).** Compared to placebo, carvedilol significantly reduced the risk of death or cardiovascular hospitalization by 33% in patients with recent or recurrent heart failure decompensation or very depressed ejection fraction (≤ 15%). (*P* = 0.002)[18] *Source:* Adapted with permission from Packer et al., *Circulation.* 2002;106(17):2194-2199.

### *Effects of Carvedilol on Heart Size*

Whereas ACE inhibitors can blunt increases in heart size following myocardial injury such as myocardial infarction, beta-blocker therapy might reverse myocardial enlargement.[19] In patients with HF-rEF, carvedilol significantly increased ejection fraction, decreased end-systolic dimension, and showed a trend toward decreased end-diastolic dimension by echocardiography (Figure 8.8). This structural effect on the heart in patients with HF-rEF supports the hypothesis that chronic excessive catecholamine stimulation contributes to the adverse consequence of ventricular enlargement.

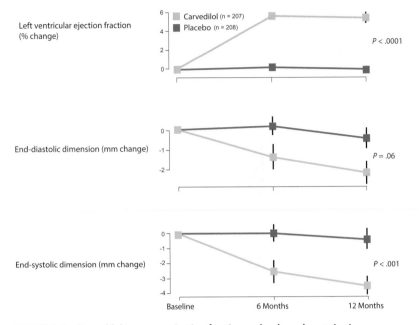

**FIGURE 8.8** **Carvedilol improves ejection fraction and reduces heart size in patients also on ACE inhibitor therapy.**[19] *Source:* Reprinted with permission from *Lancet.* 1997;349(9049):375-380.

## INITIATING β-ADRENERGIC RECEPTOR BLOCKADE IN PATIENTS WITH HEART FAILURE: START LOW AND GO SLOW!

When starting beta-blockers in patients with heart failure, low doses should be used initially, then gradually titrated to higher target doses. This minimizes potential symptoms of dizziness, fatigue, or worsening heart failure during the initiation of therapy. Typically, if a patient is tolerating a beta-blocker, double the dose every 1 to 4 weeks until target doses are attained (e.g., carvedilol titrated from 3.125 to 25 mg twice daily over a series of steps). In the IMPACT-HF trial, patients who were started on beta-blockers during initial hospitalization for HF-rEF were more likely to still be taking them as outpatients 60 days later without increased side effects.[20] Better outcomes can be achieved if target doses of beta-blockers can be reached (Figure 8.9). Carvedilol is also available in a sustained release preparation in a range of doses given once daily.[21]

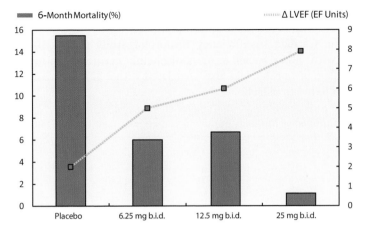

**FIGURE 8.9 Reaching target doses for carvedilol.** With increasing doses of carvedilol, 6-month mortality decreased and left ventricular ejection fraction increased (Δ LVEF).[22] *Source:* Adapted with permission Bristow et al., *Circulation.* 1996;94(11):2807-2816.

### *Potential Interactions with Other Therapies and Conditions*

Diuretic dosage may require adjustment during the early phase of beta blockade. Dizziness, if due to hypotension, can improve with a reduction in diuretics. Alternatively, shortness of breath, if due to pulmonary congestion, may require an increase in diuretics.

Chronic obstructive lung disease is common in elderly patients with heart failure, and occasionally symptoms may be exacerbated by beta-blockers. However, in the absence of true hyperresponsive airway reactivity (asthma), carvedilol is usually well tolerated and the benefits of treatment are significant.[23] Although leg claudication due to peripheral arterial disease may worsen with beta-blockers, this is uncommon with carvedilol.[23] When patients develop intolerance of beta-blockers because of hypotension or worsening heart failure despite adjustment of other medications, this may portend clinical decline and transition from Stage C to Stage D heart failure.

### OTHER BETA-BLOCKERS

The Metoprolol CR/XL Randomized Intervention Trial in Congestive Heart Failure (MERIT-HF)[24] found that compared to placebo, sustained-release metoprolol succinate, titrated to 200 mg per day, decreased mortality by 35% in patients with predominately NYHA class II and III heart failure and an ejection fraction ≤ 40% (Figure 8.10). When carvedilol was compared to immediate-release metoprolol tartrate, however, carvedilol was associated with an additional 14% decrease in risk of mortality.[25]

Thus, if metoprolol is used for HF-rEF, it should be the sustained-release, once-a-day formulation, metoprolol succinate.

In the Cardiac Insufficiency Bisoprolol Study (CIBIS II) trial in patients with either ischemic or nonischemic cardiomyopathy, a third beta-blocker, bisoprolol, was also associated with a 32% decrease in mortality compared to placebo.[26]

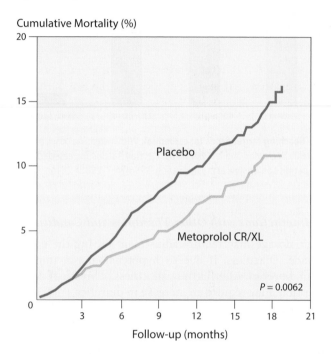

FIGURE 8.10 **Beta-blocker effects on heart failure mortality.** Metoprolol succinate compared to placebo in patients with chronic heart failure reduced the relative risk of mortality by 34%, n = 3991.[24] *Source:* Adapted with permission from *Lancet.* 1999;353(9169):2001-2007.

## Mechanisms of Improvement with ß-Adrenergic Receptor Blockade in Heart Failure

Beta-blockade can blunt the reduction in density and reduced sensitivity of β-adrenergic receptors seen with progressive heart failure.[27] Furthermore, reversal of reduced myocardial gene expression of β-receptors and SERCA2a, and of fetal patterns of myosin expression (see Chapter 4) are associated with the beneficial clinical responses to beta-blocker therapy and improved left ventricular ejection fraction.[28] The reduction in heart rate alone secondary to beta-blockade may improve myocardial energetics. This is supported by studies with ivabradine, a sinus node inhibitor (not available in the United States at this time), which slows heart rate by a non-adrenergic receptor mechanism. In the SHIFT trial in 6558 patients with an EF ≤ 35%, ivabradine reduced cardiovascular death or heart failure hospital admission by 18% when added to standard therapy in patients with resting heart rates of 70 bpm or higher.[29]

## Mineralocorticoid Receptor Antagonists

Aldosterone contributes to the progression of heart failure including promotion of myocardial fibrosis.[30] Medications known as mineralocorticoid receptor antagonists (MRAs) block aldosterone receptors. Although these medications are mild diuretics, MRAs also prevent hypokalemia associated with concomitant use of loop diuretics.[31,32] Conversely, because the available MRA agents spironolactone and eplerenone can cause hyperkalemia or renal insufficiency, they should be withheld when serum creatinine is more than 2.5 mg/dL in men or more than 2.0 mg/dL in women (or estimated glomerular filtration rate < 30 mL/min/1.73 m$^2$), and/or potassium > 5.0 mEq/L.[14]

### SPIRONOLACTONE

The RALES study randomized 1663 patients of NYHA class III or IV heart failure with left ventricular EF ≤ 35% to receive either 25 mg of spironolactone daily or placebo. After 2-years of follow up, spironolactone compared to the placebo group reduced the risk of death from any cause by 30%, and reduced the risk of hospitalization for heart failure by 35% (Figure 8.11).[32] 10% of men treated with spironolactone reported gynecomastia or breast tenderness, attributed to estrogen-like effects of spironolactone.

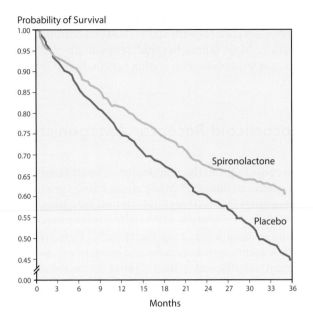

**FIGURE 8.11  Spironolactone vs. placebo in patients with NYHA class III–IV heart failure.**
*Note:* Use of spironolactone resulted in a 30% decrease in risk of mortality ($P < 0.001$).[32] *Source:* Adapted with permission from Pitt et al., *N Engl J Med.* 1999;341(10):709-717.

## EPLERENONE

The EMPHASIS trial examined the MRA eplerenone in patients with less symptomatic HF-rEF. Zannad et al. randomly assigned 2737 patients with NYHA class II heart failure to receive either eplerenone or placebo. Eplerenone reduced the risk of the primary outcome (death from cardiovascular causes or a first hospitalization for heart failure) by 37% ($P < 0.001$). Secondary endpoints (death from any cause and hospitalization for heart failure) were also reduced with eplerenone (Figure 8.12).[31] In contrast to spironolactone, eplerenone does not cause gynecomastia.

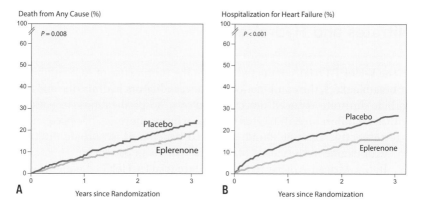

**FIGURE 8.12    Eplerenone vs. placebo in patients with systolic heart failure and mild symptoms (NYHA class II).** Eplerenone reduced risk of both death from any cause **(Panel A)** and hospitalization for heart failure **(Panel B)**. ($n$ = 2737; Death: HR 0.76, $P$ = 0.008; Heart failure hospitalization: HR 0.58, $P$ < 0.001).[31] *Source:* Adapted with permission from Zannad et al., *N Engl J Med.* 2011;364(1):11-21.

## Neutral Endopeptidase Inhibition

Extracellular neprilysin, a neutral endopeptidase enzyme (NEP), metabolizes vasoactive peptides including natriuretic peptides (e.g., ANP, BNP), bradykinin, and adrenomedullin.[33] NEP inhibition increases the levels of these substances and can offset the phenotype of progressive heart failure characterized by vasoconstriction, sodium retention, and maladaptive remodeling. In patients with HF-rEF in the PARADIGM-HF trial, a combined ARB (valsartan) and neprilysin inhibitor (sacubitril) led to a 21% further reduction in the primary composite endpoint of cardiovascular death and heart failure hospitalization compared to the ACE inhibitor enalapril.[33] All-cause mortality was reduced 16%. Although NEP inhibition is not yet available, this class of medication might complement existing neurohormonal blocker therapies in the future, and when combined with an ARB provide a substitute for ACE inhibitor therapy.

## Nitrates and Hydralazine

In the V-HeFT I trial, conducted prior to the routine use of ACE inhibitors or beta-blockers, the combination of the vasodilators hydralazine and isosorbide dinitrate reduced mortality, but not hospitalizations, in patients with heart failure already treated with digoxin and diuretics.[34] Subsequently, a retrospective analysis found enhanced benefits of isosorbide dinitrate and hydralazine in the subset of African-American patients.[35]

In the African-American Heart Failure trial (A-HeFT),[36] patients with NYHA class III and IV heart failure receiving background therapy (including ACE inhibitors or ARBs, beta-blockers, spironolactone, and diuretics), were assigned to placebo or the combination of oral isosorbide dinitrate (40 mg t.i.d.) and hydralazine (75 mg t.i.d.). Compared to the placebo group, with the addition of these therapies, overall risk of mortality was reduced by 43% ($P$ = 0.01) and the rate of first hospitalization for heart failure was reduced 33% ($P$ = 0.001). These results suggest that the combination of isosorbide dinitrate and hydralazine provides beneficial effects when added to current standard therapy in African-American patients (Figure 8.13).

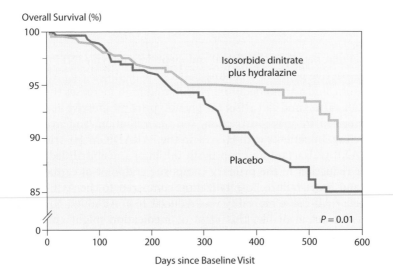

**FIGURE 8.13  The administration of isosorbide dinitrate with hydralazine to African-American patients with NYHA class III–IV heart failure reduced the risk of death by 43%.[36]**
*Source:* Adapted with permission from Taylor et al., *N Engl J Med.* 2004;351(20):2049-2057.

# Digoxin

Controversy regarding the use of digitalis preparations has persisted over the last 200 years.[37] Digitalis is a modest positive inotrope in patients with left ventricular dilation, slows the rate of conduction of atrial fibrillation at the AV node of the heart, and leads to a modest withdrawal of sympathetic tone, in part by a direct effect on the baroreceptors within the carotid sinus.[37]

The Digitalis Investigation Group (DIG) trial showed no difference in survival between patients with EF less than or equal to 45% randomized to digoxin versus placebo.[38] The combined endpoints of death or hospitalization due to heart failure, however, were significantly reduced (Figure 8.14).

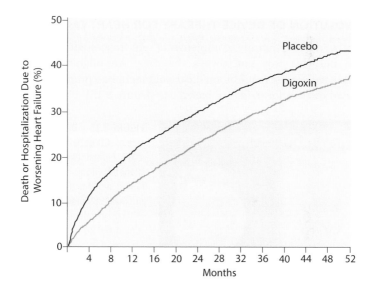

FIGURE 8.14   DIG Trial: Placebo vs. Digoxin. Incidence of death or hospitalization due to worsening heart failure comparing digoxin and placebo groups. ($P < 0.001$).[38] *Source:* Adapted with permission from *N Engl J Med.* 1997;336(8):525-533.

## DIGOXIN DOSING

Consider adding digoxin to patients in sinus rhythm with HF-rEF who remain symptomatic despite neurohormonal blockade and correction of volume overload. Because digoxin does not have an effect on overall mortality (only the combined endpoint of mortality and hospitalization), patients who are asymptomatic do not require digoxin. Optimal dosing is achieved when serum digoxin levels are $\leq 1.2$ ng/mL typically at a dose of 0.125 mg daily in patients with normal renal function.[39]

# Electrical Therapies for Heart Failure

Ventricular arrhythmias are a complication of structural heart disease, and electrical devices have impacted treatment strategies. An implantable cardioverter-defibrillator (ICD) is a pacemaker device with defibrillation capability that can electrically treat ventricular tachycardia and ventricular fibrillation. Cardiac resynchronization therapy (CRT) involves the placement of an additional lead, usually via the coronary sinus, onto the lateral wall of the left ventricle to improve left ventricular function in patients with congestive heart failure and prolonged QRS duration or pacemaker dependent bradycardia. A subcutaneous ICD (S-ICD) can treat ventricular arrhythmias without transvenous leads.

## THE EVOLUTION OF DEVICE THERAPY FOR HEART FAILURE

Currently, device therapy complements pharmacologic treatment of HF-rEF, but this was not always the case. An ongoing partnership between cardiologists and biomedical engineers has produced effective, safe, small devices for evidence-based use (Figure 8.15).

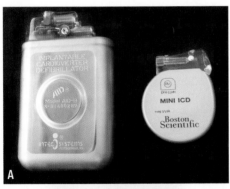

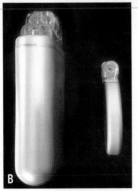

**FIGURE 8.15   Decreases in size of ICD between 1980 and 2014.** Frontal (**Panel A**) and lateral (**Panel B**) views of Intec Systems (1980) and Mini ICD (2014). The original 1980 model was 300 g and 200 cm³ in volume; the 2014 model is 60 g and 26.5 cm³. *Source:* Intec Systems ICD courtesy of Dr. Ron Miller.

## PREVENTION OF SUDDEN CARDIAC DEATH

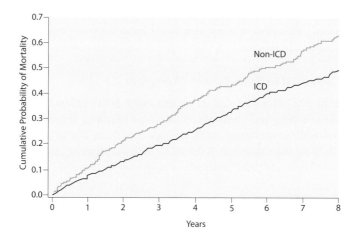

FIGURE 8.16    The MADIT II trial showed a higher probability of survival with an implantable cardiac-defibrillator (ICD). Survival with an ICD was compared to conventional therapy over an 8-year follow-up, in patients with ischemic cardiomyopathy (EF ≤ 30%) and spontaneous nonsustained ventricular tachycardia. There was a 34% reduction in the risk of death with ICD therapy during 8 years of follow-up, $P < 0.001$.[40] *Source:* Adapted with permission from Goldenberg et al., *Circulation.* 2010;122(13):1265-1271.

Initially, ICDs were only placed in high-risk patients who had been resuscitated from an episode of sudden cardiac death or sustained ventricular arrhythmia. Subsequently, clinical trials demonstrated a survival benefit in patients with a low left ventricular ejection fraction without prior history of sudden cardiac death. The Multicenter Automatic Defibrillator Implantation Trial II (MADIT II) randomized post-MI patients with persistent systolic dysfunction (LVEF ≤30%) to prophylactic ICD or conventional medical therapy.[41] Overall, there was a 34% reduction in mortality risk in those who received a prophylactic ICD (Figure 8.16), attributed to a reduction in sudden cardiac death (3.8% vs. 10.0%; $P < 0.01$). In this trial, a higher rate of heart failure (20% vs. 15%) in a subset of patients in the ICD group was attributed to routine right ventricular pacing.[40] In those programmed to minimal right ventricular

**CLASS I INDICATIONS FOR ICD FOR PRIMARY PREVENTION OF SUDDEN DEATH[42]**

1. LVEF ≤ 35% due to prior myocardial infarction at least 40 days post–myocardial infarction and NYHA functional class II or III. (Level of Evidence: A)

2. LVEF ≤ 30% due to prior myocardial infarction at least 40 days post–myocardial infarction and NYHA functional class I. (Level of Evidence: A)

3. Nonischemic dilated cardiomyopathy with LVEF ≤ 35% at least 90 days post-diagnosis and NYHA functional class II or III. (Level of Evidence: B)

pacing, the number of patients needed to treat to save 1 life was 6 (NNT = 6) based on data from 8 years of follow-up. This overall benefit occurred despite half of patients receiving their defibrillator through a higher-risk, transthoracic approach, compared to the current standard transvenous approach.

### ICD Compared to Amiodarone Therapy in HF-rEF

In the SCD-HeFT trial, 2521 patients with NYHA class II or III, and an EF ≤35%, despite maximum pharmacologic therapy, were randomized to (1) placebo, (2) amiodarone, or (3) a single-lead ICD. The primary endpoint of death from any cause was reduced by 23% in the group assigned to ICD. The risk of death with amiodarone was similar to placebo (Figure 8.17).[43]

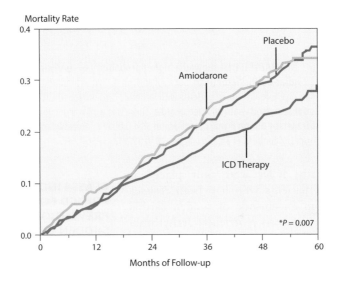

**FIGURE 8.17    SCD-HeFT: ICD versus amiodarone versus placebo therapy in mild-to-moderate heart failure patients with LVEF ≤ 35% for primary prevention of sudden death.** There was a 23% reduction in the risk of death with ICD therapy versus placebo ($P = 0.007$).[43]
*Source:* Adapted with permission from Bardy et al., *N Engl J Med.* 2005;352(3):225-237.

## CARDIAC RESYNCHRONIZATION THERAPY (CRT)

Intraventricular conduction delays on ECG (QRS duration greater than 120 ms) occur in 15% to 30% of patients with HF-rEF.[44] The resulting nonuniform spatial and temporal contraction and relaxation of the left ventricle, with potential for functional mitral regurgitation, can contribute to a loss of pump efficiency. In the absence of other ventricular impairment, the decrease in function with an intraventricular conduction delay would be small. With reduced cardiac systolic function, however, the effect of this nonuniformity can be substantial. Cardiac resynchronization therapy (CRT), by means of biventricular pacemaker stimulation, synchronizes the activation of the left ventricular free wall and septum (Figure 8.18) while improving left ventricular systolic function.[45] Electrical activation of the left ventricle is usually achieved via a transvenous electrode passed through the coronary sinus venous system of the heart or, if necessary, via a mini-thoracotomy to place a direct transthoracic epicardial lead.

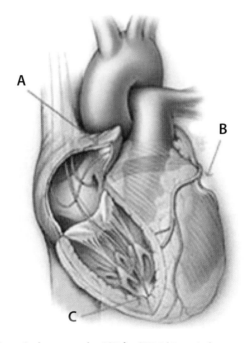

**FIGURE 8.18    Biventricular pacemaker ICD for CRT.** A biventricular pacemaker ICD for CRT typically has 3 transvenous pacing electrodes stimulating 3 locations: A, right atrium; B, left ventricle via the coronary sinus; C, right ventricle with defibrillator coil. Cardiac resynchronization therapy (CRT) is achieved by coupled activation of the left (B) and right (C) ventricular leads.

### CRT Improves Heart Failure Outcomes

The Comparison of Medical Therapy, Pacing, and Defibrillation in Heart Failure (COMPANION) trial randomly assigned 1520 patients with NYHA class III or IV, EF ≤ 35% and QRS duration ≥ 120 ms to receive one of three different types of therapy. Patients received 1) optimal pharmacologic therapy alone or in combination with cardiac-resynchronization therapy with either 2) a pacemaker or 3) a pacemaker-defibrillator.

Compared to pharmacologic therapy alone, both CRT groups showed reductions in the rate of death or hospitalization from any cause. There was a significant reduction in the death rate with combination CRT and ICD therapy ($P = 0.003$), with a trend for CRT alone ($P = 0.059$) (Figure 8.19).[46] Subsequently, CRT pacing alone without ICD was found to significantly improve survival compared to pharmacologic therapy in a similar group of patients.[47]

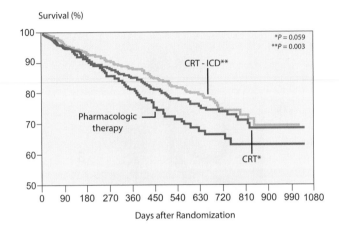

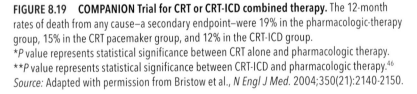

**FIGURE 8.19   COMPANION Trial for CRT or CRT-ICD combined therapy.** The 12-month rates of death from any cause—a secondary endpoint—were 19% in the pharmacologic-therapy group, 15% in the CRT pacemaker group, and 12% in the CRT-ICD group.
*$P$ value represents statistical significance between CRT alone and pharmacologic therapy.
**$P$ value represents statistical significance between CRT-ICD and pharmacologic therapy.[46]
Source: Adapted with permission from Bristow et al., N Engl J Med. 2004;350(21):2140-2150.

The MADIT-CRT trial, in less symptomatic patients, randomized 1820 NYHA class I or II patients with ischemic or nonischemic cardiomyopathy, an ejection fraction ≤ 30%, and a QRS duration ≥ 130 ms, to receive CRT with an ICD, or an ICD alone. After 2-years of follow up, 17.2% of patients who received CRT with an ICD either died or had a nonfatal heart-failure event, versus 25.3% of patients who received an ICD alone (Figure 8.20).[48] In a subgroup analysis, benefit of CRT with an ICD was confined to patients with a left bundle branch block. A decrease in both end-diastolic and systolic volumes, along with an increase in ejection fraction was also observed in the group that received CRT-ICD (Figure 8.20).[48]

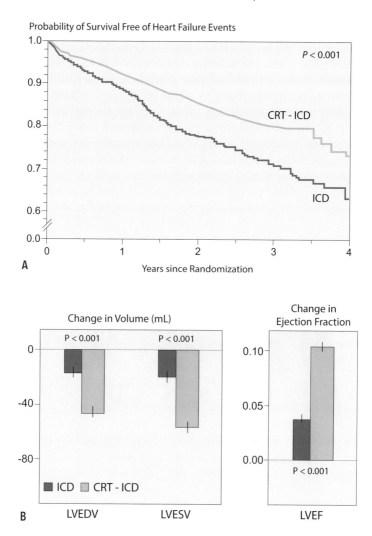

**FIGURE 8.20 (Panel A) Survival free of heart failure events rates compared between CRT-ICD and ICD alone groups. (Panel B) CRT-ICD and LV function.** There were decreases in left ventricular end-diastolic (LVEDV) and systolic (LVESV) volumes (**Panel B, left**) and increases in ejection fraction (**Panel B, right**) in patients who received CRT-ICD.[48] *Source:* Adapted with permission from Moss et al., *N Engl J Med.* 2009;361(14):1329-1338.

In a single-center study, the addition of cardiac resynchronization therapy also permitted administration of higher doses of neurohormonal blockers and lower doses of diuretics that contributed to the total subsequent reduction of morbidity and mortality.[49]

## SUBCUTANEOUS ICD

To avoid some of the complications of transvenous leads, an entirely sub-cutaneous implantable cardioverter-defibrillator has been developed for primary prevention of sudden cardiac death in patients with HF-rEF due to ventricular tachyarrhythmia. A pulse generator is placed in the left lateral chest wall and connected to an 8-cm parasternal coil electrode (Figure 8.21). In an initial study, this type of device terminated all 12 potentially life-threatening ventricular tachyarrhythmias with electrical shock therapy.[50] The subcutaneous ICD cannot provide long-term pacing, although temporary pacing post-shock therapy is available. The device lacks antitachycardia pacing capabilities that may be a limitation in patients with recurrent, monomorphic ventricular tachycardia.

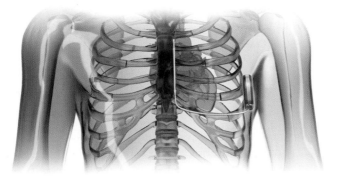

**FIGURE 8.21  Subcutaneous implantable cardio-defibrillator.** *Source:* Figure courtesy of Cameron Health.

# Atrial Fibrillation and Heart Failure

Atrial fibrillation is common in heart failure, associated with increased left atrial size,[51] and frequently results in worsening symptoms.

## ANTICOAGULATION

Anticoagulation with warfarin or oral factor Xa inhibitors (rivaroxaban, and apixaban) and direct thrombin inhibitors (dabigatran) reduces the risk of thromboembolism and stroke.[52] Anticoagulation is recommended for 3 weeks prior to and 4 weeks after cardioversion to sinus rhythm for patients with atrial fibrillation or atrial flutter of greater than 48 hours in duration, or when the duration of arrhythmia is unknown.[53] Prior anticoagulation is not mandatory before electrical cardioversion 1) in the presence of hemodynamic compromise, or 2) if transesophageal echocardiography excludes left atrial thrombus, or 3) if atrial fibrillation is less than 48 hours in duration. In these cases, anticoagulation can be initiated at the time of the procedure. The decision to continue anticoagulation indefinitely is based on risks of bleeding versus thromboembolism.[54]

## RATE AND RHYTHM THERAPIES

Amiodarone, a class III agent with a biologic half-life of 25 ± 12 days,[54] may be useful to achieve or maintain sinus rhythm. This antiarrhythmic drug helps to maintain sinus rhythm after cardioversion even with left atrial size up to 6 cm.[55] Amiodarone has a significant side effect profile (List 8.1). Sotalol and dofetilide are alternatives to amiodarone in younger patients or those with less severe left ventricular systolic dysfunction. Dronedarone is contraindicated in patients with recently decompensated heart failure and is not commonly used in heart failure.

In patients with permanent atrial fibrillation, beta-blockers and digoxin can control ventricular response rate. In general, when there is left ventricular systolic dysfunction, the calcium channel blockers diltiazem and verapamil are less well tolerated for slowing ventricular response, since fluid retention may increase. Heart failure patients with persistent atrial fibrillation may be candidates for catheter-based radiofrequency ablation or ablation of the AV node with placement of a rate-responsive biventricular permanent ventricular pacemaker.[56]

### LIST 8.1   Possible Side Effects of Amiodarone

- Pulmonary inflammation
- Abnormal LFTs
- Nausea
- Neuropathy
- Rash or photosensitivity
- Hyper- or hypothyroidism
- Asymptomatic corneal deposits

Side effects are dose-related and are uncommon at doses < 300 mg/day
Serum levels of amiodarone can be obtained, but are not useful for titration of dose. If low, they can indicate low absorption or noncompliance.[54]

# Treatment of HF-pEF

Guideline recommendations for treatment of HF-pEF are largely Level of Evidence C, based on expert opinions. Suggested treatments are both general and specifically directed at controlling the underlying diseases that give rise to diastolic heart failure (e.g., hypertension, ischemic heart disease, etc.). Part of the difficulty in defining treatment recommendations is due to the diverse mechanisms of HF-pEF including hypertensive heart disease, heart failure with morbid obesity, or HF-pEF with comorbidities.

With these caveats, therapies for HF-pEF can be divided into 3 categories:

1. Cardiovascular treatments for volume management, hypertension, atrial fibrillation (rate or rhythm control), myocardial ischemia, or valvular heart disease (Table 8.3)

2. Treatment of noncardiac comorbidities: renal, pulmonary, anemia (especially iron deficiency)

3. Healthcare systems designed to improve:

   - patient compliance (heart failure clinics, device monitoring, and home health)

   - functional status (physical therapy, cardiac rehab, and exercise prescription)

   - psychosocial adaptation

These three categories are not specific for HF-pEF, but a combined approach may be the most effective option when evidence-based treatments are less available. For example, the MRA spironolactone compared to placebo in heart failure patients with ejection fractions of 45% or greater did not affect the primary cardiovascular composite outcome but did reduce a secondary endpoint of heart failure hospitalizations.[57]

TABLE 8.3   Cardiac-specific therapies for HF-pEF.

| CARDIAC TREATMENT | DIAGNOSIS | ACTION |
|---|---|---|
| VOLUME MANAGEMENT | • History and Physical exam<br>• BNP, BUN/Cr ratio<br>• Echo<br>• Right heart catheter | • Adjust diuretics<br>• Counsel dietary Na$^+$ intake<br>• Remove NSAIDs<br>• Evaluate for primary causes of renal impairment<br>• Adjust IV fluids<br>• Ultrafiltration |
| HYPERTENSION | • Physical exam | • Increase neurohormonal blockers<br>• Add other vasodilators |
| ATRIAL FIBRILLATION | • Physical exam<br>• ECG<br>• Holter | • Rate control: increase beta blockade, digoxin, AV node ablation with pacemaker<br>• Rhythm control: amiodarone, sotalol, dofetilide, AF ablation |
| MYOCARDIAL ISCHEMIA/ VALVULAR DISEASE | • Clinical Assessment | • Medical therapy<br>• Percutaneous or surgical intervention |

# Outpatient Hemodynamic Monitoring for Congestion in HF-pEF and HF-rEF

Heart failure-related hospitalizations are most commonly due to worsening signs and symptoms of congestion. Because increases in both intracardiac and pulmonary venous pressures lead to pulmonary congestion, out-patient monitoring and treatment of these pressures may reduce heart failure related admissions and adverse outcomes.

In the CHAMPION trial, 550 patients with HF-rEF or HF-pEF and a previous hospitalization for heart failure received either standard care alone or combined with a wireless implantable hemodynamic monitoring system to measure daily pulmonary artery pressure.[58] After a 6-month follow-up, 84 heart failure-related hospitalizations were reported in the monitored group, compared to 120 in the control group (Figure 8.22).[58] Future trials that incorporate wireless monitoring of multiple physiologic signals may help establish new algorithms to improve heart failure outcomes.[59]

Cumulative Hospital Admissions

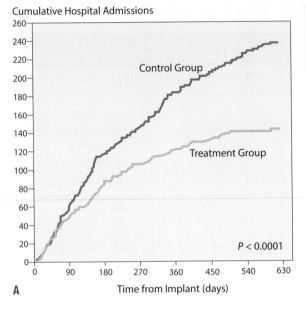

**A** Time from Implant (days)

**FIGURE 8.22
Monitoring by an implanted pulmonary artery pressure sensor system.
Panel A:** Cumulative heart failure hospital admissions reduced by 36%. **Panel B:** Patients within the monitored treatment group had a 29% lower risk of death or first heart failure hospitalization compared to those who received standard care without monitoring.[58] *Source:* Adapted with permission from Abraham et al., *Lancet.* 2011;377(9766):658-666.

Freedom from hospital admission or mortality (%)

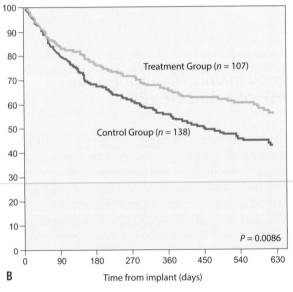

**B** Time from implant (days)

TABLE 8.4   Commonly used doses of HF medications.

| DRUG | INITIAL DOSE (MG) | TARGET DOSE (MG) | RECOMMENDED MAXIMAL DOSE (MG) | MAJOR ADVERSE REACTIONS |
|---|---|---|---|---|
| LOOP DIURETICS: | | – | | |
| furosemide | 10–40 q.d. | | 240 b.i.d. | Hypokalemia, |
| bumetanide | 0.5–1.0 q.d. | | 10 q.d. | hypotension, |
| torsemide | 10 q.d. | | 100 b.i.d. | renal insufficiency |
| ethacrynic acid | 50 q.d. | | 200 b.i.d. | |
| THIAZIDE-RELATED DIURETIC: | | | | |
| metolazone | 2.5 if needed | – | 10 q.d. | Same as loop diuretics |
| ACE INHIBITORS: | | | | |
| lisinopril | 2.5–5 q.d. | 20 q.d. | 40 b.i.d. | Hypotension, |
| enalapril | 2.5 b.i.d. | 10 b.i.d. | 20 b.i.d. | hyperkalemia, |
| captopril | 6.25–12.5 t.i.d. | 50 t.i.d. | 100 t.i.d. | renal insufficiency, cough, skin rash, angioedema, neutropenia |
| ANGIOTENSIN II RECEPTOR BLOCKERS: | | | | |
| valsartan | 40 b.i.d. | 160 b.i.d. | 160 q.d. | Dizziness, renal |
| candesartan | 4–8 q.d. | 32 q.d. | 64 q.d. | insufficiency, |
| losartan | 12.5–25 q.d. | 150 q.d. | 100 q.d. | hypotension |
| BETA-BLOCKERS: | | | | |
| carvedilol | 3.125 b.i.d. | 25 b.i.d. | 50 b.i.d. | Bradycardia, |
| metoprolol (extended release) | 12.5–25 q.d. | 200 q.d. | 200 q.d | dizziness, hypotension, |
| bisoprolol | 1.25 q.d. | 10 q.d. | 10 q.d. | worsening heart failure |
| MINERALO-CORTICOID RECEPTOR ANTAGONISTS: | | | | |
| spironolactone | 12.5–25 q.d. | 25 q.d. | 100 b.i.d. | Hyperkalemia, |
| eplerenone | 25 q.d. | 50 q.d. | | especially if administered with ACEI or ARB, renal insufficiency, gynecomastia (spironolactone only) |
| OTHER VASODILATORS: | | | | |
| hydralazine/ isosorbide dinitrate | 25/ 10 t.i.d. | 75/ 40 t.i.d. | 75/ 40 q.i.d. | Headache, dizziness |
| DIGOXIN | 0.125–0.25 q.d. | – | Serum level < 2.0 ng/mL | Cardiotoxicity, confusion, nausea, anorexia, visual disturbance |

# MICHEL MIROWSKI
## (1924–1990)

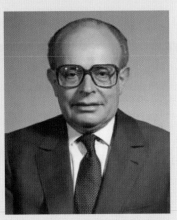

On February 14, 1980, the first implantable cardiac-defibrillator (ICD) was placed in a 57-year-old woman, an event that foretold a marked change in the management of life-threatening ventricular arrhythmias. Dr. Michel Mirowski, inspired by the loss of his mentor due to ventricular tachycardia, believed that outcomes would improve if arrhythmias were detected and treated immediately with an implantable defibrillator. Experts were skeptical that it would be possible to miniaturize a defibrillator, which at the time, was a large device weighing 30 to 40 pounds.

The first device was implanted in the abdominal wall, and a thoracotomy was also required to place defibrillator pads in direct contact with the heart. Over the following decades, the device has undergone continuous technological improvement and miniaturization (Figure 8.15). Currently, most implantation occurs transvenously, similar to a pacemaker procedure.[60,61]

# References

1. Fonarow GC, Yancy CW, Hernandez AF, Peterson ED, Spertus JA, Heidenreich PA. Potential impact of optimal implementation of evidence-based heart failure therapies on mortality. *Am Heart J.* 2011;161(6):1024-1030.

2. Vargo DL, Kramer WG, Black PK, Smith WB, Serpas T, Brater DC. Bioavailability, pharmacokinetics, and pharmacodynamics of torsemide and furosemide in patients with congestive heart failure. *Clin Pharmacol Ther.* 1995;57(6):601-609.

3. Kumar R, Singh VP, Baker KM. The intracellular renin-angiotensin system: a new paradigm. *Trends Endocrinol Metab.* 2007;18(5):208-214.

4. Weber MA. Safety issues during antihypertensive treatment with angiotensin converting enzyme inhibitors. *Am J Med.* 1988;84(4A):16-23.

5. Brunner-La Rocca HP, Vaddadi G, Esler MD. Recent insight into therapy of congestive heart failure: focus on ACE inhibition and angiotensin-II antagonism. *J Am Coll Cardiol.* 1999;33(5):1163-1173.

6. Effect of enalapril on survival in patients with reduced left ventricular ejection fractions and congestive heart failure. The SOLVD Investigators. *N Engl J Med.* 1991;325(5):293-302.

7. Packer M, Poole-Wilson PA, Armstrong PW, Cleland JG, Horowitz JD, Massie BM, et al. Comparative effects of low and high doses of the angiotensin-converting enzyme inhibitor, lisinopril, on morbidity and mortality in chronic heart failure. ATLAS Study Group. *Circulation.* 1999;100:2312-2318.

8. St. John Sutton M, Pfeffer MA, Plappert T, et al. Quantitative two-dimensional echocardiographic measurements are major predictors of adverse cardiovascular events

after acute myocardial infarction. The protective effects of captopril. *Circulation.* 1994;89(1):68-75.

9. Granger CB, McMurray JJ, Yusuf S, et al. Effects of candesartan in patients with chronic heart failure and reduced left-ventricular systolic function intolerant to angiotensin-converting-enzyme inhibitors: the CHARM-Alternative trial. *Lancet.* 2003;362(9386):772-776.

10. Pfeffer MA, Braunwald E, Moyé LA, et al. Effect of captopril on mortality and morbidity in patients with left ventricular dysfunction after myocardial infarction. Results of the survival and ventricular enlargement trial. The SAVE Investigators. *N Engl J Med.* 1992;327(10):669-677.

11. Pfeffer MA, McMurray JJ, Velazquez EJ, et al. Valsartan, captopril, or both in myocardial infarction complicated by heart failure, left ventricular dysfunction, or both. *N Engl J Med.* 2003;349(20):1893-1906.

12. Gruppo Italiano per lo Studio della Sopravvivenza nell'infarto Miocardico. GISSI-3: effects of lisinopril and transdermal glyceryl trinitrate singly and together on 6–week mortality and ventricular function after acute myocardial infarction. *Lancet.* 1994;343(8906):1115-1122.

13. ISIS-4 (Fourth International Study of Infarct Survival) Collaborative Group. ISIS-4: a randomised factorial trial assessing early oral captopril, oral mononitrate, and intravenous magnesium sulphate in 58,050 patients with suspected acute myocardial infarction. *Lancet.* 1995;345(8951):669-685.

14. Yancy CW, Jessup M, Bozkurt B, et al. 2013 ACCF/AHA guideline for the management of heart failure: a report of the American College of Cardiology Foundation/American Heart Association Task Force on Practice Guidelines. *J Am Coll Cardiol.* 2013;62(16):e147-e239.

15. Krum H, Massie B, Abraham WT, et al. Direct renin inhibition in addition to or as an alternative to angiotensin converting enzyme inhibition in patients with chronic systolic heart failure: rationale and design of the Aliskiren Trial to Minimize OutcomeS in Patients with HEart failuRE (ATMOSPHERE) study. *Eur J Heart Fail.* 2011;13(1):107-114.

16. Frishman WH. Carvedilol. *N Engl J Med.* 1998;339(24):1759-1765.

17. Packer M, Bristow MR, Cohn JN, et al. The effect of carvedilol on morbidity and mortality in patients with chronic heart failure. U.S. Carvedilol Heart Failure Study Group. *N Engl J Med.* 1996;334(21):1349-1355.

18. Packer M, Fowler MB, Roecker EB, et al. Effect of carvedilol on the morbidity of patients with severe chronic heart failure: results of the carvedilol prospective randomized cumulative survival (COPERNICUS) study. *Circulation.* 2002;106(17):2194-2199.

19. Randomised, placebo-controlled trial of carvedilol in patients with congestive heart failure due to ischaemic heart disease. Australia/New Zealand Heart Failure Research Collaborative Group. *Lancet.* 1997;349(9049):375-380.

20. Gattis WA, O'Connor CM, Gallup DS, Hasselblad V, Gheorghiade M. Predischarge initiation of carvedilol in patients hospitalized for decompensated heart failure: results of the Initiation Management Predischarge: Process for Assessment of Carvedilol Therapy in Heart Failure (IMPACT-HF) trial. *J Am Coll Cardiol.* 2004;43(9):1534-1541.

21. Udelson JE, Pressler SJ, Sackner-Bernstein J, Massaro J, Ordronneau P, Lukas MA, Hauptman PJ. Adherence with once daily versus twice daily carvedilol in patients with heart failure: the Compliance And Quality of Life Study Comparing Once-Daily Controlled-Release Carvedilol CR and Twice-Daily Immediate-Release Carvedilol IR in Patients with Heart Failure (CASPER) Trial. *J Card Fail.* 2009;15(5):385-393.

22. Bristow MR, Gilbert EM, Abraham WT, et al. Carvedilol produces dose-related improvements in left ventricular function and survival in subjects with chronic heart failure. MOCHA Investigators. *Circulation.* 1996;94(11):2807-2816.

23. Kotlyar E, Keogh AM, Macdonald PS, Arnold RH, McCaffrey DJ, Glanville AR. Tolerability of carvedilol in patients with heart failure and concomitant chronic obstructive pulmonary disease or asthma. *J Heart Lung Transplant.* 2002;21(12): 1290-1295.

24. Effect of metoprolol CR/XL in chronic heart failure: Metoprolol CR/XL Randomised Intervention Trial in Congestive Heart Failure (MERIT-HF). *Lancet.* 1999;353(9169): 2001-2007.

25. Poole-Wilson PA, Swedberg K, Cleland JG, et al. Comparison of carvedilol and metoprolol on clinical outcomes in patients with chronic heart failure in the Carvedilol Or Metoprolol European Trial (COMET): randomised controlled trial. *Lancet.* 2003;362(9377):7-13.

26. The Cardiac Insufficiency Bisoprolol Study II (CIBIS-II): a randomised trial. *Lancet.* 1999;353(9146):9-13.

27. Gilbert EM, Abraham WT, Olsen S, et al. Comparative hemodynamic, left ventricular functional, and antiadrenergic effects of chronic treatment with metoprolol versus carvedilol in the failing heart. *Circulation.* 1996;94(11):2817-2825.

28. Lowes BD, Gilbert EM, Abraham WT, et al. Myocardial gene expression in dilated cardiomyopathy treated with beta-blocking agents. *N Engl J Med.* 2002;346(18): 1357-1365.

29. Swedberg K, Komajda M, Böhm M, et al. Ivabradine and outcomes in chronic heart failure (SHIFT): a randomised placebo-controlled study. *Lancet.* 2010;376(9744): 875-885.

30. Pitt B. Should chronic heart failure patients with reduced left-ventricular ejection fraction receive angiotensin-receptor blockers? *Nat Clin Pract Cardiovasc Med.* 2005;2(2):70-71.

31. Zannad F, McMurray JJ, Krum H, et al. Eplerenone in patients with systolic heart failure and mild symptoms. *N Engl J Med.* 2011;364(1):11-21.

32. Pitt B, Zannad F, Remme WJ, et al. The effect of spironolactone on morbidity and mortality in patients with severe heart failure. Randomized Aldactone Evaluation Study Investigators. *N Engl J Med.* 1999;341(10):709-717.

33. McMurray JJ, Packer M, Desai AS, et al. Angiotensin-neprilysin inhibition versus enalapril in heart failure. *N Engl J Med.* 2014;371(11):993-1004.

34. Loeb HS, Johnson G, Henrick A, Smith R, Wilson J, Cremo R, Cohn JN. Effect of enalapril, hydralazine plus isosorbide dinitrate, and prazosin on hospitalization in patients with chronic congestive heart failure. The V-HeFT VA Cooperative Studies Group. *Circulation.* 1993;87(6 Suppl):VI78-VI87.

35. Carson P, Ziesche S, Johnson G, Cohn JN. Racial differences in response to therapy for heart failure: analysis of the vasodilator-heart failure trials. Vasodilator-Heart Failure Trial Study Group. *J Card Fail.* 1999;5(3):178-187.

36. Taylor AL, Ziesche S, Yancy C, et al. Combination of isosorbide dinitrate and hydralazine in blacks with heart failure. *N Engl J Med.* 2004;351(20):2049-2057.

37. Kelly RA, Smith TW. Digoxin in heart failure: implications of recent trials. *J Am Coll Cardiol.* 1993;22(4 Suppl A):107A-112A.

38. The Digitalis Investigation Group. The effect of digoxin on mortality and morbidity in patients with heart failure. *N Engl J Med.* 1997;336(8):525-533.

39. Adams KF Jr, Gheorghiade M, Uretsky BF, Patterson JH, Schwartz TA, Young JB. Clinical benefits of low serum digoxin concentrations in heart failure. *J Am Coll Cardiol.* 2002;39(6):946-953.

40. Goldenberg I, Gillespie J, Moss AJ, et al. Long-term benefit of primary prevention with an implantable cardioverter-defibrillator: an extended 8–year follow-up study of the Multicenter Automatic Defibrillator Implantation Trial II. *Circulation.* 2010;122(13):1265-1271.

41. Moss AJ, Zareba W, Hall WJ, Klein H, Wilber DJ, Cannom DS, et al.; Multicenter Automatic Defibrillator Implantation Trial II Investigators. Prophylactic implantation of a defibrillator in patients with myocardial infarction and reduced ejection fraction. *N Engl J Med* 2002;346:877-883.

42. Epstein AE, Dimarco JP, Ellenbogen KA, et al. ACC/AHA/HRS 2008 guidelines for Device-Based Therapy of Cardiac Rhythm Abnormalities: executive summary. *Heart Rhythm.* 2008;5(6):934-955.

43. Bardy GH, Lee KL, Mark DB, et al. Amiodarone or an implantable cardioverter-defibrillator for congestive heart failure. *N Engl J Med.* 2005;352(3):225-237.

44. Werling C, Weisse U, Siemon G, et al. Biventricular pacing in patients with ICD: how many patients are possible candidates? *Thorac Cardiovasc Surg.* 2002;50(2):67-70.

45. Nelson GS, Berger RD, Fetics BJ, Talbot M, Spinelli JC, Hare JM, Kass DA. Left ventricular or biventricular pacing improves cardiac function at diminished energy cost in patients with dilated cardiomyopathy and left bundle-branch block. *Circulation.* 2000;102(25):3053-3059.

46. Bristow MR, Saxon LA, Boehmer J, et al. Cardiac-resynchronization therapy with or without an implantable defibrillator in advanced chronic heart failure. *N Engl J Med.* 2004;350(21):2140-2150.

47. Cleland JG, Daubert JC, Erdmann E, et al. The effect of cardiac resynchronization on morbidity and mortality in heart failure. *N Engl J Med.* 2005;352(15):1539-1549.

48. Moss AJ, Hall WJ, Cannom DS, et al. Cardiac-resynchronization therapy for the prevention of heart-failure events. *N Engl J Med.* 2009;361(14):1329-1338.

49. Schmidt S, Hürlimann D, Starck CT, et al. Treatment with higher dosages of heart failure medication is associated with improved outcome following cardiac resynchronization therapy. *Eur Heart J.* 2014;35(16):1051-1060.

50. Bardy GH, Smith WM, Hood MA, et al. An entirely subcutaneous implantable cardioverter-defibrillator. *N Engl J Med.* 2010;363(1):36-44.

51. Psaty BM, Manolio TA, Kuller LH, et al. Incidence of and risk factors for atrial fibrillation in older adults. *Circulation.* 1997;96(7):2455-2461.

52. Pink J, Pirmohamed M, Hughes DA. Comparative effectiveness of dabigatran, rivaroxaban, apixaban, and warfarin in the management of patients with nonvalvular atrial fibrillation. *Clin Pharmacol Ther.* 2013;94(2):269-276.

53. January CT, Wann LS, Alpert JS, et al. 2014 AHA/ACC/HRS Guideline for the Management of Patients With Atrial Fibrillation: Executive Summary: A Report of the American College of Cardiology/American Heart Association Task Force on Practice Guidelines and the Heart Rhythm Society. *Circulation.* 2014;130(23):2071-2104.

54. Goodman LS, Gilman A, Brunton LL. *Goodman & Gilman's Manual of Pharmacology and Therapeutics.* New York: McGraw-Hill Medical; 2008.

55. Brodsky MA, Allen BJ, Capparelli EV, Luckett CR, Morton R, Henry WL. Factors determining maintenance of sinus rhythm after chronic atrial fibrillation with left atrial dilatation. *Am J Cardiol.* 1989;63(15):1065-1068.

56. Ganesan AN, et al. Role of AV nodal ablation in cardiac resynchronization in patients with coexistent atrial fibrillation and heart failure a systematic review. *J Am Coll Cardiol.* 2012;59(8):719-726.

57. Pitt B, Brooks AG, Roberts-Thomson KC, Lau DH, Kalman JM, Sanders P. Spironolactone for heart failure with preserved ejection fraction. *N Engl J Med.* 2014;370(15):1383-1392.

58. Abraham WT, et al. Wireless pulmonary artery haemodynamic monitoring in chronic heart failure: a randomised controlled trial. *Lancet.* 2011;377(9766):658-666.

59. Boehmer JP/National Institutes of Health. Evaluation of Multisensor Data in Heart Failure Patients With Implanted Devices (MultiSENSE). 2014 [March 10, 2014]; Available from: http://clinicaltrials.gov/ct2/show/NCT01128166.

60. Kastor JA. Michel Mirowski and the automatic implantable defibrillator. *Am J Cardiol.* 1989;63(15):1121-1126.

61. Kastor JA, Moss AJ, Mower MM, Weisfeldt ML. Michel Mirowski: a man with a mission. *Pacing Clin Electrophysiol.* 1991;14(5 Pt 2):864-865.

# CHAPTER 9

# Stage C: Therapies for Acute Decompensated Heart Failure

## FAST FACTS

- The "3 Fs" of heart failure assessment–Fit, Function, and Factors–help to evaluate the heart failure patient at the time of acute decompensation and identify contributing factors.

- Approximately half of patients admitted with decompensated heart failure have an ejection fraction > 40% (HF-pEF).

- Intravenous diuretics, either intermittent or continuous, can be used for acute circulatory congestion.

- Ultrafiltration is an alternate method for treating volume overload in patients with decompensated heart failure, especially in the presence of anasarca.

- Consider intravenous inotropes for acute decompensation of HF-rEF, if diuretic or vasodilator therapy is limited by hypotension or worsening renal function.

- Mechanical devices for circulatory support may be needed for hemodynamic rescue.

*A man "about 60. . . his legs were anasarcous, his belly much swelled, and an evident fluctuation of water. His breathing very bad, an irregular pulse, and unable to lie down. His easiest posture was standing with his body leaning over a chair, in which situation he would continue many hours together, labouring for breath, with the sweat trickling down his face very profusely;*

*the urine in very small quantity. Diuretics of every kind I could think of were used with very little or no advantage."*

—William Withering, 1785[1]

## Applying the "3 Fs" to Decompensated Heart Failure

Decompensated heart failure is an acute, symptomatic, life-threatening event amplified by neurohumoral activation. The same principles of heart failure assessment at initial presentation also apply to acute decompensated heart failure and guide subsequent management:

Fit: Does the presentation fit the diagnosis of decompensated heart failure?

Function: Is systolic or diastolic function abnormal?

Factors: What factors caused the acute decompensation and are any of them treatable?

### FIT

The "fit" with acute decompensated heart failure is supported by history, physical, and chest x-ray findings consistent with congestion or low perfusion. Lab evidence of an elevated natriuretic peptide level can supplement this initial set of findings (see Chapter 2). Vital signs and renal indices help quantitate the severity of the presentation. Oxygen supplementation and assisted ventilation with mask therapies (e.g., BiPAP) can improve hypoxemia. Rarely, respiratory insufficiency requires intubation and mechanical ventilation.

### FUNCTION

Echocardiography, if not recently performed, can assess left and right ventricular systolic and diastolic function and associated echo-Doppler findings. Systolic function can dynamically change and findings treated accordingly (see below). In a multicenter OPTIMIZE-HF registry of 41,267 patients admitted with decompensated heart failure, over half (51.2%) had HF-pEF (EF > 40%). In-hospital mortality was 2.9% for HF-pEF versus 3.9% for HF-rEF.[2]

## FACTORS

Decompensated heart failure with an acute coronary syndrome requires special consideration for early revascularization (Figure 9.1). Myocardial ischemia as a contributing factor is suggested by a history of chest pain, abnormal electrocardiogram, or elevated troponin. There are many other factors (List 9.1), and a comprehensive approach to decompensated heart failure involves assessment of etiologies and precipitating factors while stabilizing hemodynamics and fluid balance. Treating precipitating factors associated with circulatory stress, such as infection, may be important to resolve decompensated findings. Identification of patient noncompliance with diet and medication is also important for subsequent prevention of recurrent decompensation.

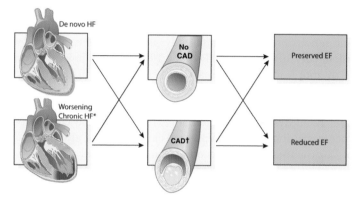

**FIGURE 9.1    The role of coronary artery disease in decompensated heart failure.** The presence or absence of coronary artery disease (**middle panels**) intersects with all four heart failure presentations.(*) Advanced HF is a subset of chronic HF. CAD (†) = coronary artery disease with or without acute coronary syndromes.[3] *Source:* Adapted with permission from Gheorghiade M, Pang PS, *J Am Coll Cardiol.* 2009;53(7):557-573.

**LIST 9.1    Common Factors that Precipitate Hospitalization for Heart Failure**

- Acute myocardial ischemia
- Change in valve function
- Concurrent infections (e.g., pneumonia, viral illnesses)
- Uncorrected high blood pressure
- Atrial fibrillation and other arrhythmias
- Recent addition of negative inotropic drugs (e.g., verapamil, nifedipine, diltiazem, beta-blockers)
- Pulmonary embolus
- Nonsteroidal anti-inflammatory drugs
- Excessive alcohol or illicit drug use
- Endocrine abnormalities (e.g., diabetes mellitus, hyperthyroidism, hypothyroidism)
- Noncompliance with medical regimen, sodium and/or fluid restriction

**SUBSEQUENT MANAGEMENT**

Once the storm of acute decompensation has been calmed, repeat observations of patient status are needed to evaluate the accuracy of initial assessments and efficacy of therapies. Following acute clinical improvement, implementation of evidence-based guidelines improves long-term outcomes (see Chapter 8).

## Hemodynamic Profiles in Decompensated Heart Failure

Two conditions are common in acute heart failure: fluid congestion and tissue hypoperfusion. Congestion arising from elevated pulmonary and systemic venous pressures results in dyspnea, orthopnea, jugular venous distension, edema, and ascites. Hypoperfusion with a low cardiac output occurs in more advanced cases or when patients are intravascularly depleted due to over-diuresis or associated dehydrating illness. Hypoperfusion can contribute to fatigue, dizziness, narrow pulse pressure, and renal dysfunction. Therefore, reversing fluid congestion and, when necessary, increasing a depressed cardiac output are essential components for the treatment of decompensated heart failure states.

Stevenson described 4 resting hemodynamic profiles based on the presence or absence, respectively, of hypoperfusion (Cold or Warm) and/or congestion (Wet or Dry) (Figure 9.2).[4] Classification of patients with decompensated heart failure as Warm and Wet, Cold and Dry, or Cold and Wet, can then guide therapies to return them to Warm and Dry, which represents the "normal baseline" in compensated heart failure. Most patients with congestion are Warm and Wet and can be treated with intravenous diuretics and oral vasodilators. Patients who are Cold and Dry may respond to cautious rehydration, but may become Wet. Patients who are Cold and Wet are more severely ill and often require intravenous (IV) vasodilator or inotropic drug therapy.[4]

Rapid Assesment of Hemodynamic Status

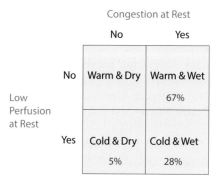

FIGURE 9.2 **Four resting hemodynamic profiles based on congestion and perfusion status used for initial assessment of patients presenting with decompensated heart failure.** The Warm and Dry patient (upper left quadrant) is considered "normal" or stabilized with ongoing treatment for heart failure. Percentage in each category based on patients admitted to Brigham and Women's Hospital with a diagnosis of HF ($n = 452$).[5]

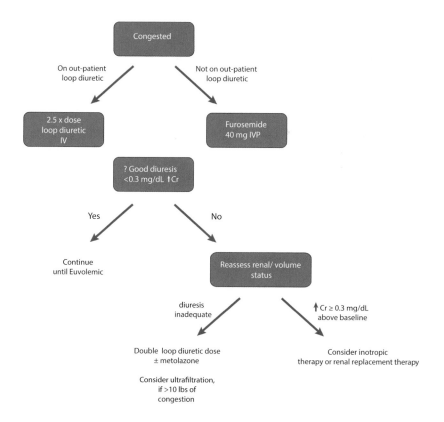

FIGURE 9.3 **A diuretic treatment algorithm for acute decompensated circulatory congestion.**

# Volume Management

The majority of decompensated heart failure patients present with fluid overload and pulmonary congestion provoking acute symptoms. Thus, relief of congestion is essential to the management of decompensated heart failure (Figure 9.3). However, diuretics can have both desirable and undesirable effects (Figure 9.4), so optimal dosing is important.

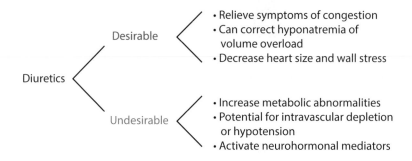

Diuretics

Desirable
- Relieve symptoms of congestion
- Can correct hyponatremia of volume overload
- Decrease heart size and wall stress

Undesirable
- Increase metabolic abnormalities
- Potential for intravascular depletion or hypotension
- Activate neurohormonal mediators

FIGURE 9.4    Effects of diuretics in heart failure.

### DIURETIC OPTIMIZATION STRATEGIES EVALUATION (DOSE) STUDY

In the Diuretic Optimization Strategies Evaluation study, patients with acute decompensated heart failure received intravenous furosemide in a 2 × 2 factorial design: via bolus every 12 hours or continuous infusion; and at low-dose or high-dose therapy (Figure 9.5).[6] Low-dose therapy consisted of a total daily intravenous dose equal to the previous oral dose. High-dose therapy was 2.5 × previous oral dose. From baseline to 72 hours, high-dose furosemide resulted in greater net fluid loss, weight loss, and improvement in dyspnea (Figure 9.5). However, there was no significant difference in the change of serum creatinine between bolus and continuous infusion, or between high- and low-dose diuretics.[6]

Change in Weight (lbs)

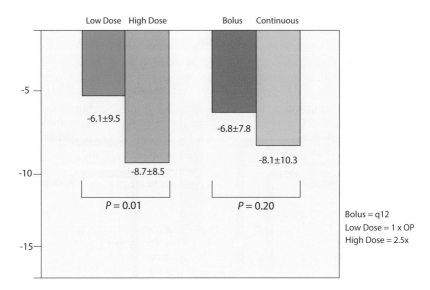

**FIGURE 9.5   Weight loss at 72 hours in the DOSE trial.** High dose (2.5 × outpatient loop-diuretic dose) resulted in greater diuresis. Bolus versus continuous intravenous diuretic administration did not lead to a significant difference in diuresis. OP, outpatient; *n* = 308.[6]
*Source:* Adapted with permission from Felker et al., *N Engl J Med.* 2011;364(9):797-805.

## ULTRAFILTRATION

As heart failure progresses, reduced response to diuretics is common.[7] Although most patients can be treated with diuretics alone, ultrafiltration can also alleviate excess volume and improve diuretic sensitivity (Figure 9.6).[8] Compared with diuretics, ultrafiltration provides a predictable way to achieve euvolemia with minimal electrolyte abnormalities and neuro-humoral activation.[9] However, when renal function is deteriorating, ultrafiltration may contribute to continued worsening of renal function, and in this setting, high-dose intravenous diuretics supplemented by vasoactive therapy may be more appropriate (see Chapter 10).[10]

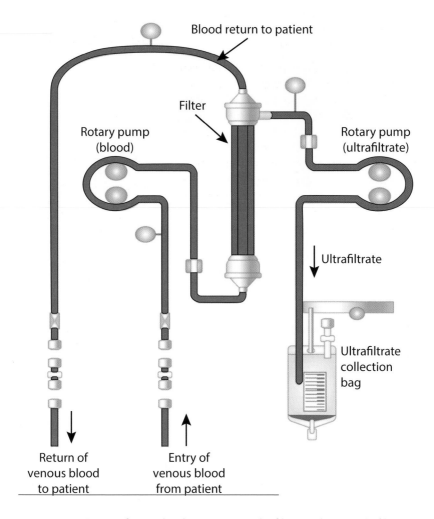

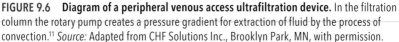

**FIGURE 9.6** **Diagram of a peripheral venous access ultrafiltration device.** In the filtration column the rotary pump creates a pressure gradient for extraction of fluid by the process of convection.[11] *Source:* Adapted from CHF Solutions Inc., Brooklyn Park, MN, with permission.

Vascular access may be from peripheral or central venous catheters. Hematocrit, electrolytes, BUN, and creatinine are monitored every 12–24 hours. To gain predictability of fluid loss and reduce electrolyte abnormalities, loop diuretics can be withheld on days when a patient is receiving ultrafiltration. A nephrology consultation should be considered for patients with marked renal impairment (serum creatinine ≥3.0 mg/dL), as dialysis may be a better option to correct volume overload and metabolic abnormalities in these patients.

### Effects of Ultrafiltration on Fluid Loss, Electrolyte Balance, and Neurohormonal Activation

Costanzo et al. in the UNLOAD trial observed both greater weight loss and net fluid loss over a 48-hour period with ultrafiltration compared to standard intravenous loop diuretic treatment (Figure 9.7).[12] Patients had at least 2 physical findings of fluid congestion and a creatinine less than 3.0 mg/dL. Ninety-day rehospitalization for heart failure, a secondary trial endpoint, was reduced by 50% in the ultrafiltration group.

**ULTRAFILTRATION MAY BE BENEFICIAL IN THE FOLLOWING SITUATIONS:**
- Marked volume overload, including patients with anasarca
- Patients with decompensated heart failure and stable reduced renal function with creatinine < 3.0 mg/dL, including significant right ventricular dysfunction
- Patients with fluid retention symptoms refractory to intravenous diuretics

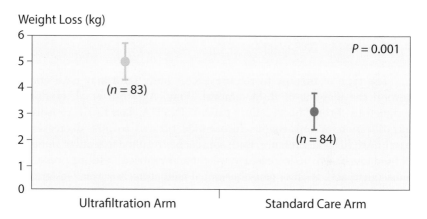

**Weight Loss (kg)**

FIGURE 9.7 **Weight loss with ultrafiltration.** Mean weight loss at 48 hours with ultrafiltration vs. standard care in patients with decompensated heart failure. Weight loss with ultrafiltration was 5.0 ± 0.68 kg vs. standard care 3.1 ± 0.75 kg. Error bars indicate 95% confidence intervals (CIs).[12] *Source:* Adapted with permission from Costanzo et al., *J Am Coll Cardiol.* 2007;49(6):675-683.

Ali et al. measured the amount of the electrolytes sodium, potassium, and magnesium in loop diuretic induced urine versus ultrafiltrate in patients with heart failure. Per unit volume, ultrafiltration removed a significantly greater amount of sodium, while reducing the loss of potassium and magnesium (Figure 9.8).[13] This difference accounts for a lower incidence of hypokalemia in patients treated with ultrafiltration compared with intravenous diuretics.[12]

Urine vs. UF Electrolytes (mg/dL)

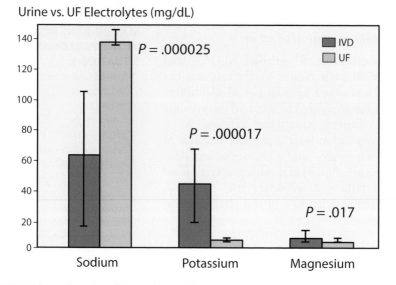

FIGURE 9.8   **Electrolyte shifts with ultrafiltration (UF) or with intravenous loop diuretics (IVD).** UF removed significantly more sodium and less potassium and magnesium per deciliter (dL) versus loop diuretic–promoted urine (IVD).[13] *Source:* Adapted with permission from Ali et al., *Congest Heart Fail.* 2009;15(1):1-4.

The type of therapy to remove excess body fluid may have effects beyond the amount of fluid removal alone. Agostoni et al. randomly assigned 16 chronic heart failure patients (NYHA class II–III) to isolated ultrafiltration or intravenous furosemide titrated to 50% decreases in baseline right atrial pressure. Both approaches resulted in similar amounts of fluid loss based on decreases in weight and ventricular filling pressures. Subsequent activation of neurohormonal mediators, however, was greater in the furosemide compared to the ultrafiltration group. Over 3 months, those who received ultrafiltration maintained a reduced body weight, compared to those who received intravenous furosemide (Figure 9.9).[9]

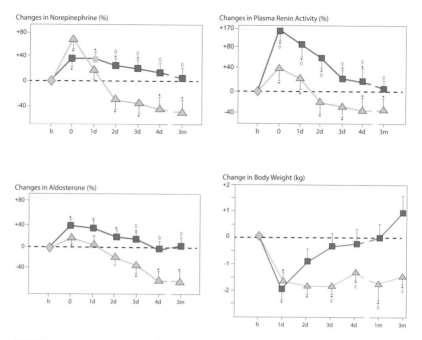

**FIGURE 9.9** Percent changes of circulating levels of norepinephrine, plasma renin activity, and aldosterone (%) and body weight (kg) following one 8-hour ultrafiltration, (*n* = 8) or intravenous furosemide (*n* = 8) treatment resulting in 50% reductions in right atrial pressure and then followed for 3 months. *Symbols:* Blue squares, IV furosemide; gold triangles, ultrafiltration. Timepoints on X axis: b, baseline (first and only day of treatment); 0, immediately after ultrafiltration or furosemide treatment; d, days; m, months. Statistical symbols: * $P < 0.01$ vs. baseline, ◊ $P < 0.01$ vs. other therapy.[9] *Source:* Adapted with permission from Agostoni et al., *Am J Med.* 1994;96(3):191-199.

## Intravenous Vasoactive Drug Therapy and Acute Heart Failure

Compared to a normal individual, the patient with compensated heart failure has a reduced cardiac reserve for responding to circulatory stressors such as fluid overload, infection, ischemia, or arrhythmia. To treat a decompensated patient with worsening heart failure, short-term intravenous vasoactive therapy may be required. Drugs with vasodilator or positive myocardial inotropic effects can reduce ventricular filling pressures and increase cardiac output beyond the effects from endogenous catecholamines alone. Temporary augmentation of myocardial function may avoid a downhill spiral of respiratory failure, progressive multiorgan dysfunction, and death while the reversible causes of cardiac decompensation are treated. Nevertheless, vasodilator/inotropic therapy should be used cautiously, as it may promote other adverse cardiac events, including arrhythmias, hypotension, and renal dysfunction.[14,15]

## NITRATES AND NITROPRUSSIDE (VASODILATORS)

Similar to oral nitrates, intravenous vasodilator therapy with nitric oxide donors, nitroprusside or nitroglycerin, can improve circulatory function by reducing preload and afterload without direct effect on myocardial contractility.[16]

Both agents act through increased production of nitric oxide. Nitroprusside generates nitric oxide spontaneously whereas nitroglycerin requires free sulfhydryl groups from the cellular biochemical environment. Nitric oxide activates a soluble guanylate cyclase which catalyses the formation of cyclic guanosine monophosphate (cGMP) from guanosine triphosphate (GTP). Once formed, cGMP acts as an intracellular secondary messenger to decrease intracellular calcium and vascular smooth muscle tone.[17]

Nitroprusside has a "balanced" action on dilating both arteries and veins. Nitroglycerin's action is primarily venodilation. Nevertheless, both lead to decreases in mean arterial and venous pressures.[18] Nitroglycerin is less likely to shunt blood flow from ischemic myocardium and is preferable in acute myocardial ischemia syndromes, such as heart failure with angina pectoris or myocardial infarction (MI).[19]

Gaseous nitric oxide acting as a pulmonary vasodilator can be administered as inhaled therapy for the treatment of right heart failure in the setting of increased pulmonary vascular resistance and reduced left ventricular filling pressures. This is generally done in patients receiving mechanical ventilation.

## NESIRITIDE (VASODILATOR/DIURETIC)

Nesiritide is an intravenous form of the naturally occurring B-type natriuretic peptide. As such, it has balanced venous and arterial vasodilator properties, in addition to mild renal diuretic effects.

In patients with decompensated heart failure, 3 hours after initiation of therapy, nesiritide compared to intravenous nitroglycerin (median dose 13 mcg/min) was found to have a greater effect to reduce pulmonary capillary wedge pressure and symptoms of dyspnea (Figure 9.10).[20] In patients undergoing open-heart surgery, use of nesiritide compared to placebo was associated with less renal dysfunction, a reduced length of stay, and a lower mortality.[21]

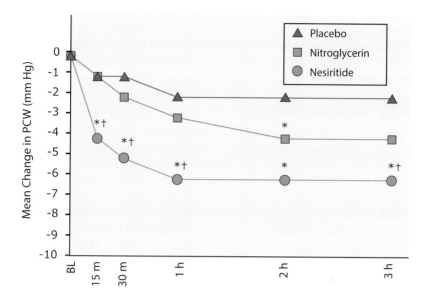

**FIGURE 9.10   Comparison of Nesiritide and IV Nitroglycerin.** Changes from baseline of pulmonary capillary wedge pressure following placebo, intravenous nitroglycerin, or nesiritide. Asterisk (*) indicates $P < 0.05$ for nesiritide or nitroglycerin compared with placebo. Dagger (†) indicates $P < 0.05$ for nesiritide compared with nitroglycerin.[20] *Source:* Adapted with permission from *JAMA.* 2002;287(12):1531-1540.

A retrospective meta-analysis of trials using nesiritide in acute heart failure, however, suggested that renal function could be impaired with nesiritide.[15] Subsequently, a large, 7000-patient trial, ASCEND–HF, did not find an increase in serum creatinine or 30-day mortality compared to placebo.[22] A trend to improve dyspnea with the drug did not reach statistical significance in this trial.

When nesiritide is used, the risk of hypotension and associated worsening renal function may be reduced by avoiding doses greater than 0.01 mcg/kg/min, or by omitting a bolus initiation dose.

## MILRINONE (INOTROPE/VASODILATOR)

The phosphodiesterase inhibitor, milrinone, acts to increase intracellular cAMP in both heart and vascular smooth muscle cells by blocking its catabolism. This results in both increased cardiac contractility and vasodilatation, which together are effective at reducing elevated left- and right-heart filling pressures and increasing cardiac output in patients with HF-rEF.[16] Unlike other

**MILRINONE**
- Phosphodiesterase III inhibitor
- Increase intracellular cAMP in both heart and vascular muscle
- Results in increased cardiac contractility and vasodilation

intravenous agents used in acute heart failure syndromes, milrinone has a longer biologic half-life of 2–3 hours that is prolonged further with renal insufficiency.[23] Because of this, milrinone requires a loading dose to have a rapid onset of action. When stopped, it will persist for hours within the circulation.

## DOBUTAMINE (INOTROPE)

Dobutamine is a $\beta_1$ adrenergic receptor agonist resulting in increased myocyte cAMP and cardiac contractility. As a moderate $\beta_2$-agonist, it will result in modest vascular smooth muscle vasodilatation. Dobutamine is a racemic compound, existing as equal amounts of two optical isomers with the same chemical structure. One isomer acts as a mild α-agonist and the other acts as a mild α-antagonist. These two α effects tend to yield a net mild vasodilation.[24] Thus, dobutamine is a positive inotropic medication that increases cardiac output with minimal change in blood pressure and moderately decreases venous filling pressures. In an individual patient, however, its effects on blood pressure might be variable in part, depending on the level of activation of the patient's α-receptors by endogenous sympathetic norepinephrine prior to using the drug.

**DOBUTAMINE**

- Potent $\beta_1$ adrenergic receptor agonist resulting in increased heart c-AMP
- Mild $\beta_2$-agonist
- 50:50 mixture of mild α-agonist and antagonist isomers

## DOPAMINE (INOTROPE/VASOCONSTRICTOR)

Dopamine has multiple dose-dependent mechanisms of action.[25] At low doses (< 3 mcg/kg/min), it acts on renovascular dopaminergic receptors to increase renal blood flow and may have a diuretic effect. At moderate doses (3–5 mcg/kg/min), dopamine activates dopaminergic and β-adrenergic receptors, and so is also a positive inotrope. At higher doses (> 5 mcg/kg/min), it acts as a potent arterial and venous vasoconstrictor via release of endogenous preformed stores of norepinephrine from presynaptic sympathetic nerve terminals,[26] a pharmacologic "tyramine-like" effect. In advanced hypotensive chronic heart failure patients, who may have depleted endogenous stores of norepinephrine, adding intravenous pharmacologic norepinephrine (Levophed®) directly (instead of using higher doses of dopamine) can help maintain an adequate systemic blood pressure. The need for dopamine (or norepinephrine) in a patient with decompensated heart failure can signal the presence of coexisting infection.

# Comparative Hemodynamic Effects of Intravenous Medications

Most of the vasoactive intravenous medications used in heart failure have more than one mode of action. Thus, it becomes important to understand the multiplicity of effects so that combination therapy results in added benefit and effects do not cancel each other.

## NITROPRUSSIDE VS. MILRINONE

Milrinone, but not nitroprusside, increases cardiac contractility as measured by peak rate of rise of left ventricular pressure during isovolumic systole (peak +dp/dt). As vasodilators, both nitroprusside and milrinone decrease mean aortic and left ventricular end-diastolic pressures. At individually matched mean aortic pressures, however, greater increases in stroke work index and falls in left ventricular filling pressure are achieved with milrinone compared to nitroprusside (Figure 9.11).

**DOPAMINE**
- Dopaminergic and β-agonist at low to moderate doses
- At high dose (> 5 mcg/kg/min), α-agonist secondary to release of endogenous pre-synaptic norepinephrine

**STROKE WORK**
- Stroke Work = Stroke volume × (Mean Arterial Pressure – Ventricular End Ventricular Diastolic Pressure)
- Stroke Work Index: [g × m/m$^2$] refers to the concept of the work of ejection expressed as Units of Energy/BSA. It relates to the area within a ventricular pressure – volume loop.

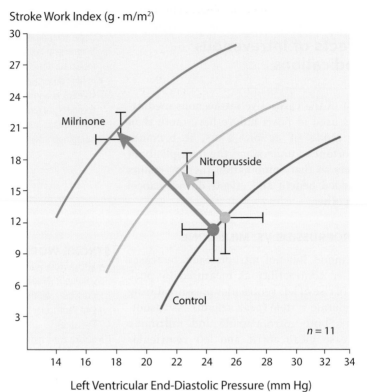

**FIGURE 9.11 Effects of intravenous nitroprusside and milrinone on LV performance (Stroke Work Index).** Graphic display of changes in stroke work index and left ventricular end-diastolic pressure at doses of medications that resulted in matched decreases in mean aortic pressure (the other variable of therapy). Colored lines show shifts in Frank-Starling type curves.[16] *Source:* Adapted with permission from Jaski et al., *J Clin Invest.* 1985;75(2):643-649.

Alternatively, the inotropic vasodilator effect of milrinone blunts decreases in mean arterial pressure compared to a pure vasodilator effect alone. When milrinone and nitroprusside are compared at doses that produce the same increase in cardiac index (approximately 50%), decreases in left-heart filling pressures are similar (Figure 9.12); however, mean arterial pressure is relatively preserved with milrinone.[16]

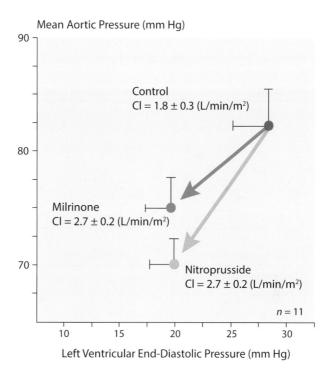

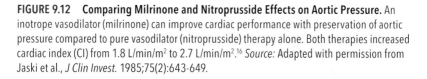

**FIGURE 9.12    Comparing Milrinone and Nitroprusside Effects on Aortic Pressure.** An inotrope vasodilator (milrinone) can improve cardiac performance with preservation of aortic pressure compared to pure vasodilator (nitroprusside) therapy alone. Both therapies increased cardiac index (CI) from 1.8 L/min/m² to 2.7 L/min/m².[16] *Source:* Adapted with permission from Jaski et al., *J Clin Invest.* 1985;75(2):643-649.

## DOBUTAMINE VS. MILRINONE

Dobutamine and milrinone are both positive inotropes with vasodilator effects. Yet, there are important differences between these agents in hemodynamic indices of heart rate, stroke volume, LV filling pressure, mean arterial pressure, contractility (peak +dp/dt), and systemic vascular resistance (Figure 9.13).[27] At peak doses, both dobutamine and milrinone increase heart rate approximately 10 bpm and stroke volume 50%. Left ventricular filling pressure falls modestly with dobutamine, but more with milrinone (dobutamine −29%; milrinone −46%). Mean arterial pressure remains unchanged with dobutamine, but decreases about 10 mm Hg with milrinone. Systemic vascular resistance falls more with milrinone (dobutamine −29%; milrinone −51%). Left ventricular contractility (peak +dp/dt) increases with both drugs, but more with dobutamine (dobutamine +50%; milrinone +30%). In summary, at high doses, dobutamine is a more potent inotrope, and milrinone a more potent vasodilator (Figure 9.14).[27] These agents also have different effects on myocardial oxygen consumption, which is increased by dobutamine, but not by milrinone (Figure 9.15).[28]

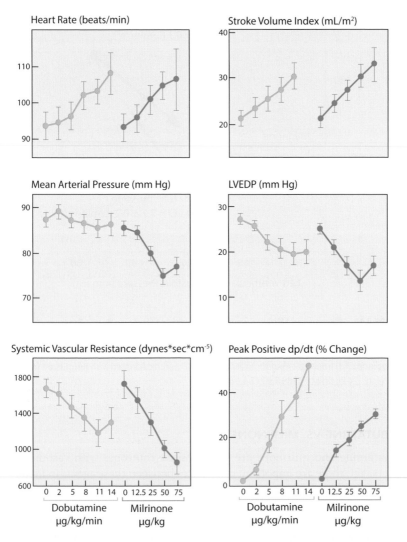

**FIGURE 9.13    Intravenous dobutamine compared to milrinone (n = 15).** Middle and lower panels show where the greatest differences are present. At high doses, dobutamine leads to greater increases in contractility (peak +dp/dt). Milrinone leads to greater decreases in left ventricular end-diastolic pressure (LVEDP) and afterload (systemic vascular resistance) (see text).[27] *Source:* Adapted with permission from Colucci et al., *Circulation.* 1986;73(3 Pt 2):III175-III183.

## Contractility

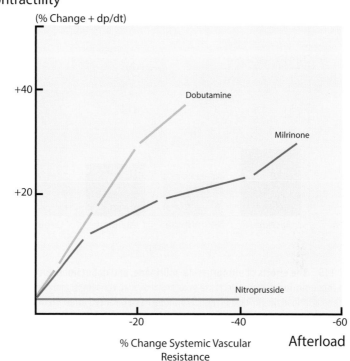

FIGURE 9.14 **Changes in contractility versus afterload seen with nitroprusside, milrinone, and dobutamine.** Contractility (shown on the vertical axis as the percent change in +dp/dt) and afterload (shown on the horizontal axis as percent change in systemic vascular resistance). Nitroprusside has no effect on contractility but acts as a potent vasodilator (decreased systemic vascular resistance). Milrinone leads to the greatest fall in calculated systemic vascular resistance with an intermediate effect on increasing myocardial contractility. Finally, high dose dobutamine has the greatest effect on contractility with some vasodilator properties.[27] *Source:* Adapted with permission from Colucci et al., *Circulation.* 1986;73(3 Pt 2):III175-III183.

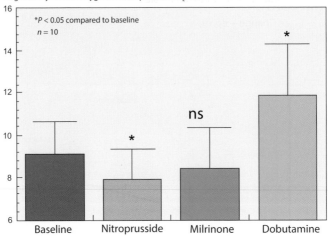

Regional Myocardial Oxygen Consumption (mL O$_2$/min)

**FIGURE 9.15    The effects of nitroprusside, milrinone, and dobutamine on myocardial oxygen consumption.** Nitrates decrease myocardial oxygen consumption by decreasing preload and afterload due to vasodilation. Milrinone has a balanced effect on myocardial oxygen consumption acting as a vasodilator (similar to nitrates) offset by increases in contractility. Dobutamine will increase contractility and lead to a moderate increase in myocardial oxygen consumption.[28] *Source:* Adapted with permission from Monrad et al., *Circulation.* 1986;73(3 Pt 2): III168-III174.

## DOPAMINE VS. DOBUTAMINE

The metabolic cost of using dopamine to increase blood pressure and cardiac output is an increase in myocardial oxygen consumption due to increases in contractility and systemic vascular resistance.[29] When dopamine and dobutamine are compared, dobutamine yields a greater increase in cardiac index at a lower cost of increased myocardial oxygen consumption (the heart rate × systolic blood pressure product can be used as a surrogate for myocardial oxygen consumption) (Figure 9.16, Panel A). Dopamine also results in a greater increase in premature ventricular contractions (Figure 9.16, Panel B).

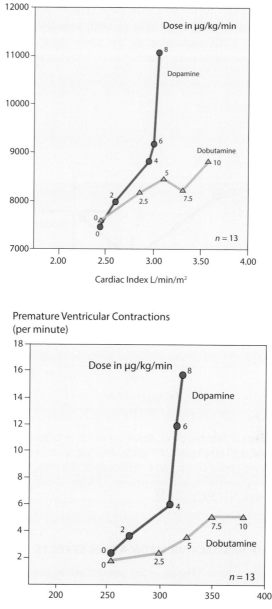

**FIGURE 9.16** **(Panel A) The impact of dopamine and dobutamine on myocardial oxygen consumption.** The product of heart rate and systolic blood pressure on the y axis is an indicator of myocardial oxygen consumption. (**Panel B**) Premature ventricular contractions associated with dopamine and dobutamine.[29] *Source:* Adapted with permission Leier et al., *Circulation.* 1978;58(3 Pt 1):466-475.

Dopamine and dobutamine have opposite effects on left ventricular filling pressure at the 10 mcg/kg/min dose (Figure 9.17).[30] Filling pressures decrease with dobutamine due to both vasodilation and positive inotropic effects. With dopamine at the same dose, vasoconstriction mechanisms predominate over positive inotropic effects, and filling pressures increase.[30]

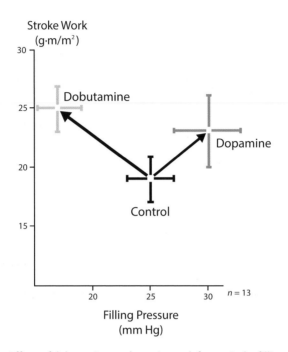

**FIGURE 9.17    Effects of dobutamine vs. dopamine on left ventricular filling pressure. Both drugs infused at 10 mcg/kg/min.** A Frank-Starling type curve showing changes in stroke work versus ventricular filling pressure. At these doses, dopamine vasoconstriction predominates and increases left heart filling pressure.[30] *Source:* Adapted with permission from Loeb et al., *Circulation.* 1977;55(2):375-378.

## COMPARATIVE VASOACTIVE MEDICATION EFFECTS

A Frank-Starling curve (Figure 9.18) presentation can depict expected changes in cardiac output versus filling pressures with specific pharmacologic interventions. Medications that increase contractility or decrease afterload will lead to an upward shift in the curve, whereas those that increase afterload will lead to a downward shift in the Frank-Starling curve. For example, pure vasoconstrictors like phenylephrine increase blood pressure, but also increase filling pressure and decrease cardiac output. Diuretics without direct cardiac or vascular actions will reduce filling pressures while staying on the same Frank-Starling curve.

## Cardiac Output

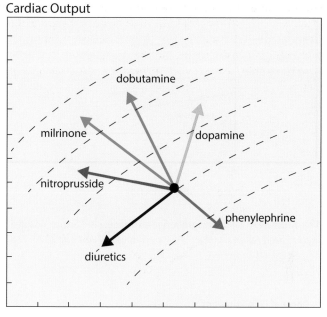

## Filling Pressures

**FIGURE 9.18** **Frank-Starling curves demonstrating the effects of intravenous medications on left ventricular performance.**[31] *Source:* Adapted from Jaski BE, *Basics of Heart Failure.* Springer Science + Business Media B.V.; 2000: 222, with permission.

### *The Acute Heart Failure Diagram*

An approach to IV pharmacologic therapy in patients with decompensated heart failure and HF-rEF can be displayed graphically (Figure 9.19). On the vertical axis is an index of left ventricular afterload–systolic blood pressure. On the horizontal axis is an index of left ventricular preload–pulmonary capillary wedge pressure (PCWP). Left-heart filling pressures can be estimated based on clinical or echocardiographic criteria or measured with a Swan-Ganz catheter, if needed. An initial pharmacologic approach is indicated in each sector demarcated by lines at different levels of systolic blood pressure. For example, if PCWP is > 18 mm Hg but systolic blood pressure (SBP) is < 80 mm Hg, then dopamine is the drug of choice. If blood pressure is normal or high, pure vasodilator therapy (nitrate/nesiritide) is usually effective. Dobutamine and milrinone are suitable in intermediate sectors. The doses of IV medications for heart failure are summarized in Table 9.1.

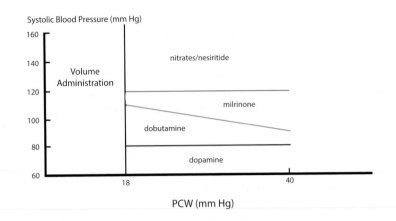

**FIGURE 9.19  Acute heart failure diagram.** See text for details.[31] *Source:* Adapted from Jaski BE, *Basics of Heart Failure.* Springer Science + Business Media B.V.; 2000: 225, with permission.

**TABLE 9.1    Doses of IV medications.**[31]

| AGENT | DOSE | MAJOR HEMODYNAMIC EFFECTS |
|---|---|---|
| Nitroprusside | 10–400 mcg/min | Vasodilation |
| Nitroglycerin | 10–400 mcg/min | Vasodilation |
| Nesiritide | 0.005–0.01 mcg/kg/min | Vasodilation |
| Milrinone | 50 mcg/kg over 10 min | Inotrope, Vasodilation |
|  | 0.25–0.75 mcg/kg/min |  |
| Dobutamine | 2–14 mcg/kg/min | Inotrope, Vasodilation |
| Dopamine | 1–3 mcg/kg/min | Inotrope, Vasodilation; |
|  | 3–20 mcg/kg/min | Inotrope, Vasoconstriction |
| Norepinephrine/epinephrine | 0.5–20 mcg/min | Inotrope, Vasoconstriction |
| Phenylephrine | 10–100 mcg/min | Vasoconstriction |

# Mechanical Circulatory Support

When acute heart failure results in hemodynamic compromise, neuro-hormonal inotropic stimulation (endogenous or exogenous) can improve heart function. However, the increase in cardiac contractility also incurs the risk of myocardial ischemia. Mechanical assist devices supplement myocardial contractility reserve with hydraulic energy derived from external sources. Mechanical assistance increases total circulatory power to allow the maintenance of adequate tissue perfusion, while at the same time reducing the utilization of cardiac energy stores and thus increasing the available reserve (Figure 9.20). Compared to pharmacologic therapy, technical expertise and caution are needed to minimize the risk of complications associated with placing intravascular devices.

Circulatory Power (energy/time)

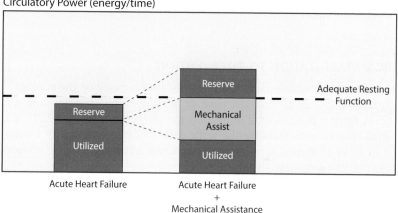

FIGURE 9.20 **Hemodynamics of mechanical circulatory assistance.** Mechanical assist maintains adequate resting function and restores a measure of myocardial reserve.[31] *Source:* Adapted from Jaski BE, *Basics of Heart Failure.* Springer Science + Business Media B.V.; 2000: 233, with permission.

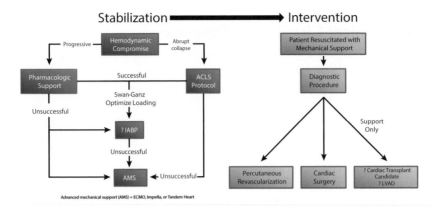

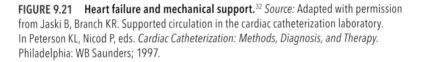

**FIGURE 9.21** **Heart failure and mechanical support.**[32] *Source:* Adapted with permission from Jaski B, Branch KR. Supported circulation in the cardiac catheterization laboratory. In Peterson KL, Nicod P, eds. *Cardiac Catheterization: Methods, Diagnosis, and Therapy.* Philadelphia: WB Saunders; 1997.

## FROM STABILIZATION TO INTERVENTION

The need for mechanical circulatory assistance is based on the etiology of cardiac failure as well as the pace of hemodynamic deterioration and moves from a process of stabilization to intervention (Figure 9.21). The initial treatment to stabilize the acute patient is conventional IV therapy or, in cases of abrupt cardiovascular collapse, advanced cardiac life support (ACLS) protocols are appropriate.[33]

There are several clinical factors to consider in caring for the patient with hemodynamic compromise. Intravascular depletion should be considered initially in any patient with severe hemodynamic compromise. Hemodynamic stabilization may include insertion of an intra-aortic balloon pump or advanced mechanical support (Figure 9.22). Stabilization can permit diagnostic procedures and intracoronary therapeutic interventions to be performed more safely.[34]

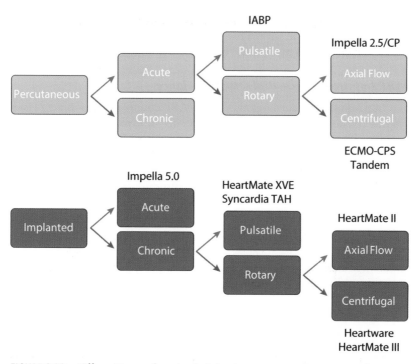

**FIGURE 9.22    Different types of mechanical circulatory support.** Percutaneous devices are for acute support, whereas surgically implanted may be for acute or chronic support. IABP, intra-aortic balloon pump; TAH, total artificial heart; ECMO, extracorporeal mechanical oxygenation; CPS, cardiopulmonary support.

### INTRA-AORTIC BALLOON PUMP (IABP)

Intra-aortic balloon counterpulsation may be indicated in patients with acute decompensated heart failure despite intravenous vasoactive therapy, especially in patients with MI and cardiogenic shock.[35] Percutaneous advanced mechanical support may be an option for the patient refractory to intra-aortic balloon pump (IABP).[36]

> **INTRA-AORTIC BALLOON PUMP**
> An intravascular balloon that is inflated and deflated in the descending thoracic aorta from a percutaneous catheter in the femoral artery that supports the systemic and coronary circulations.

### *Mechanics of IABP Support*

Timed with cardiac diastole, IABP inflation displaces blood volume within the aorta to increase total systemic and myocardial blood flow. During IABP support, diastolic blood pressure typically exceeds systolic blood pressure. This increased coronary perfusion pressure during diastole improves myocardial oxygen delivery when coronary vascular impedance to flow is low compared to systole. Deflation of the balloon during cardiac systole reduces volume within the aorta and, therefore, decreases left ventricular afterload and myocardial oxygen consumption.

### IABP Improves Myocardial Oxygen Balance

In patients with cardiogenic shock, IABP counterpulsation decreases systolic tension–time index (TTI), a measure of myocardial oxygen consumption, and augments diastolic pressure–time index (DPTI), an index of the coronary perfusion gradient (DPTI–LVDP) (Figure 9.23). This decrease in myocardial oxygen consumption and increase in coronary perfusion can improve left ventricular dysfunction associated with myocardial ischemia.[37–39]

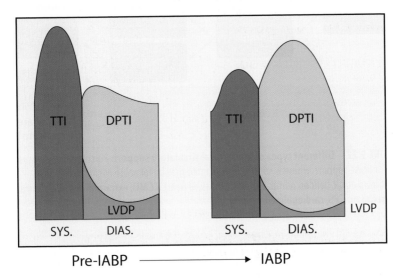

**FIGURE 9.23  IABP support improves left ventricular dysfunction associated with myocardial ischemia.** IABP decreases myocardial oxygen consumption (represented by TTI) and increases coronary perfusion (represented by DPTI). Abbreviations: IABP, intra-aortic balloon pump counterpulsation; LVDP, left ventricular diastolic pressure; SYS, systolic; DIAS, diastolic; TTI, tension–time index; DPTI, diastolic pressure–time index. See text for discussion.[40] Source: Adapted with permission from Hanlon-Pena PM, Quaal SJ, *Am J Crit Care.* 2011;20(4):323-333.

### IABP for Cardiogenic Shock with Myocardial Infarction and Early Revascularization

Traditionally, cardiogenic shock associated with myocardial infarction has been treated with IABP either immediately before or after percutaneous revascularization. The results of the IABP-SHOCK II trial, however, have challenged this approach. In 598 randomized patients with acute myocardial infarction and cardiogenic shock undergoing attempted early revascularization, routine use of an IABP (86.6% placed following revascularization) did not have a significant effect on 30-day mortality (39.7% in the IABP group and 41.3% in the control group; $P$ = NS). Patients had a median ejection fraction of 35%, and IV catecholamines were used in 90% of both groups. It is uncertain if these results would apply to patients not considered eligible for randomization. Application of more robust mechanical circulatory support devices (see below) could impact the high mortality in both groups.[41]

## ADVANCED PERCUTANEOUS MECHANICAL SUPPORT

Recent years have seen the development of more advanced mechanical support devices that are still inserted via peripheral access (Table 9.2).

### INDICATIONS FOR IABP AND HEART FAILURE
- Cardiogenic shock despite inotropic therapy
- Acute MI complicated by mitral regurgitation or ventricular septal defect
- Acute myocarditis associated with cardiogenic shock
- Bridge to transplant

### RELATIVE OR ABSOLUTE CONTRAINDICATIONS TO IABP USE
- Aortic dissection or aneurysm
- Severe aortic valve regurgitation
- Obstructive peripheral vascular disease
- Little or no native cardiac output (consider advanced mechanical support)

TABLE 9.2   Advanced percutaneous mechanical support devices.

| DEVICE AND PERCUTANEOUS ACCESS POINTS | CIRCULATORY SUPPORT | BIV SUPPORT | COST |
|---|---|---|---|
| **IABP:** Counterpulsation in the descending thoracic and abdominal aorta. | + | No | $ |
| **Impella 2.5/CP:** Continuous flow from the LV to the ascending aorta with an axial pump placed across the AV. | ++ | No | $$$ |
| **Tandem Heart:** Continuous flow from the left atria (via transseptal approach) to the iliac artery with external centrifugal pump. | +++ | No | $$$ |
| **Percutaneous Extra Corporeal Membrane Oxygenation (ECMO):** Continuous flow from central systemic veins/RA to iliac artery with external centrifugal pump and oxygenator. | +++ | Yes | $$ |

BiV, biventricular.

Seyfarth et al. compared the safety and efficacy of circulatory support between the Impella 2.5 (Figure 9.24) and the traditional IABP in patients with myocardial infarction placed following percutaneous revascularization with a mean baseline cardiac index of 1.7 L/min/m$^2$ in both groups. Within the group that received Impella 2.5, cardiac index improved by 0.49 L/min/m$^2$, compared to only a 0.11 L/min/m$^2$ increase in the group that received IABP support.[43] A more recently released Impella CP percutaneous pump may provide up to a 4 L/min cardiac output support.

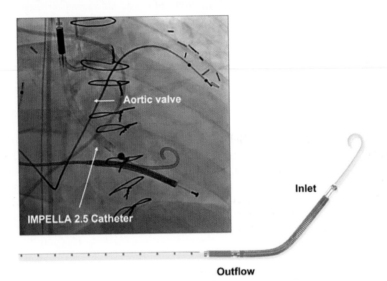

**Outflow**

FIGURE 9.24    **Impella 2.5 positioned across the aortic valve.** Also present are ICD/pacemaker leads in the right ventricle and through the coronary sinus to the left ventricle.[42] *Source:* Adapted with permission from Dixon et al., *JACC Cardiovasc Interv.* 2009;2(2):91-96.

## FULMINANT MYOCARDITIS TREATED WITH ECMO

Fulminant myocarditis (FM) is an uncommon but potentially fatal condition most commonly of viral origin characterized by widespread myocardial inflammation leading to severe decompensated heart failure or cardiogenic shock.[44] Rapidly progressive biventricular dysfunction or malignant arrhythmias can precipitate sudden circulatory collapse or progressive multisystem organ failure.[45] Publications from large series report mortality up to 58%.[46] In some cases, the severity of myocardial stunning and associated hemodynamic compromise render conventional therapies, including inotropes and intra-aortic balloon counterpulsation (IABP), ineffective. Mechanical circulatory support including percutaneous cardiopulmonary support via extracorporeal membrane oxygenation (ECMO)[47] or left ventricular assist device (LVAD) implantation can serve as a bridge to recovery (Figures 9.25, 9.26).[48] Remarkably, if patients survive the acute phase of the illness, long-term prognosis is excellent.[49]

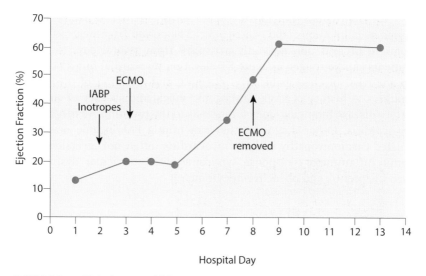

**FIGURE 9.25    Clinical course of fulminant myocarditis secondary to Echovirus 30 (determined with convalescent titers).** A previously healthy, 26-year-old male presented with a 2-day history of pleuritic chest pain, dyspnea, hypotension, fevers, and nonproductive cough. Initial left ventricular ejection fraction by echocardiography was 12%. Coronary angiography showed normal coronary arteries. Patient was treated with IABP and ECMO. Ejection fraction and complete clinical recovery was manifest over 2 weeks.[50] *Source:* Adapted with permission from Nayak KR, Jaski BE, *J Invasive Cardiol.* 2006;18(9):E253-E255.

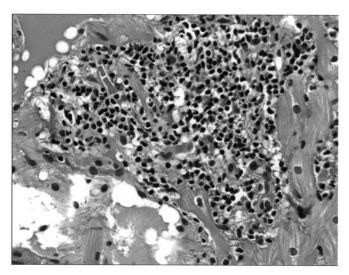

**FIGURE 9.26    Right ventricular biopsy from the patient described in Figure 9.25** showing widespread mononuclear cell infiltrates with myocytolysis without the presence of viral inclusion bodies, eosinophils, or giant cells.[50] *Source:* Adapted with permission from Nayak KR, Jaski BE, *J Invasive Cardiol.* 2006;18(9):E253-E255.

Clinical manifestations that occur with FM include fatigue, fever, dyspnea, palpitations, and chest pain.[44] The period from onset of symptoms to presentation generally may vary from several days to weeks. Patients can be triaged as acute ST-elevation myocardial infarctions due to the triad of chest pain, ECG changes, and elevation of myocardial markers. A history of fever, cardiogenic shock, and absence of coronary artery disease by angiography often leads to the presumptive diagnosis of myocarditis. Other diagnoses that can mimic FM include new-onset dilated cardiomyopathy without myocarditis (often not reversible), systemic inflammatory response syndrome with ventricular dysfunction (see Chapter 6), and pheochromocytoma.

# References

1. Withering W. An account of the foxglove, and some of its medical uses with practical remarks on dropsy, and other diseases. London: M Swinney for GGJ and J Robinson; 1785.

2. Fonarow GC, Gattis Stough W, Abraham WT, et al. Characteristics, treatments, and outcomes of patients with preserved systolic function hospitalized for heart failure: a report from the OPTIMIZE-HF Registry. *J Am Coll Cardiol.* 2007;50(8):768-777.

3. Gheorghiade M, Pang PS. Acute heart failure syndromes. *J Am Coll Cardiol.* 2009;53(7):557–573.

4. Stevenson LW. Tailored therapy to hemodynamic goals for advanced heart failure. *Eur J Heart Fail.* 1999;1(3):251-257.

5. Nohria A, Tsang SW, Fang JC, et al. Clinical assessment identifies hemodynamic profiles that predict outcomes in patients admitted with heart failure. *J Am Coll Cardiol.* 2003;41(10):1797-1804.

6. Felker GM, Lee KL, Bull DA, et al. Diuretic strategies in patients with acute decompensated heart failure. *N Engl J Med.* 2011;364(9):797-805.

7. Brater DC. Diuretic therapy. *N Engl J Med.* 1998;339(6):387-395.

8. Costanzo MR, Saltzburg M, O'Sullivan J, Sobotka P. Early ultrafiltration in patients with decompensated heart failure and diuretic resistance. *J Am Coll Cardiol.* 2005;46(11):2047-2051.

9. Agostoni P, Marenzi G, Lauri G, et al. Sustained improvement in functional capacity after removal of body fluid with isolated ultrafiltration in chronic cardiac insufficiency: failure of furosemide to provide the same result. *Am J Med.* 1994;96(3):191-199.

10. Bart BA, Goldsmith SR, Lee KL, et al. Cardiorenal Rescue Study in Acute Decompensated Heart Failure: Rationale and Design of CARRESS-HF, for the Heart Failure Clinical Research Network. *J Cardiac Fail.* 2012;18(3):176-182.

11. Felker GM, Mentz RJ. Diuretics and ultrafiltration in acute decompensated heart failure. *J Am Coll Cardiol.* 2012;59(24):2145-2153.

12. Costanzo MR, Guglin ME, Saltzburg MT, et al. Ultrafiltration versus intravenous diuretics for patients hospitalized for acute decompensated heart failure. *J Am Coll Cardiol.* 2007;49(6):675-683.

13. Ali SS, Olinger CC, Sobotka PA, Dahle TG, Bunte MC, Blake D, Boyle AJ. Loop diuretics can cause clinical natriuretic failure: a prescription for volume expansion. *Congest Heart Fail.* 2009;15(1):1-4.

14. Cuffe MS, Califf RM, Adams KF Jr, et al. Short-term intravenous milrinone for acute exacerbation of chronic heart failure: a randomized controlled trial. *JAMA.* 2002;287(12):1541-1547.

15. Sackner-Bernstein JD, Skopicki HA, Aaronson KD. Risk of worsening renal function with nesiritide in patients with acutely decompensated heart failure. *Circulation.* 2005;111(12):1487-1491.

16. Jaski BE, Fifer MA, Wright RF, et al. Positive inotropic and vasodilator actions of milrinone in patients with severe congestive heart failure. Dose-response relationships and comparison to nitroprusside. *J Clin Invest.* 1985;75(2):643-649.

17. Harrison DG, Bates JN. The nitrovasodilators. New ideas about old drugs. *Circulation.* 1993;87(5):1461-1467.

18. Breisblatt WM, Navratil DL, Burns MJ, Spaccavento LJ. Comparable effects of intravenous nitroglycerin and intravenous nitroprusside in acute ischemia. *Am Heart J.* 1988;116:465-472.

19. Mann T, et al. Effect of nitroprusside on regional myocardial blood flow in coronary artery disease. Results in 25 patients and comparison with nitroglycerin. *Circulation.* 1978;57(4):732-738.

20. Publication Committee for the VMAC Investigators (Vasodilatation in the Management of Acute CHF). Intravenous nesiritide vs nitroglycerin for treatment of decompensated congestive heart failure: a randomized controlled trial. *JAMA.* 2002;287(12):1531-1540.

21. Mentzer RM Jr, Oz MC, Sladen RN, Graeve AH, Hebeler RF Jr, Luber JM Jr, Smedira NG; NAPA Investigators. Effects of perioperative nesiritide in patients with left ventricular dysfunction undergoing cardiac surgery:the NAPA Trial. *J Am Coll Cardiol.* 2007;49(6):716-726.

22. O'Connor CM, Starling RC, Hernandez AF, et al. Effect of nesiritide in patients with acute decompensated heart failure. *N Engl J Med.* 2011;365(1):32-43.

23. Colucci WS, Jaski BE, Fifer MA, Wright RF, Braunwald E. Milrinone: a positive inotropic vasodilator. *Trans Assoc Am Physicians.* 1984;97:124-133.

24. Leier CV, Unverferth DV. Drugs five years later. Dobutamine. *Ann Intern Med.* 1983;99(4):490-496.

25. Goldberg LI. Dopamine—clinical uses of an endogenous catecholamine. *N Engl J Med.* 1974;291(14):707-710.

26. Farmer JB. Indirect sympathomimetic actions of dopamine. *J Pharm Pharmacol.* 1966;18(4):261-262.

27. Colucci WS, Wright RF, Jaski BE, Fifer MA, Braunwald E. Milrinone and dobutamine in severe heart failure: differing hemodynamic effects and individual patient responsiveness. *Circulation.* 1986;73(3 Pt 2):III175-III183.

28. Monrad ES, Baim DS, Smith HS, Lanoue AS. Milrinone, dobutamine, and nitroprusside: comparative effects on hemodynamics and myocardial energetics in patients with severe congestive heart failure. *Circulation.* 1986;73(3 Pt 2): III168-III174.

29. Leier CV, Heban PT, Huss P, Bush CA, Lewis RP. Comparative systemic and regional hemodynamic effects of dopamine and dobutamine in patients with cardiomyopathic heart failure. *Circulation.* 1978;58(3 Pt 1):466-475.

30. Loeb HS, Bredakis J, Gunner RM. Superiority of dobutamine over dopamine for augmentation of cardiac output in patients with chronic low output cardiac failure. *Circulation.* 1977;55(2):375-378.

31. Jaski BE. *Basics of Heart Failure: A Problem Solving Approach.* Boston: Kluwer Academic Publishers; 2000.

32. Jaski B, Branch KR. Supported circulation in the cardiac catheterization laboratory. In Peterson KL, Nicod P, eds. *Cardiac Catheterization: Methods, Diagnosis, and Therapy.* Philadelphia: WB Saunders; 1997.

33. Grauer KC, Daniel L. *ACLS Certification Preparation and a Comprehensive Review.* 3d ed. St. Louis: Mosby-Year Book; 1993.

34. Kapur NK. Circulatory support devices in the catheterization laboratory: evolution or revolution? *J Invasive Cardiol.* 2013;25(2):62-63.

35. Prondzinsky R, Unverzagt S, Russ M, et al. Hemodynamic effects of intra-aortic balloon counterpulsation in patients with acute myocardial infarction complicated by cardiogenic shock: the prospective, randomized IABP shock trial. *Shock.* 2012;37(4):378-384.

36. Reichman RT, Joyo CI, Dembitsky WP, et al. Improved patient survival after cardiac arrest using a cardiopulmonary support system. *Ann Thorac Surg.* 1990;49(1):101-104; discussion 104-105.

37. Moulopoulos SD, Topaz S, Kolff WJ. Diastolic balloon pumping (with carbon dioxide) in the aorta—a mechanical assistance to the failing circulation. *Am Heart J.* 1962;63:669-675.

38. Gewirtz H, Ohley W, Williams DO, Sun Y, Most AS. Effect of intraaortic balloon counterpulsation on regional myocardial blood flow and oxygen consumption in the presence of coronary artery stenosis: observations in an awake animal model. *Am J Cardiol.* 1982;50(4):829-837.

39. Leinbach RC, Buckley MJ, Austen WG, Petschek HE, Kantrowitz AR, Sanders CA. Effects of intra-aortic balloon pumping on coronary flow and metabolism in man. *Circulation.* 1971;43(5 Suppl):I77-I81.

40. Hanlon-Pena PM, Quaal SJ. Intra-aortic balloon pump timing: review of evidence supporting current practice. *Am J Crit Care.* 2011;20(4):323-333; quiz 334.

41. Thiele H, Zeymer U, Neumann FJ, et al. Intraaortic balloon support for myocardial infarction with cardiogenic shock. *N Engl J Med.* 2012;367(14):1287-1296.

42. Dixon SR, Henriques JPS, Mauri L, et al. A prospective feasibility trial investigating the use of the Impella 2.5 system in patients undergoing high-risk percutaneous coronary intervention (The PROTECT I Trial): initial U.S. experience. *JACC Cardiovasc Interv.* 2009;2(2):91-96.

43. Seyfarth M, Sibbing D, Bauer I, et al. A randomized clinical trial to evaluate the safety and efficacy of a percutaneous left ventricular assist device versus intra-aortic balloon pumping for treatment of cardiogenic shock caused by myocardial infarction. *J Am Coll Cardiol.* 2008;52(19):1584-1588.

44. Feldman AM, McNamara D. Myocarditis. *N Engl J Med.* 2000;343(19):1388-1398.

45. Leprince P, Combes A, Bonnet N, et al. Circulatory support for fulminant myocarditis: consideration for implantation, weaning and explantation. *Eur J Cardiothorac Surg.* 2003;24(3):399-403.

46. Aoyama N, Izumi T, Hiramori K, et al. National survey of fulminant myocarditis in Japan: therapeutic guidelines and long-term prognosis of using percutaneous cardiopulmonary support for fulminant myocarditis (special report from a scientific committee). *Circ J.* 2002;66(2):133-144.

47. Dembitsky WP, Moore CH, Holman WL, et al. Successful mechanical circulatory support for noncoronary shock. *J Heart Lung Transplant.* 1992;11(1 Pt 1):129-135.

48. Rockman HA, Adamson RM, Dembitsky WP, Bonar JW, Jaski BE. Acute fulminant myocarditis: long-term follow-up after circulatory support with left ventricular assist device. *Am Heart J.* 1991;121(3 Pt 1):922-926.

49. McCarthy RE 3rd, Boehmer JP, Hruban RH, et al. Long-term outcome of fulminant myocarditis as compared with acute (nonfulminant) myocarditis. *N Engl J Med.* 2000;342(10):690-695.

50. Nayak KR, Jaski BE. Mechanical circulatory support in fulminant myocarditis: case report with brief review and use of novel anterograde limb perfusion device. *J Invasive Cardiol.* 2006;18(9):E253-E255.

# CHAPTER 10

# Stage C: Cardiorenal Syndrome

*"Which comes first? The chicken, or the egg?"*

## The Cardiorenal Syndrome: Definition and Characteristics

Cardiorenal syndrome (CRS) can be defined as a disorder of the heart and kidneys with acute or chronic dysfunction of one organ associated with acute or chronic dysfunction of the other.[1] One or more of three specific features are usually present: heart failure with coexisting renal disease

**UNDERLYING MECHANISMS IN THE CARDIORENAL SYNDROME**

- Exaggerated abnormal renin-angiotensin-aldosterone system activation
- Imbalance in nitric oxide/reactive oxygen species homeostasis
- Inflammation, including high levels of cytokines
- Sympathetic nervous system activation

(cardiorenal failure), worsening renal function (developing during the treatment of acute decompensated heart failure), and/or diuretic resistance.[2]

## THE CARDIORENAL SYNDROME CLASSIFICATION BY SUBTYPES

Ronco et al. categorized CRS into 5 subtypes depending on the primary dysfunctional organ and chronicity of the syndrome (Table 10.1, Figure 10.1).[1] Renal dysfunction is the primary organ involvement in types 3 and 4, which are designated as "renocardiac" syndromes. Management and prognosis can depend on which organ is determined as the primary cause of the syndrome. Forman and coworkers reported a 27% incidence of cardiorenal syndrome in patients hospitalized for heart failure.[3] Worsening renal function (WRF) was defined as an increase in serum creatinine of >0.3 mg/dL from baseline. A history of heart failure or diabetes, admission creatinine >1.5 mg/dL, and systolic blood pressure >160 mm Hg predicted higher risk of WRF. WRF was associated with increased in-hospital mortality, complications, and duration of hospitalization.[3]

**TABLE 10.1    Subtype classification of CRS.[1]**

| TYPE 1 ACUTE CARDIORENAL SYNDROME | Rapid worsening of cardiac function leading to acute kidney injury. |
|---|---|
| TYPE 2 CHRONIC CARDIORENAL SYNDROME | Chronic abnormalities in cardiac function causing progressive chronic kidney disease. |
| TYPE 3 ACUTE RENOCARDIAC SYNDROME | Abrupt and primary worsening of kidney function leading to acute cardiac dysfunction. |
| TYPE 4 CHRONIC RENOCARDIAC SYNDROME | Primary chronic kidney disease contributing to decreased cardiac function, ventricular hypertrophy, diastolic dysfunction, and/or increased risk of adverse cardiovascular events. |
| TYPE 5 SECONDARY CARDIORENAL SYNDROME | Presence of combined cardiac and renal dysfunction due to acute or chronic systemic disorders.[4] |

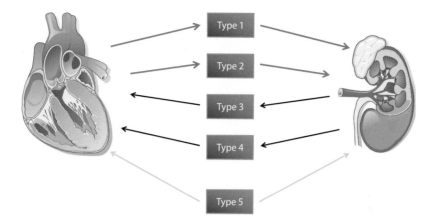

**FIGURE 10.1 The 5 subtypes of CRS identified by Ronco et al.** The interaction between the heart and kidneys may occur as a result of either primary cardiac dysfunction (**red arrows**) or renal dysfunction (**black arrows**) or both (**gold arrows**).[1] *Source:* Adapted with permission from Ronco et al., *J Am Coll Cardiol.* 2008;52(19):1527-1539.

## Measuring Renal Function

The National Kidney Foundation has divided renal function and impairment into 5 progressive stages based on estimated glomerular filtration rate (eGFR) (Table 10.2). In this system, chronic kidney disease (CKD) is defined as a reduction of glomerular filtration rate (GFR) $<60$ mL/min/1.73 $m^2$ for at least 3 months and includes Stages 3, 4, and 5.[54] Stages 1 and 2 refer to normal or only mildly reduced eGFR.

**TABLE 10.2 Stages of chronic kidney disease (CKD) from the National Kidney Foundation.**[5]

| CKD STAGES | eGFR | DESCRIPTION OF REDUCTION IN GFR |
|---|---|---|
| 1 | $\geq 90$ | Normal (no dysfunction) |
| 2 | 60–89 | Mild |
| 3 | 30–59 | Moderate |
| 4 | 15–29 | Severe |
| 5 | $<15$ | Kidney failure |

Historically, GFR was measured by 24-hour urine collection and blood measurements of a filtered marker such as creatinine. Currently, estimated GFR (eGFR) may be calculated from validated equations for adults derived from a single measurement of a blood-level marker, typically creatinine or cystatin C (Table 10.3). Estimated GFR is corrected for body surface area and expressed compared to the average-sized man as mL/min/1.73 m$^2$. In 2011, 92% of laboratories reporting eGFR used the 4-variable MDRD equation.[6]

TABLE 10.3 Common equations derived using endogenous filtration markers to calculate eGFR in adults. Abbreviations: BUN, blood urea nitrogen; CCr, creatinine clearance; Cr, creatinine; CysC, cystatin C; eGFR, estimated GFR; SCr, serum creatinine (mg/dL); SCys, serum cystatin C (mg/L).

| EQUATION NAME (EGFR UNITS) | VARIABLES | VALIDATION MARKERS |
|---|---|---|
| Cockcroft-Gault Creatinine Clearance[a] (mL/min)[7] | SCr, age, body mass, gender | CCr from 24-hr urine collection |
| Original Modification of Diet in Renal Disease[b] (MDRD) – 6 variables[8] (mL/min/1.73 m$^2$) | SCr, age, race (black or non-black), gender, BUN, albumin levels | 24-hr urinary clearance of constantly infused $^{125}$I-iothalamate |
| Revised MDRD[c] 4 variables[9] (mL/min/1.73 m$^2$) | SCr, age, race (black or non-black), gender | 24-hr urinary clearance of constantly infused $^{125}$I-iothalamate |
| Chronic Kidney Disease Epidemiology Collaboration[d] (CKD-EPI)[10] (mL/min/1.73 m$^2$) | SCr, age, race (black or non-black), gender | Urinary or plasma clearance of insulin or $^{125}$I-iothalamate |
| CKD-EPI cystatin C[e] (mL/min/1.73 m$^2$)[11] | SCys, gender | Urinary clearance of $^{125}$I-iothalamate |
| CKD-EPI creatinine-cystatin C[f] (mL/min/1.73 m$^2$)[11] | SCr, SCys, race (black or non-black), gender | Urinary clearance of $^{125}$I-iothalamate |

**Legend:** Each equation (method) has certain metabolic parameters that affect validity

[a]Cockcroft-Gault Creatinine Clearance: Serum Cr is affected by patient muscle mass and renal tubular secretion.

[b]Original MDRD – 6: Equation is valid when GFR < 60 mL/min/1.73 m$^2$.

[c]MDRD – 4: Equation is valid when GFR < 60 mL/min/1.73 m$^2$.

[d]Equation more sensitive to changes in GFR with baseline preserved renal function (GFR > 60 mL/min/1.73 m$^2$).

[e]CysC production is not dependent on muscle mass and is completely metabolized in the kidney without excretion or reuptake.

[f]CKD-EPI creatinine-cystatin C: CysC production is not dependent on muscle mass and is completely metabolized in the kidney without excretion or reuptake.

## CREATININE VERSUS CYSTATIN C

Creatinine is a low-molecular-weight metabolite (113 Da [Daltons]) derived from the breakdown of skeletal muscle creatine phosphate. This waste product is widely used as a biomarker of kidney function and commonly used to calculate eGFR values. However, estimated creatinine clearance can overestimate true GFR if decreased cellular production reduces serum creatinine significantly (e.g., cachexia, age, malnutrition, female gender, and dietary protein restriction). Failure to take these factors into account can lead to the underdiagnosis of CKD.

Recently, cystatin C has become an alternative marker for eGFR. The relatively large protein molecule (13,250 Da), a cysteine protease inhibitor, is produced at a constant rate by nucleated cells. It is freely filtered by the glomerulus and not secreted, but reabsorbed with complete catabolism by proximal tubules. Therefore, calculated eGFR using serum cystatin C versus creatinine alone may be more reflective of actual renal filtration function.[12]

# Association of Abnormal GFR and Heart Failure Mortality

Currently, approximately 26 million adults in the United States have a GFR < 60 mL/min/1.73 m$^2$ (Stages 3–5 CKD).[12] Hillege and coworkers[13] studied renal function as a predictor for mortality in heart failure in outpatients with a left ventricular ejection fraction (LVEF) ≤35% (Figure 10.2). Impaired renal function was independent of impaired LVEF, yet strongly associated with mortality in patients with heart failure and correlated with plasma levels of N-terminal atrial natriuretic peptide (ANP).

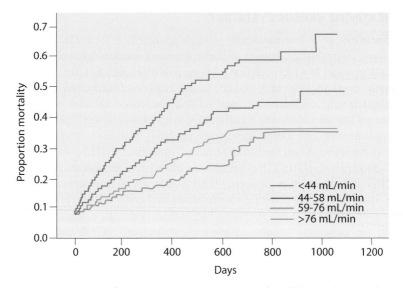

**FIGURE 10.2 Renal dysfunction associated with increased morbidity and mortality in outpatients with class III/IV heart failure.** Kaplan-Meier mortality curves for quartiles of baseline creatinine clearance (GFRc) as shown in the lower right corner. The GFRc was calculated using Cockroft-Gault equation. (NYHA class: III [*n* = 1138]; III/IV [*n* = 607]; IV [*n* = 161].) After a median follow-up of 277 days, 18% of patients had died. Impaired renal function was a stronger predictor of mortality than indices of impaired cardiac function (LVEF and NYHA class) and was also associated with increasing levels of N-terminal ANP. Patients in the lowest quartile of GFRc (< 44 mL/min) had almost 3 times the risk of mortality than patients with the highest renal function (GFRc > 76 mL/min).[13] *Source:* Adapted with permission from Hillege et al., *Circulation.* 2000;102(2):203-210.

## IMPAIRED RENAL FUNCTION IN HOSPITALIZED HEART FAILURE PATIENTS

From the ADHERE database, $n$ = 105,388, Heywood and coworkers calculated GFR using the 4-variable MDRD in hospitalized heart failure patients with a mean serum creatinine of 1.8 ± 1.6 mg/dL. Moderate to severe renal dysfunction (Stage 3-5 CKD) was identified in 59.3% of males and 67.6% of females. In-hospital mortality increased as renal function decreased from normal renal function (Stage 1 CKD) to severe dysfunction (Stage 4 CKD) and kidney failure (Stage 5 CKD) from 1.9% to 7.6% and 6.5%, respectively.[14]

# Factors Affecting GFR

The majority of physiological variables have a predictable effect on GFR (Table 10.4). Changes in central venous pressure have a variable effect discussed below.

TABLE 10.4    Physiological variables affecting GFR.

| VARIABLE | ACUTE EFFECT ON GFR |
|---|---|
| ↑ Mean arterial pressure | ↑ |
| ↑ Renal blood flow | ↑ |
| ↑ Central venous pressure | ↓↑ |
| ↑ Renal sympathetic pre-glomerular vasoconstriction | ↓ |
| ↑ Renal angiotensin II post-glomerular vasoconstriction | ↑ |
| ↑ Exogenous nephron toxins | ↓ |

## CENTRAL VENOUS PRESSURE (CVP) AND GFR

*In vitro* animal experiments demonstrate that an isolated increase in renal vein pressure (equal to CVP *in vivo*) leads to worsening GFR.[15] In patients with cardiorenal syndrome, however, causality may be uncertain, because a primary change in either (central) venous pressure or kidney function can secondarily affect the other. In patients with cardiovascular disease undergoing right heart catheterization, the relationship between CVP and renal function is bimodal, with worse renal function at both very low and high filling pressures.[16] At low levels of CVP (and presumably cardiac output), Damman and coworkers observed a gradual concordant increase in CVP and GFR (Figure 10.3). At CVP >6 mm Hg, however, renal function decreased as CVP further increased. This effect was more pronounced in patients with a preserved (not decreased) cardiac output. In part, this may relate to a high CVP leading to a decrease in renal vascular pressure gradient (arterial pressure - venous pressure), although CVP may also be a surrogate indicator for a range of neurohumoral and inflammatory processes. When CVP is lowered (during relief of congestion) in individual cases, variable effects on renal function are seen suggesting that the overall inverse association between CVP and GFR can be altered by multiple feedback pathways.[15]

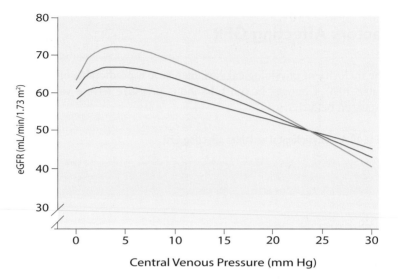

**FIGURE 10.3  Curvilinear relationships between eGFR versus CVP at three different levels of cardiac index (colored lines).** Data from right heart catheterization ($n = 2577$; mean eGFR for all 3 groups = $65 \pm 24$ mL/min/1.73 m², with a cardiac index = $2.9 \pm 0.81$ L/min/m², and CVP = $5.9 \pm 4.3$ mm Hg, $P < 0.0001$). **Red line** indicates cardiac index < 2.5 L/min/m²; **green line** indicates cardiac index 2.5 to 3.2 L/min/m²; orange line indicates cardiac index > 3.2 L/min/m². A very low CVP was associated with a decrease in eGFR in all 3 groups. High CVP was more closely associated with impaired renal function in patients with a higher cardiac index **(orange line)**.[16] *Source:* Adapted with permission from Damman et al., *J Am Coll Cardiol.* 2009;53(7):582-588.

# Management of Heart Failure with Impaired Kidney Function

Decompensated cardiac systolic dysfunction may be associated with acute increases in serum creatinine.[1,3] Positive intravenous inotropes such as dobutamine may help restore renal function for days to weeks (Figure 10.4). By itself, however, this therapy is a temporary solution, and the requirement for inotropic support may identify a patient in transition from Stage C to Stage D heart failure.

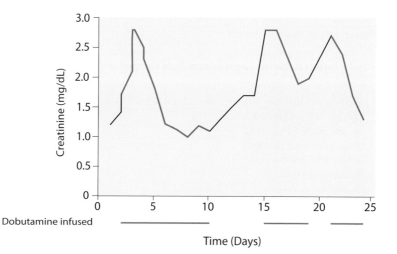

Dobutamine infused

Time (Days)

**FIGURE 10.4    Example of a patient with recurrent in-hospital renal dysfunction.**
Infusions of dobutamine (**red**) improved creatinine levels. However, when the patient was not on inotropic support (**black segments**), worsening renal function recurred.

## TARGET RATES OF FLUID REMOVAL TO PRESERVE RENAL FUNCTION

There is always a risk of worsening renal function during therapeutic fluid removal in the acute heart failure patient. Certain factors may be present at baseline and others need to be assessed after initiation of therapy (List 10.1). When risk factors are present, consider decreasing the diuretic dose or decreasing ultrafiltration fluid removal rates. Although allowing plasma refill from the extravascular space to replenish intravascular volume helps maintain renal function, other clinical factors are also important.[17] These considerations may be offset by the need to treat initial volume overload aggressively to avert acute life threatening complications including respiratory failure requiring mechanical ventilation. In high-risk patients, temporary inotropic support may blunt the potential for fluid removal therapy to worsen renal function. As noted above, in the presence of a high initial central venous pressure, therapy that leads to decongestion and lowers CVP alone may lead to improved renal function.[18] If renal function worsens despite persistent

**THERAPEUTIC OPTIONS FOR WORSENING RENAL FUNCTION IN THE CARDIORENAL PATIENT**

• Assess for new cardiac or renal causes including intravascular depletion
• IV inotropes in patients with LV or RV systolic dysfunction
• Achieve euvolemia via diuretics, ultrafiltration, or dialysis
• Wean renin-angiotensin-aldosterone inhibitors (especially in patients with HF-pEF)

congestion, reassessing the patient's circulatory status with right heart catheterization may be useful.

**LIST 10.1  Factors that Affect Target Rates of Fluid Removal in Heart Failure**

**Baseline factors that may warrant slower target rates of fluid removal**
> Low systolic blood pressure
> Low glomerular filtration rate
> Low central venous pressure
> Low initial volume overload
> Diabetes mellitus
> Proteinuria
> Small body size

**Once therapy is initiated, other factors that may suggest a need for slower target rates of fluid removal**
> Creatinine rise
> Decreases in systolic blood pressure / hypotension
> Urine output < 125 cm³/6 hr
> Hemoconcentration

## PHARMACOLOGIC THERAPY VERSUS ULTRAFILTRATION FOR CARDIORENAL SYNDROME WITH WORSENING RENAL FUNCTION (WRF)

In the Cardiorenal Rescue Study in Acute Decompensated Heart Failure (CARRESS-HF) trial, algorithm-based diuretic and vasoactive therapy (Tables 10.5 and 10.6) was compared to ultrafiltration in acute decompensated heart failure patients with WRF. In this trial, WRF was defined as an increase in creatinine $\geq 0.3$ mg/dL between 12 weeks before and 10 days after admission. Compared to ultrafiltration, a high-dose, up-titrated, continuous infusion of loop diuretics (with the addition of metolazone, vasoactive therapy, or both) led to a similar weight loss with a better preservation of renal function assessed at 96 hours after randomization. One factor that could have contributed to this outcome included a higher number of patients receiving intravenous inotropes in the pharmacologic therapy (12%) versus the ultrafiltration treated groups (3%).

TABLE 10.5    Stepped pharmacologic care treatment algorithm for WRF: CARRESS-HF.[19]

**Based urine output (UO) goals assessed daily at randomization, 24, 48, and 96 hours**

| | |
|---|---|
| UO > 5 L/d | Reduce current diuretic regimen if desired |
| UO 3–5 L/d | Continue current diuretic regimen |
| UO < 3 L/d | See diuretic grid (Table 10.6) |

**Additional recommendations at each daily assessment**

**24-hour assessment**

UO recommendations as above

Advance to next step on grid if UO < 3 L/d

**48-hour assessment**

UO recommendations as above

Advance to next step on grid if UO < 3 L/d

Consider dopamine or dobutamine at 2 µg/kg/min if SBP < 110 mm Hg and EF < 40% or RV systolic dysfunction

Consider nitroglycerin or nesiritide if SBP > 120 mm Hg (any EF) and severe symptoms

**72- and 96-hour assessments**

Advance to next step on grid if UO < 3 L/d

Consider dopamine or dobutamine at 2 µg/kg/min if SBP < 110 mm Hg and EF < 40% or right ventricular systolic dysfunction

Consider nitroglycerin or nesiritide if SBP > 120 mm Hg (any EF) and severe symptoms

Consider hemodynamic guided IV therapy, LVAD, dialysis, or ultrafiltration crossover

TABLE 10.6    DIURETIC GRID for CARRESS-HF[19] protocol.

| INITIAL STEP BASED ON OUTPATIENT THERAPY | | SUGGESTED DOSE | |
|---|---|---|---|
| STEP | THERAPY | DAILY LOOP DOSE (MG FUROSEMIDE OR EQUIVALENT) | THIAZIDE |
| A | ≤ 80 mg | 40 mg IV bolus + 5 mg/h | None |
| B | 81–160 mg | 80 mg IV bolus + 10 mg/h | 5 mg metolazone once daily |
| C | 161–240 mg | 80 mg IV bolus + 20 mg/h | 5 mg metolazone twice daily |
| D | > 240 mg | 80 mg IV bolus + 30 mg/h | 5 mg metolazone twice daily |

## TRANSIENT VERSUS PERSISTENT WORSENING RENAL FUNCTION

In an analysis derived from the Vasodilation in the Management of Acute Congestive Heart Failure (VMAC) trial, Aronson and coworkers characterized in-hospital WRF as persistent versus transient.[20] Persistent renal dysfunction was defined as an increase in serum creatinine ≥ 0.5 mg/dL persisting at day 30 postadmission. Compared to transient WRF (returning to levels <0.5 mg/dL above the level at admission), only persistent WRF was associated with a worse long-term outcome (Figure 10.5).

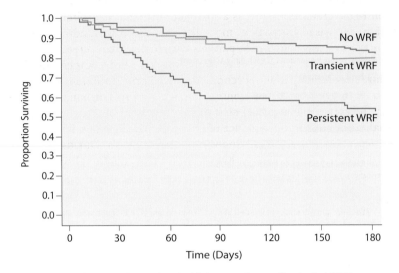

**FIGURE 10.5**   **Persistent WRF associated with increased mortality.** In the VMAC trial, hospitalized acute heart failure syndrome (AHFS) patients with dyspnea at rest were categorized into 3 groups: without WRF, with transient WRF, or with persistent WRF (see text). The 6-month mortality rates in patients without WRF, with transient WRF, and with persistent WRF were 17.3%, 20.5%, and 46.1%, respectively (no WRF vs. transient WRF: $P = 0.68$; no WRF vs. persistent WRF: $P < 0.0001$). Baseline mean serum creatinine (SCr) without WRF, with transient WRF, and with persistent WRF were $1.5 \pm 0.9$ mg/dL, $1.7 \pm 0.7$ mg/dL, and $2.1 \pm 1.4$ mg/dL, respectively. Patients with persistent WRF showed a mean increase in SCr levels of $1.17 \pm 1.05$ mg/dL at 30 days compared to baseline. ($n = 467$, $P < 0.001$).[20] *Source:* Adapted with permission from Aronson D, Burger AJ, *J Card Fail.* 2010;16(7):541-547.

## INTRAVASCULAR VOLUME DURING DECONGESTIVE THERAPY

Hemoconcentration during heart failure treatment implies intravascular volume reduction and aggressive decongestion. Hemoconcentration can occur in heart failure patients when intravascular volume loss augmented by diuresis or ultrafiltration exceeds the refill rate into the intravascular space (from extravascular fluid and exogenous oral or IV sources). Testani and coworkers[21] examined the relationship between hemoconcentration and survival in the setting of WRF. They defined hemoconcentration based on increases of blood hematocrit, total protein, or albumin concentrations between admission and discharge. WRF was defined as a 20% decrease in calculated eGFR. In heart failure patients undergoing diuresis, the occurrence of hemoconcentration (intravascular volume reduction) was associated with greater fluid removal, weight loss, and worsening renal function. Despite this, however, patient long-term survival was improved in the hemoconcentration group (Figure 10.6). In a subsequent three-trial retrospective analysis, Testani and coworkers[21] used BUN:creatinine ratio as a surrogate for renal neurohormonal activation. Increased in-hospital mortality associated with admission renal insufficiency was confined to patients with higher BUN:creatinine ratios.

Thus, the mechanism of renal dysfunction in decompensated heart failure may affect patient outcome. Impaired renal function, if accompanied by irreversible kidney injury or marked neurohormonal activation, may indicate a worse prognosis. During treatment, if transient impaired renal function is a consequence of intravascular depletion from effective decongestion alone, it may imply a better prognosis. During treatment, the distinction between true kidney injury and functional renal impairment can be challenging.[22]

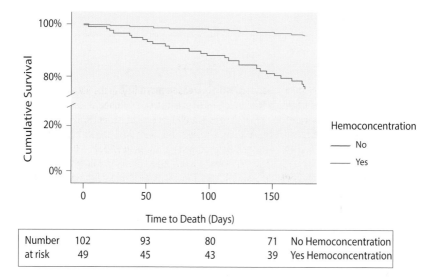

**FIGURE 10.6    Hemoconcentration improves long-term survival in patients despite association with WRF.** Hospitalized heart failure patients' survival curves with or without hemoconcentration. All patients had WRF. Patients who met the combined criteria for the presence of hemoconcentration after adjustment for baseline characteristics had an improved long-term survival compared to those in whom it was absent ($P < 0.001$). This occurred despite association of hemoconcentration with an in-hospital decrease in GFR compared to those without hemoconcentration. Bottom panel shows number of patients in each group at time zero and surviving over the time period.[21] *Source:* Adapted with permission from Testani et al., *Circulation.* 2010;122(3):265-272.

## HYPONATREMIA AND VASOPRESSIN

Approximately 20% of patients hospitalized for heart failure are hyponatremic defined by a serum sodium value of 135 mEq/L or less.[23] This electrolyte abnormality derives from high levels of vasopressin (antidiuretic hormone) in the progressive neurohumoral activation of heart failure (see Chapter 4). In a study of 5347 consecutive hospitalized patients with a diagnosis of HF, hyponatremia was associated with an increased length of stay, worsening renal function, and in-hospital mortality.[23]

In hypervolemic or euvolemic patients, the oral vasopressin antagonist tolvaptan is approved for the treatment of severe hyponatremia (≤ 125 mEq/L) or markedly symptomatic hyponatremia that has resisted correction with fluid restriction at an oral dose of 15 mg increasing to 60 mg daily, as needed to achieve the desired level of serum sodium (Figure 10.7).[24] Alternatively, intravenous conivaptan can be used.[25]

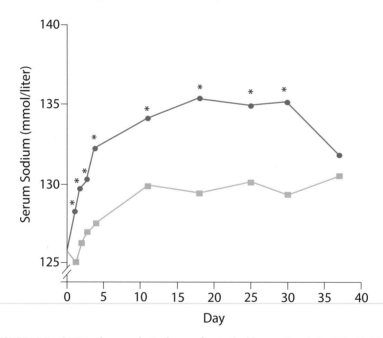

**FIGURE 10.7    SALT-1, pharmacologic therapy for marked hyponatremia (< 125 mEq/L).**
Change in serum sodium versus time in patients receiving oral tolvaptan (**green**) or placebo (**orange**) (n = 99). Approximately one-third of patients in this series were hyponatremic on the basis of heart failure. *P < 0.05.[24] Source: Adapted with permission from Schrier et al., N Engl J Med. 2006;355(20):2099-2112.

Vasopressin antagonist therapy should be initiated in the hospital, where serum sodium and the patient's intravascular volume status can be monitored. Although this therapy can increase serum sodium levels—with associated improvements in cognitive function, diuresis, and improved hemodynamics—the effect on endpoints of morbidity and mortality are uncertain. Too rapid correction of hyponatremia (e.g., >12 mEq/L/24 hours) can cause central nervous system osmotic demyelination with associated symptoms.[26]

## FUTURE STRATEGIES TO DETERMINE EUVOLEMIA

In an individual patient, it may be challenging to determine the state of "euvolemia" associated with optimal long-term outcome. Whereas the physical exam can detect when a patient is "wet," it is insensitive for assessing when that same patient is "euvolemic" or becoming "dry." When patients are taking medications associated with fluid retention (e.g., calcium channel blockers), persistent edema may be present despite intravascular depletion. Returning a patient to a euvolemic state should be desirable even if associated with transient renal impairment. Excessive fluid removal, however, may lead to excessive neurohumoral activation, acute tubular necrosis, and poor patient outcomes. During treatment of fluid overload, laboratory markers of renal function can be monitored, but these biomarkers may be nonspecific and delayed in onset for assessing true euvolemia.

In the future, novel biomarkers may have a beneficial role to help predict acute kidney injury and guide management.[27] Biomarkers such as neutrophil gelatinase-associated lipocalin (NGAL) have been shown to predict acute kidney injury 24 to 48 hours before an increase in creatinine is observed.[28] In addition, cutaneous electrical bioimpedence and other signals may give an estimate of body fluids and dry weight, thus aiding clinicians to determine true patient euvolemia.[29-31]

Finally, catheter-based renal artery sympathetic denervation may also play a role in the future treatment of cardiorenal syndrome, because activation of both efferent and afferent sympathetic renal nerves have been found to play a role in the pathogenesis and progression of kidney dysfunction in heart failure patients.[32]

# References

1. Ronco C, Haapio M, House AA, Anavekar N, Bellomo R. Cardiorenal syndrome. *J Am Coll Cardiol.* 2008;52(19):1527-1539.

2. Liang K, Williams AW, Greene EL, Redfield MM. Acute decompensated heart failure and the cardiorenal syndrome. *Crit Care Med.* 2008;36(1 Suppl):S75-S88.

3. Forman DE, Butler J, Wang Y, et al. Incidence, predictors at admission, and impact of worsening renal function among patients hospitalized with heart failure. *J Am Coll Cardiol.* 2004;43(1):61-67.

4. McCullough PA, Kellum JA, Mehta RL, et al. Cardiorenal Syndrome Type 5: Clinical Presentation, Pathophysiology and Management Strategies from the Eleventh Consensus Conference of the Acute Dialysis Quality Initiative (ADQI). *Contrib Nephrol.* 2013;182:174-194.

5. Levey AS, Coresh J, Balk E, et al. National Kidney Foundation practice guidelines for chronic kidney disease: evaluation, classification, and stratification. *Ann Intern Med.* 2003;139(2):137-147.

6. Matsushita K, Mahmoodi BK, Woodward M, et al. Comparison of risk prediction using the CKD-EPI equation and the MDRD study equation for estimated glomerular filtration rate. *JAMA.* 2012;307(18):1941-1951.

7. Cockcroft DW, Gault MH. Prediction of creatinine clearance from serum creatinine. *Nephron.* 1976;16:31–41.

8. Levey AS, Bosch JP, Lewis JB, Greene T, Rogers N, Roth D. A more accurate method to estimate glomerular filtration rate from serum creatinine: a new prediction equation. Modification of Diet in Renal Disease Study Group. *Ann Intern Med.* 1999;130(6):461-470.

9. Levey AS, Coresh J, Greene T, et al. Using standardized serum creatinine values in the modification of diet in renal disease study equation for estimating glomerular filtration rate. *Ann Intern Med.* 2006;145(4):247-254.

10. Levey AS, Stevens LA, Schmid CH, et al. A new equation to estimate glomerular filtration rate. *Ann Intern Med.* 2009;150(9):604-612.

11. Inker LA, et al. Estimating glomerular filtration rate from serum creatinine and cystatin C. *N Engl J Med.* 2012;367(1):20-29.

12. McMurray MD, JE Trivax, McCullough PA. Serum cystatin C, renal filtration function, and left ventricular remodeling. *Circ Heart Fail.* 2009;2(2):86-89.

13. Hillege HL, Girbes AR, de Kam PJ, et al. Renal function, neurohormonal activation, and survival in patients with chronic heart failure. *Circulation.* 2000;102(2):203-210.

14. Heywood JT, et al. High prevalence of renal dysfunction and its impact on outcome in 118,465 patients hospitalized with acute decompensated heart failure: a report from the ADHERE database. *J Card Fail.* 2007;13(6):422-430.

15. Firth JD, Raine AE, Ledingham JG. Raised venous pressure: a direct cause of renal sodium retention in oedema? *Lancet.* 1988;1(8593):1033-1035.

16. Damman K, van Deursen VM, Navis G, Voors AA, van Veldhuisen DJ, Hillege HL. Increased central venous pressure is associated with impaired renal function and mortality in a broad spectrum of patients with cardiovascular disease. *J Am Coll Cardiol.* 2009;53(7):582-588.

17. Raichlin E, Haglund NA, Dumitru I, et al. Worsening renal function in patients with acute decompensated heart failure treated with ultrafiltration: predictors and outcomes. *J Card Fail.* 2013;19(12):787-794.

18. Mullens W, Abrahams Z, Grancis GD, et al. Importance of venous congestion for worsening of renal function in advanced decompensated heart failure. *J Am Coll Cardiol.* 2009;53(7):589-596.

19. Bart BA, Goldsmith SR, Lee KL, et al. Cardiorenal rescue study in acute decompensated heart failure: rationale and design of CARRESS-HF, for the Heart Failure Clinical Research Network. *J Card Fail.* 2012;18(3):176-182.

20. Aronson D, Burger AJ. The relationship between transient and persistent worsening renal function and mortality in patients with acute decompensated heart failure. *J Card Fail.* 2010;16(7):541-547.

21. Testani JM, Chen J, McCauley BD, Kimmel SE, Shannon RP. Potential effects of aggressive decongestion during the treatment of decompensated heart failure on renal function and survival. *Circulation.* 2010;122(3):265-272.

22. Brandimarte F, Vaduganathan M, Mureddu GF, et al. Prognostic implications of renal dysfunction in patients hospitalized with heart failure: data from the last decade of clinical investigations. *Heart Fail Rev.* 2013;18(2):167-176.

23. Shchekochikhin DY, Schrier RW, Lindenfeld J, Price LL, Jaber BL, Madias NE. Outcome differences in community- versus hospital-acquired hyponatremia in patients with a diagnosis of heart failure. *Circ Heart Fail.* 2013;6(3):379-386.

24. Schrier RW, Gross P, Gheorghiade M, et al. Tolvaptan, a selective oral vasopressin V2-receptor antagonist, for hyponatremia. *N Engl J Med.* 2006;355(20):2099-2112.

25. Udelson JE, Smith WB, Hendrix GH, et al. Acute hemodynamic effects of conivaptan, a dual V(1A) and V(2) vasopressin receptor antagonist, in patients with advanced heart failure. *Circulation.* 2001;104(20):2417-2423.

26. Konstam MA, Gheorghiade M, Burnett JC Jr, et al. Effects of oral tolvaptan in patients hospitalized for worsening heart failure: the EVEREST Outcome Trial. *JAMA.* 2007;297(12):1319-1331.

27. Goldstein SL, Jaber BL, Faubel S, et al. AKI transition of care: a potential opportunity to detect and prevent CKD. *Clin J Am Soc Nephrol.* 2013;8(3):476-483.

28. Ronco C, Cruz D, Noland BW. Neutrophil gelatinase-associated lipocalin curve and neutrophil gelatinase-associated lipocalin extended-range assay: a new biomarker approach in the early diagnosis of acute kidney injury and cardio-renal syndrome. *Semin Nephrol.* 2012;32(1):121-128.

29. National Institutes of Health. *Evaluation of Multisensor Data in Heart Failure Patients With Implanted Devices (MultiSENSE).* March 10, 2014; Available from: http://clinicaltrials.gov/ct2/show/NCT01128166.

30. Liebo MJ, Katra RP, Chakravarthy N, Libbus I, Tang WHW. Noninvasive wireless bioimpedance monitoring tracks patients with healthcare utilization following discharge from acute decompensated heart failure: Results from the ACUTE pilot study. *J Card Fail.* 2013;19(8):S88-S89.

31. Auricchio A, Brugada J, Ellenbogen KA, et al. Assessment of a novel device-based diagnostic algorithm to monitor patient status in moderate-to-severe heart failure: rationale and design of the CLEPSYDRA study. *Eur J Heart Fail.* 2010;12(12): 1363-1371.

32. Sobotka PA, Krum H, Böhm M, Francis DP, Schlaich MP. The role of renal denervation in the treatment of heart failure. *Curr Cardiol Rep.* 2012;14(3):285-292.

# CHAPTER 11

# Stage D Heart Failure: Options and Opportunities

*"Diseases desperate grown / By desperate appliance are relieved / Or not at all."*

–William Shakespeare, Hamlet, Act IV, Scene 3

## Who Is the Stage D Heart Failure Patient?

Stage D heart failure, also known as advanced heart failure, represents the group of patients with refractory symptoms that fail to stabilize despite hospital admission. Identifying when a patient has crossed the threshold to advanced heart failure can be challenging. Families or caregivers may have difficulty recognizing gradual changes in physical and mental status. Nevertheless, the occurrences of multiple hospital admissions, cardiorenal syndrome, the need to reduce doses of neurohormonal blocker medications, recurrent ventricular arrhythmias, and laboratory markers of disease progression, including hyponatremia or anemia, may herald a shift to advanced disease and poor prognosis.[1] The need for chronic inotropic support implies a particularly poor prognosis (Figure 11.1). Patient frailty and the lack of psychosocial support further reduce the ability of these patients to cope with both cardiac and noncardiac limitations. Aggressive measures such as heart transplant or left ventricular assist device are more likely to benefit the Stage D patient whose overall disability is predominantly due to heart failure alone. When there is multisystem involvement, palliative care may be more appropriate.

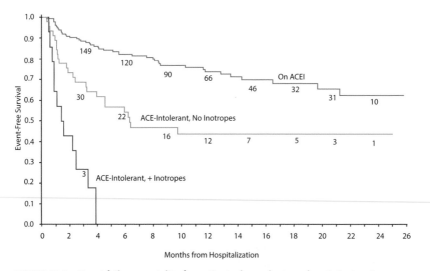

**FIGURE 11.1   Heart failure mortality for patients dependent on chronic inotropic support.** ACE inhibitor intolerance and a need for inotropes both identify heart failure patients with a worse prognosis.[2] *Source:* Adapted with permission from Kittleson et al., *J Am Coll Cardiol.* 2003;41(11):2029-2035.

Stage D patients, in general, have symptoms at rest or with simple activities of daily living and a poor 1-year prognosis. Several clinical criteria suggest that heart failure has progressed to Stage D (List 11.1). Most patients have been hospitalized for heart failure in the preceding 12 months. Even for the Stage D patient, a careful evaluation is warranted to confirm the diagnosis of heart failure as the etiology of a patient's symptoms. Precipitating factors should be identified and, if possible, treated. The measures that have been outlined for patients in Stages A, B, and C should be reviewed for potential treatment options.

**EXPECTED TIME COURSE FOR HEART FAILURE MORTALITY 50%**[3]
- Cardiogenic shock (chronic heart failure with rapidly progressive end-organ dysfunction, acute MI, post-cardiotomy shock)– **In-hospital mortality > 50%**
- Chronic heart failure dependent on IV inotropes–**3-6 Months**
- Stage D systolic dysfunction heart failure–**12 Months**

LIST 11.1   **Clinical Criteria that Suggest Stage D**

- Unacceptable symptoms despite maximum medical or device therapy
- Treadmill testing: peak $VO_2 \leq 14$ mL/kg/min or $\leq 50\%$ age-gender predicted maximum
- Weight loss due to cardiac cachexia
- Recurrent symptomatic ventricular arrhythmias
- Recurrent CHF hospitalizations within 6 months
- Progressive cardiorenal syndrome
- Intolerance of neurohormonal blockers at target levels
- Requirement for chronic inotropic support

# Palliative Care

Palliative care should be considered for patients with severe, persistent symptoms who do not qualify for or do not desire ventricular replacement options, such as heart transplantation or left ventricular assist devices. Palliative care is associated with improved patient and family satisfaction in care and symptom management and decreased hospital readmissions, procedures, interventions, and cost.[4] Palliative care includes many treatments not usually considered as part of heart failure care (Table 11.1). Consultations for palliation may result in referral to hospice that will usually be an at-home program. Surprisingly, in advanced heart failure patients, hospice has been associated with an increase in survival compared to those who did not receive hospice care.[4]

**TABLE 11.1    Palliative Therapies for Stage D Symptoms.**[4]

| | CLASS OF RECOMMENDATIONS* | | | | |
|---|---|---|---|---|---|
| SYMPTOMS | I | IIA | IIB | III | INSUFFICIENT |
| DYSPNEA | Loop diuretics with or without thiazides<br><br>Nitrates<br><br>Low-dose opioids | Inotropes<br><br>Ultrafiltration (if diuretic resistant)<br><br>Walking aids<br><br>Breathing training<br><br>Exercise training<br><br>Hawthorn extract | Oxygen (without hypoxia) | Benzodiazapines | Acupuncture/ acupressure |
| PAIN | Opioids<br><br>Bone pain: bisphosphonates<br><br>Anginal pain: nitrates, β blockers, Ca²⁺ channel blockers, ranolazine, coronary revascularization | | Acupuncture<br><br>Exercise training<br><br>Music | Nonsteroidal anti-inflammatory drugs | |
| DEPRESSION | Selective serotonin reuptake inhibitors, serotonin-norepinephrine reuptake inhibitors, tricyclic antidepressants | Psychological interventions: cognitive behavioral therapy, counseling, or supportive therapy | Exercise | | Acupuncture |
| FATIGUE | | Treat secondary causes (anemia, infection, sleep apnea, etc)<br><br>Stimulants<br><br>Exercise training<br><br>Hawthorn extract | | Increased rest and reduction of physical activity | Anti-inflammatory agents<br><br>L-carnitine<br><br>Nutritional supplements or appetite stimulants |

*Recommendations for palliative care based on Benefit compared to Risk of Treatment:

**Class I:** Conditions for which there is evidence for and/or general agreement that the procedure or treatment is useful and effective.

**Class IIa:** The weight of evidence or opinion is in favor of the procedure or treatment.

**Class IIb:** Usefulness/efficacy is less well established by evidence or opinion.

**Class III:** Conditions for which there is evidence and/or general agreement that the procedure or treatment is not useful/effective and in some cases may be harmful.

**Insufficient:** Insufficient evidence to make recommendation.

# Cardiac Transplant

Cardiac transplant has become a widely accepted treatment for advanced heart disease. Even so, the psychosocial requirements and long term immunosuppressive therapy associated with the procedure require careful patient selection and preparation.

## REFERRAL OR CONSIDERATION FOR CARDIAC TRANSPLANT

Consider patients for evaluation for cardiac transplant when they develop Stage D findings—despite comprehensive Stage C therapies. Significant noncardiac comorbidities or inability to comply with a complex medical regimen may contraindicate transplant. Most cardiac transplant candidates are 70 years or younger in age.

One clinical finding in particular suggests the need for transplant evaluation. The occurrence of cardiac cachexia defined as a nonintentional weight loss of at least 7.5% over six months is an ominous finding associated with a 39% one-year mortality[5] and an independent risk factor for death.

Measurement of patient oxygen consumption during cardiopulmonary exercise testing (see Chapter 2) can provide useful prognostic information to aid with the timing of listing for cardiac transplant. A peak $O_2$ consumption of $\leq 14$ mL/kg/min can indicate a poor one-year prognosis with only continued medical therapy and no cardiac transplant (Figure 11.2).[6] Especially in patients younger than 40 years old, percent predicted peak $O_2$ consumption ($PPVO_2$) may be more accurate.[7] In these patients, the finding of a $PPVO_2$ (corrected for age, body weight, and sex) $\leq 50\%$ is a worse prognostic indicator than using a fixed value threshold of $\leq 14$ mL/kg/min (Figure 11.3). Conversely, a $PPVO_2 > 50\%$ has been associated with a one- and two-year survival of 98% and 90%, respectively. Both peak $O_2$ consumption and $PPVO_2$ can be used in clinical practice.

Cumulative Survival (%)

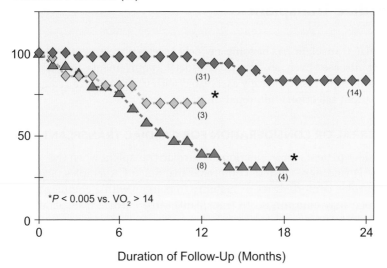

Duration of Follow-Up (Months)

**FIGURE 11.2 Cardiopulmonary exercise testing: Peak VO₂ and prognosis.** A peak VO$_2$ value of ≤ 14 mL/kg/min (red triangles and yellow diamonds) predicts a poor survival. Some patients were accepted as transplant candidates (yellow diamonds [n = 35]) and some patients were rejected for transplant (red triangles [n = 27]). Patients with VO$_2$ > 14 mL/kg/min (blue diamonds [n = 52]) were not considered for transplant.[6] *Source:* Adapted with permission from Mancini et al., *Circulation.* 1991;83(3):778-786.

Because heart failure patients have reduced exercise capacity, the modified Naughton treadmill protocol (which increases workload at a slower rate than the standard Bruce protocol) may give a better estimate of peak oxygen consumption. In the modified Naughton protocol, each stage increases estimated O$_2$ consumption by 1 MET (3.5 mL O$_2$/kg/min) (Table 11.2).

Treadmill testing can also provide a baseline index for the amount of functional improvement a patient can expect after heart transplant based on the assessment of oxygen consumption and duration of graded exercise in patients with heart failure.[8,9]

**TABLE 11.2    Example of modified Naughton protocol useful for exercise testing in patients with heart failure.** Stage X of this protocol is equivalent to Stage 3 of the Bruce Protocol.[10]

| STAGE (2-MINUTE INCREMENTS) | SPEED (MPH) | GRADE (%) |
|:---:|:---:|:---:|
| I | 1.0 | 0 |
| II | 1.5 | 0 |
| III | 2.0 | 3.5 |
| IV | 2.0 | 7.0 |
| V | 2.0 | 10.5 |
| VI | 3.0 | 7.5 |
| VII | 3.0 | 10.0 |
| VIII | 3.0 | 12.5 |
| IX | 3.4 | 12.0 |
| X | 3.4 | 14.0 |

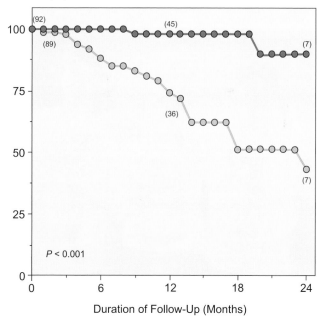

**FIGURE 11.3    Percent predicted peak $O_2$ consumption (PPVO$_2$) as a determinant of prognosis in younger patients.** Those with a PPVO$_2 \leq 50\%$ (yellow [n = 89]) had a poor prognosis compared to those with a PPVO$_2 > 50\%$ (blue [n = 92]).[7] *Source:* Adapted with permission from Stelken et al., *J Am Coll Cardiol.* 1996;27(2):345-352.

## FUNCTIONAL RECOVERY AFTER HEART TRANSPLANT

Improvement in functional capacity is an important aspect of quality of life after heart transplant. The majority of patients are NYHA class IV at the time of heart transplant.

After transplant, most patients are returned to a New York Heart Association class I functional status, although peak exercise capacity and oxygen consumption are still less than matched controls.[9] On average, peak $O_2$ consumption with exercise improves over the first 6 months after heart transplantation.[9] Greater increases in peak $O_2$ consumption will be achieved by patients who participate in a structured cardiac-rehabilitation program.[11]

Following heart transplant, patients have an increased resting heart rate of 80–120 bpm. This reflects the denervated state of the heart and the absence of parasympathetic innervation that normally lowers the resting heart rate. Nevertheless, with exercise, further increases in heart rate are achieved by the delivery of catecholamines to the heart via the circulation. In a multivariate analysis, younger age, higher peak heart rate, lower body mass index, and better diastolic function were independent predictors of peak $O_2$ consumption with exercise after transplant.[12] In younger recipients without significant comorbidities, remarkable physical endurance achievements can be achieved (Figure 11.4).

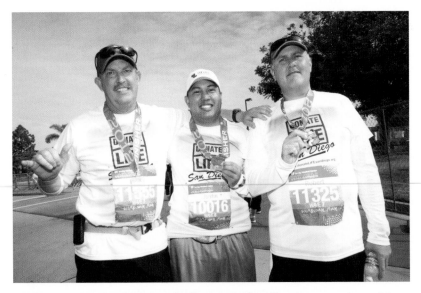

**FIGURE 11.4   Functional recovery after heart transplant.** Three heart transplant recipients (ages 52, 29, and 45 years) after completing the first of 3 half marathons in 2012. Recipients were 1.8, 2.8, and 3.3 years post heart transplant, respectively.

**History of Cardiac Transplant Procedures and Immunosuppressive Therapies**

| Year | Event |
|------|-------|
| 1906 | Carrel: Proposed heart transplant techniques |
| 1960 | Shumway: Dog model of orthotopic transplant |
| 1967 | Bernard: Successful heart transplant in man |
| 1968 | Shumway: Successful heart transplant in the United States |
| 1972 | Endomyocardial biopsy |
| 1977 | Distant donor heart procurement |
| 1980 | Cyclosporine-A |
| 1991 | Tacrolimus |
| 1998 | Mycophenolate mofetil |
| 2003 | Sirolimus/everolimus |

## CAUSE OF DEATH FOLLOWING CARDIAC TRANSPLANT

Cardiac transplant is currently an established therapeutic intervention limited by the availability of donor organs. The number of heart transplants worldwide reported to the International Society of Heart and Lung Transplant (ISHLT) has plateaued at 4096 in 2011. The ISHLT registry unadjusted 1-year and estimated 5-year survival rates were 84% and 73% for the 2006 to 2011 cohort.[13] Median survival from the 1992–2001 era was 10.7 years (Figure 11.5).[13] Current options for long-term immunosuppression include the use of mycophenolate mofetil, tacrolimus, sirolimus, and everolimus.[14]

Primary etiologies of patient death following heart transplant vary as the postoperative time lengthens.[13] During the first month, graft failure due to either nonimmune mechanisms or rejection with or without inflammatory myocardial cell infiltrates predominates.[13] The ISHLT has established a grading system for acute cellular rejection (Figure 11.6). Between 1 month and 12 months, infection and rejection are major reasons for patient death. After 1 year, graft coronary atherosclerosis, malignancy, and nonspecific graft failure become leading causes of death. Characteristic malignancies for the patient on chronic immunosuppression include lymphoma, lung cancer, and rapidly progressive skin cancers.[15]

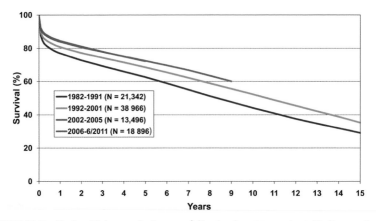

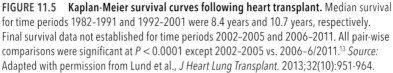

**FIGURE 11.5 Kaplan-Meier survival curves following heart transplant.** Median survival for time periods 1982–1991 and 1992–2001 were 8.4 years and 10.7 years, respectively. Final survival data not established for time periods 2002–2005 and 2006–2011. All pair-wise comparisons were significant at $P < 0.0001$ except 2002–2005 vs. 2006-6/2011.[13] *Source:* Adapted with permission from Lund et al., *J Heart Lung Transplant.* 2013;32(10):951-964.

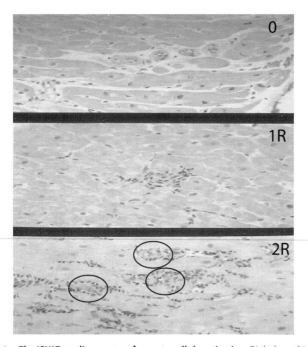

**FIGURE 11.6 The ISHLT grading system for acute cellular rejection.** Right-heart biopsy samples post cardiac transplant:
Grade 0 – no rejection.
Grade 1 R, mild – Interstitial and/or perivascular infiltrate with up to one focus of myocyte damage.
Grade 2 R, moderate – two or more foci (ovals) of infiltrate with associated myocyte damage.
Grade 3 R, severe (not shown) – diffuse infiltrate with multifocal myocyte damage, with or without edema, hemorrhage, or vasculitis.

# Left Ventricular Assist Device (LVAD)

The use of LVADs has become an accepted therapy for advanced heart failure patients either as a bridge or as an alternative to cardiac transplant (destination therapy). With the patient at rest, the systemic circulation flows almost entirely from the left ventricular apex through the LVAD (serving as a pump in series) to the aorta with only intermittent left ventricular parallel ejection of blood through the native aortic valve. With greater contractility and loading of the left ventricle with exercise, however, blood from the left ventricle reaches the aorta both through the LVAD and also via a consistently in-parallel circuit through the native aortic valve.[16]

Older pulsatile flow LVADs were restricted by large size and limited durability. In comparison, current rotational smaller pumps provide continuous blood flow (Figure 11.7). Routinely, nonpulsatile brachial artery pressure can be estimated with a blood pressure cuff and cutaneous Doppler flow probe. Nevertheless, in approximately 50% of patients, residual left ventricular contraction can contribute phasically to LVAD flow, allowing accurate blood pressure measurement with an automated cuff.[17]

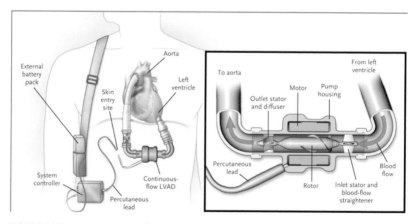

**FIGURE 11.7    HeartMate II Left Ventricular Assist Device (LVAD).** This implanted device provides continuous axial flow to the systemic circulation. Inset showing the components and direction of blood flow.[18] *Source:* Adapted with permission from Miller et al., *N Engl J Med.* 2007;357(9):885-896.

As of 2014, the largest worldwide experience for LVAD therapy has been with the continuous axial flow HeartMate II pump (Figure 11.7) with over 18,000 implants (personal communication, Thoratec Corporation, Pleasanton, CA). The device consists of an inflow conduit surgically attached to the left ventricular apex and an outflow conduit anastomosed to the ascending aorta. Oxygenated blood from the lungs passes through the left ventricle, and is continuously drawn from the ventricular apex into the internal axial-flow blood pump, through the inflow conduit. It is then pumped (by the spinning of the rotor via the outflow conduit) into the ascending aorta where it enters the systemic circulation. The pump itself is placed within the abdominal wall or peritoneal cavity. A percutaneous lead, via an electrical cable, connects the pump to an external systemic controller and battery packs worn on supporting clothing.

**BRIDGE TO TRANSPLANT: INCLUSION CRITERIA – LVAD (HEARTMATE II)**

- Eligible for transplant
- Body surface area (BSA) ≥ 1.2 m²
- New York Heart Association (NYHA) class IV heart symptoms
- On inotropic support, if tolerated, with progressive end-organ dysfunction

## BRIDGE TO TRANSPLANT

Miller et al. assessed the HeartMate II continuous flow pumps LVAD as a bridge to heart transplant in 133 patients. The primary composite endpoint was survival with transplant, cardiac recovery, or continued LVAD support still eligible for transplant. At 6 months post device implantation, 75% of the patients had achieved one of these outcomes (Figure 11.8).[18]

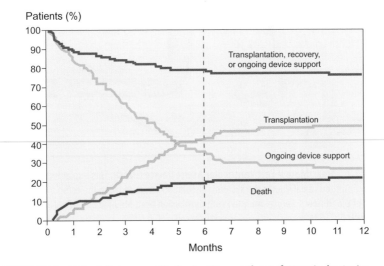

**FIGURE 11.8   Patient Outcomes with the Continuous-Flow Left Ventricular Assist Device.** LVAD was implanted as an intended bridge to transplant. Over three-quarters of patients (blue line) were living at 6 months with little change at 12 months.[18] *Source:* Adapted with permission from Miller et al., *N Engl J Med.* 2007;357(9):885-896.

## LVAD DESTINATION THERAPY

For many with Stage D heart failure, heart transplant may not be a viable option due to contraindications to immunosuppressive therapy and a limited number of donor organs. For these patients, LVADs can serve as a permanent or destination therapy. In the REMATCH trial, 129 patients with NYHA class IV heart failure were randomly assigned to receive either a pulsatile LVAD or optimal medical management. Compared to the group that received medical therapy, LVADs reduced the 2-year risk of death from any cause by 48%.[19]

Subsequently, Slaughter et al. compared the two LVAD design models (pulsatile vs. continuous-flow devices) for efficacy when used as a destination therapy. In this study, 134 patients received a HeartMate II continuous-flow device, while 66 patients received the pulsatile-flow device used in the previous REMATCH trial (Figure 11.9). After a 2-year follow up, adverse events and device failures were significantly less, and survival greater, in the group that received the continuous-flow support.[20] One- and 2-year survival rates with the continuous-flow pump were 68% and 58%, respectively.

**INCLUSION CRITERIA— LVAD DESTINATION THERAPY**

- Ineligible for cardiac transplant
- Patients with advanced and unacceptable heart failure symptoms (NYHA class IIIB or class IV) despite maximum medical and pacemaker/defibrillation therapy
- Left ventricular ejection fraction ≤ 25%
- Peak $VO_2$ consumption < 14 mL/kg/min or < 50% of predicted $VO_{2max}$ with attainment of anaerobic threshold (AT, RER > 1.0), if not contraindicated due to IV inotropes, angina or physical disability
- Body surface area (BSA) > 1.2 m$^2$

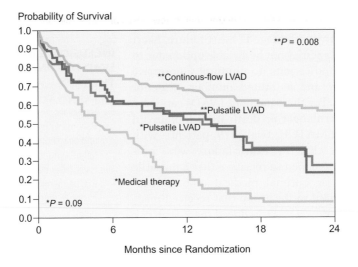

**FIGURE 11.9** **Comparing patient survival from 2 randomized trials following LVAD implantation.** Comparison between survival over time for patients implanted with either a continuous- or pulsatile-flow device, or patients receiving optimal medical therapy. Note: Curves labeled (*) represent data from the 2001 REMATCH Trial,[19] and *P = 0.09 refers to that comparison. Curves labeled (**) represent data from the 2009 HMII Destination Therapy trial by Slaughter et al., and **P = 0.008 refers to that study's data.[20] Survival outcomes with the pulsatile LVAD were very similar despite being from different trials. The 2-year survival with the HMII of 58% is compared to that with medical therapy of 8%.[21] *Source:* Adapted with permission from Fang JC, *N Engl J Med.* 2009;361(23):2282-2285.

## COMPLICATIONS OF LVAD THERAPY

Following LVAD implantation, the patient can be considered to have a combined LVAD-heart complex[16] and potential problems can arise from either component. Important limitations of the LVAD include possible mechanical failure of the device, neurologic complications, infection, and postoperative bleeding. Patients can have persistent right-heart failure despite optimal LVAD function. Adverse events, especially need for pump replacement, are significantly less with the continuous-flow device than the earlier use of a pulsatile pump design (Table 11.3). The presence of aortic insufficiency represents a unique problem for patients with an LVAD, which can lead to recirculation of blood flow through the pump without contribution to systemic perfusion. When needed, aortic valve closure in LVAD-supported patients is safe and well tolerated either at the time of LVAD implant or subsequently.[22]

TABLE 11.3    Adverse events of continuous flow versus pulsatile flow LVAD.[20]

| EVENT TYPE | CONTINUOUS-FLOW LVAD (n = 133) (211 PATIENT–YEARS) | | PULSATILE-FLOW LVAD (n = 59) (41 PATIENT–YEARS) | |
|---|---|---|---|---|
| | NO. (%) | NO. OF EVENTS/ PATIENT–YR | NO. (%) | NO. OF EVENTS/ PATIENT–YR |
| PUMP REPLACEMENT | 12 (9) | 0.06 | 20 (34) | 0.51 |
| STROKE | 24 (18) | 0.13 | 8 (14) | 0.22 |
| ISCHEMIC | 11 (8) | 0.06 | 4 (7) | 0.10 |
| HEMORRHAGIC | 15 (11) | 0.07 | 5 (8) | 0.12 |
| LVAD-RELATED INFECTION | 47 (35) | 0.48 | 21 (36) | 0.90 |
| LOCAL NON-LVAD INFECTION | 65 (49) | 0.76 | 27 (46) | 1.33 |
| SEPSIS | 48 (36) | 0.39 | 26 (44) | 1.11 |
| BLEEDING | | | | |
| BLEEDING REQUIRING PRBC | 108 (81) | 1.66 | 45 (76) | 2.45 |
| BLEEDING REQUIRING SURGERY | 40 (30) | 0.23 | 9 (15) | 0.29 |
| OTHER NEUROLOGIC EVENT | 29 (22) | 0.17 | 10 (17) | 0.29 |
| RIGHT HEART FAILURE | | | | |
| MANAGED WITH EXTENDED USE OF INOTROPES | 27 (20) | 0.14 | 16 (27) | 0.46 |
| MANAGED WITH RVAD | 5 (4) | 0.02 | 3 (5) | 0.07 |
| CARDIAC ARRHYTHMIA | 75 (56) | 0.69 | 35 (59) | 1.31 |
| RESPIRATORY FAILURE | 50 (38) | 0.31 | 24 (41) | 0.80 |
| RENAL FAILURE | 21 (16) | 0.10 | 14 (24) | 0.34 |
| HEPATIC DYSFUNCTION | 3 (2) | 0.01 | 0 | 0.00 |
| LVAD THROMBOSIS | 5 (4) | 0.02 | 0 | 0.00 |
| REHOSPITALIZATION | 107 (94) | 2.64 | 42 (96) | 4.25 |

## PREOPERATIVE RISK EVALUATIONS FOR LVAD

A preoperative risk score has been developed in over 1000 patients receiving the HeartMate II LVAD from a multivariate analysis that found higher 90-day mortality in older patients, those with more severe hypoalbuminemia, renal dysfunction, and elevated prothrombin time.[23] In a single center study, Adamson et al. retrospectively assessed the outcomes of patients with NYHA class IV implanted with the HeartMate II LVAD divided into two groups: group 1 ≥70 years versus group 2 <70 years.[24]

Survival to 24 months was similar between the 2 groups. Older patients showed the same improvement in quality of life metrics and had a similar frequency of adverse events. Thus, in *selected* older patients, LVAD support as destination therapy may provide similar benefit as for younger recipients (Figure 11.10).[24]

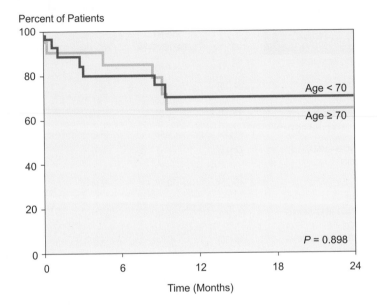

**FIGURE 11.10   Kaplan-Meier Analysis of Survival after LVAD implantation stratified by age of patient.** Comparison between the group of patients ≥ 70 years (*n* = 30) vs. those < 70 years (*n* = 25) that received LVAD at Sharp Memorial Hospital.[24] *Source:* Adapted with permission from Adamson et al., *J Am Coll Cardiol.* 2011;57(25):2487-2495.

The Interagency Registry for Mechanically Assisted Circulatory Support (INTERMACS) classification divides patients who may benefit from LVAD placement into subgroups based on clinical scenario and operative risk (Profile 1–7), with Profile 1 having the highest operative risk (Table 11.4). The classification also suggests an optimal time frame for the intervention for each subgroup.

**TABLE 11.4   INTERMACS Classification of Candidates for LVAD therapy.**[25] Interagency Registry for Mechanically Assisted Circulatory Support (INTERMACS) patient profiles and timeframe for LVAD intervention. *May not require an LVAD if other interventions could lead to reversal of clinical profiles: For example, revascularization, temporary percutaneous support device; Presence of life threatening ventricular arrhythmias may accelerate the time frame for intervention.

| INTERMACS PROFILE DESCRIPTION | TIME FRAME FOR INTERVENTION /LVAD* |
|---|---|
| **Profile 1:** Critical cardiogenic shock–*"Crash and Burn"* | Within hours |
| **Profile 2:** Progressive decline on **inotropic support**–*"Sliding on Inotropes"* | Within a few days |
| **Profile 3:** Stable but inotrope dependent–*"Dependent Stability"* | Over a period of weeks |
| **Profile 4:** Resting symptoms–Recurrent **advanced heart failure** | Over a period of weeks to a few months |
| **Profile 5:** Exertion intolerant | Variable |
| **Profile 6:** Exertion limited–*"Walking Wounded"* | Variable |
| **Profile 7:** Advanced NYHA III–Patients are clinically stable and indulging in meaningful activity, limited to mild physical exertion with a history of decompensation | Not currently indicated |

Boyle et al. assessed patient outcomes following LVAD placement based on 3 simplified groupings of preoperative INTERMACS profiles: Group 1, progressive cardiogenic shock despite inotropes (INTERMACS Profile 1); Group 2, inotrope-dependent (INTERMACS Profile 2 or 3); and Group 3, not on inotropes (INTERMACS Profiles 4 to 7). The sicker patients in Group 1 had a lower survival to hospital discharge (70.4%) compared with Group 2 (93.8%) or Group 3 (95.8%). However, after hospital discharge, long-term survival rates for patients in the intermediate Group 2 began to decline and approached the lower survival in Group 1, while the less sick Group 3 maintained a high survival rate (Figure 11.11). Although the study is consistent with all groups achieving better survival with LVAD than their expected survival with medical therapy, it suggests that LVAD patient selection should, if possible, identify candidates for therapy before they reach the stage of inotrope-dependent heart failure.[26]

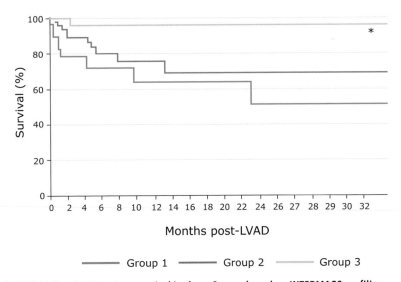

**FIGURE 11.11    LVAD post-op survival in three Groups based on INTERMACS profiling.**
Group 1 (progressive cardiogenic shock despite inotropes), Group 2 (inotrope-dependent) and Group 3 (not on inotropes). Note: See text for groupings of INTERMAC profile categories. Asterisk (*) indicates $P < 0.05$ in Group 3 vs. Group 1.[26] *Source:* Adapted with permission from Boyle et al., *J Heart Lung Transplant.* 2011;30(4):402-407.

## OTHER LVADS

The HeartWare LVAD, an alternative continuous-flow LVAD with a centrifugal design (Figure 11.12), was found noninferior to the HeartMate II as a bridge to transplant device in a national registry, the ADVANCE trial.[27] Aaronson et al. compared 140 patients implanted with the HeartWare device to 499 patients enrolled in INTERMACS as the control. Within the INTERMACS group, 95% of the patients were implanted with continuous-flow pumps. After a 180-day follow-up, the primary endpoint, survival after implantation, transplant or recovery, occurred in 90.7% of patients who received the HeartWare and 90.1% of patients in the INTERMACS registry.[27]

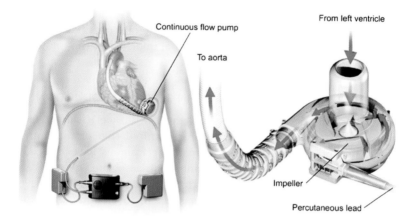

**FIGURE 11.12   HeartWare left ventricular assist device.**[27] *Source:* Adapted with permission from Aaronson et al., *Circulation.* 2012;125(25):3191-3200.

## NEW TECHNOLOGY

It is anticipated that human trials will begin soon with approved LVAD platforms that can be totally internally implanted and powered by wireless transcutaneously charged batteries. This will eliminate the current percutaneous drivelines, which are inconvenient and an ongoing portal for infection.

# Investigational Therapy

## STEM CELL THERAPY

The regeneration of heart tissue via resident, endogenous, or exogenous stem cells, or myoblasts, has been an area of intense basic and clinical research. Although interventions such as bone marrow transplantation provide supporting evidence for the use of cellular therapeutic strategies, challenges remain when applying these treatments for cardiovascular disease. Cardiac tissue possesses a highly structured cellular architecture. The heart is constantly changing and responding to various stimuli, injury, and dynamic demands, inducing the heart to change its geometric shape (see Chapter 4). Overall, controlled trials have shown small but not consistent improvements in cardiac function with administration of cardiac progenitor cells via intravenous, intracoronary, or intramural ventricular routes.[28] When stem cell mechanisms are better understood, it is conceivable that entire immune-identical or nonantigenic heart organs could be created ex vivo for individual implants, with minimal or no need for immunosuppressive therapies.

## GENE THERAPY TO AUGMENT PROTEIN SERCA2a PRODUCTION

Historically, gene therapies have been plagued with skepticism and ethical concerns regarding the potential for manipulation of the human genome. Recent advances in gene transfer techniques have helped to address these concerns. The recombinant adeno-associated virus (rAAV) has been one of the most successful transfer agents because it is derived from common viruses that already have some history of previous exposure to 90% of adults. Unlike earlier intact adenovirus vectors, rAAV vectors are entirely synthetic, nonreplicating, have minimal immunogenicity, and establish stable long-term transgene expression. They allow introduction of functional DNA into the myocyte nucleus as a circular exosome without integration into the cell's chromosomes.[29]

A common feature in patients with advanced systolic dysfunction (HF-rEF) of multiple etiologies is reduced mRNA and protein expression of the calcium cycling protein, sarco(endo)plasmic reticulum (SR) $Ca^{2+}$ ATPase2a (SERCA2a) (see Chapter 4).[30] In animal models of heart failure, restoration of intracellular calcium trafficking via SERCA2a gene transfer using rAAV vectors, restores contractile deficiency, reduces myocardial oxygen consumption, and decreases ventricular arrhythmias.[31]

Recent clinical trials in heart failure patients have allowed similar correction of SERCA2a deficiencies by gene transfer in patients with NYHA class III or IV heart failure.[32] In a small dose ranging study, the Calcium Up-Regulation by Percutaneous Administration of Gene Therapy In Cardiac Disease (CUPID) trial, 39 patients were randomized to receive a single dose of intracoronary rAAV-SERCA2a or placebo.[33] In patients who received the highest dose of the gene transfer therapy, over a 12-month period, ejection fraction trended higher and clinical events were lower (Figure 11.13). No significant safety issues related to gene therapy were found. Currently, larger trials are in progress to assess whether these findings can be confirmed.

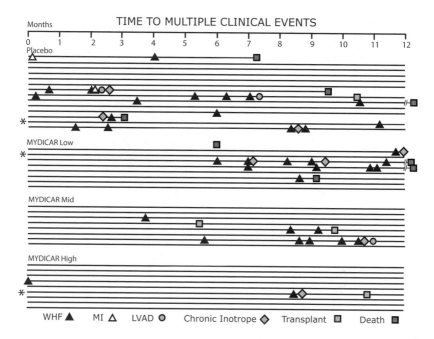

**FIGURE 11.13    SERCA2a gene therapy (MYDICAR) and reduction of clinical events based on dose response.** Fewer events in the MYDICAR high-dose arm (bottom) were seen. Intermediate or delayed onset of clinical events were seen in the low- and mid-dose MYDICAR patients compared to placebo. Clinical events are depicted by symbols, and events occurring after 12 months are indicated after a hash sign (///). Each line represents a single patient whose cumulative follow-up of the active observation period plus long-term follow-up is depicted. An asterisk at the beginning of a line represents a patient with anti-AAV1 neutralizing antibody titer that was < 1:2 during screening but ≥ 1:2 at baseline. WHF indicates worsening heart failure; MI, myocardial infarction; LVAD, left ventricular assist device.[33] *Source:* Adapted with permission from Jessup et al., *Circulation.* 2011;124(3):304-313.

# NORMAN EDWARD SHUMWAY, MD, PhD
### (1923–2006)

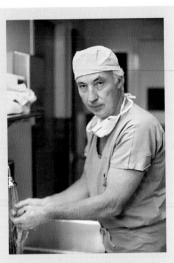

*"Inspirational leader and guiding spirit who made heart transplants a reality."*

—Senator Bill Frist, MD

On January 6, 1968 at Stanford University in Palo Alto, CA, after more than 10 years of experimental heart transplant surgery in animals, Dr. Norman Shumway performed the first human heart transplant in the United States, shortly after the world's first human heart transplantation was conducted by Dr. Christian Barnard in South Africa.

Despite the high death rate of early heart transplant surgeries, Dr. Shumway remained dedicated to the procedure through years in which many surgical centers stopped attempting it. Under his direction, Stanford rose to become the international leader in heart transplant. He and his team refined the operation, introduced the use of transvenous cardiac biopsy to recognize rejection, and pioneered the use of immune-suppressive medications such as cyclosporine to prevent organ rejection. His center's development of an effective method of distant donor heart transportation using topical hypothermia markedly increased the number of organs available for cardiac transplant.

Colleagues knew Dr. Shumway as a dedicated mentor with a unique sense of humor. He trained many of today's leaders in cardiac transplant, including one of his children, who is a heart transplant surgeon at the University of Minnesota. His many honors include being given the title "Honorary President for Life" by the International Society for Heart and Lung Transplantation.

# References

1. Teuteberg JJ, Lewis EF, Nohria A, et al. Characteristics of patients who die with heart failure and a low ejection fraction in the new millennium. *J Card Fail.* 2006;12(1): 47-53.

2. Kittleson M, Hurwitz S, Shah MR, et al. Development of circulatory-renal limitations to angiotensin-converting enzyme inhibitors identifies patients with severe heart failure and early mortality. *J Am Coll Cardiol.* 2003;41(11):2029-2035.

3. Stevenson LW, Kormos RL. Mechanical cardiac support 2000: current applications and future trial design. *J Heart Lung Transplant.* 2001;20(1):1-38.

4. Adler ED, Goldfinger JZ, Kalman J, Park ME, Meier DE. Palliative care in the treatment of advanced heart failure. *Circulation.* 2009;120(25):2597-2606.

5. Anker SD, Ponikowski P, Varney S, et al. Wasting as independent risk factor for mortality in chronic heart failure. *Lancet.* 1997;349(9058):1050-1053.

6. Mancini DM, Eisen H, Kussmaul W, Mull R, Edmunds LH, Jr., Wilson JR. Value of peak exercise oxygen consumption for optimal timing of cardiac transplantation in ambulatory patients with heart failure. *Circulation.* 1991;83(3):778-786.

7. Stelken AM, Younis LT, Jennison SH, et al. Prognostic value of cardiopulmonary exercise testing using percent achieved of predicted peak oxygen uptake for patients with ischemic and dilated cardiomyopathy. *J Am Coll Cardiol.* 1996;27(2):345-352.

8. Jaski BE. *Basics of Heart Failure: A Problem Solving Approach.* Boston: Kluwer Academic Publishers; 2000.

9. Jaski BE, Lingle RJ, Kim J, et al. Comparison of functional capacity in patients with end-stage heart failure following implantation of a left ventricular assist device versus heart transplantation: results of the experience with left ventricular assist device with exercise trial. *J Heart Lung Transpl.* 1999;18(11):1031-1040.

10. Fletcher GF, Balady GJ, Amsterdam EA, et al. Exercise standards for testing and training: a statement for healthcare professionals from the American Heart Association. *Circulation.* 2001;104(14):1694-1740.

11. Kobashigawa JA, Leaf DA, Lee N, et al. A controlled trial of exercise rehabilitation after heart transplantation. *N Engl J Med.* 1999;340(4):272-277.

12. Roten L, Schmid JP, Merz F, et al. Diastolic dysfunction of the cardiac allograft and maximal exercise capacity. *J Heart Lung Transplant.* 2009;28(5):434-439.

13. Lund LH, Edwards LB, Kucheryavaya AY, et al. The Registry of the International Society for Heart and Lung Transplantation: thirtieth official adult heart transplant report—2013; focus theme: age. *J Heart Lung Transplant.* 2013;32(10):951-964.

14. Mentzer RM, Jr., Jahania MS, Lasley RD. Tacrolimus as a rescue immunosuppressant after heart and lung transplantation. The U.S. Multicenter FK506 Study Group. *Transplantation.* 1998;65(1):109-113.

15. Adamson R, Obispo E, Dychter S, et al. High incidence and clinical course of aggressive skin cancer in heart transplant patients: a single-center study. *Transplant Proc.* 1998;30(4):1124-1126.

16. Jaski BE, Kim J, Maly RS, et al. Effects of exercise during long-term support with a left ventricular assist device. Results of the experience with left ventricular assist device with exercise (EVADE) pilot trial. *Circulation.* 1997;95(10):2401-2406.

17. Bennett MK, Roberts CA, Dordunoo D, Shah A, Russell SD. Ideal methodology to assess systemic blood pressure in patients with continuous-flow left ventricular assist devices. *J Heart Lung Transplant.* 2010;29(5):593-594.

18. Miller LW, Pagani FD, Russell SD, et al. Use of a continuous-flow device in patients awaiting heart transplantation. *N Engl J Med.* 2007;357(9):885-896.

19. Rose EA, Gelijns AC, Moskowitz AJ, et al. Long-term use of a left ventricular assist device for end-stage heart failure. *N Engl J Med.* 2001;345(20):1435-1443.

20. Slaughter MS, Rogers JG, Milano CA, et al. Advanced heart failure treated with continuous-flow left ventricular assist device. *N Engl J Med.* 2009;361(23):2241-2251.

21. Fang JC. Rise of the machines—left ventricular assist devices as permanent therapy for advanced heart failure. *N Engl J Med.* 2009;361(23):2282-2285.

22. Adamson RM, Dembitsky WP, Baradarian S, et al. Aortic valve closure associated with HeartMate left ventricular device support: technical considerations and long-term results. *J Heart Lung Transplant.* 2011;30(5):576-582.

23. Cowger J, Sundareswaran K, Rogers JG, et al. Predicting survival in patients receiving continuous flow left ventricular assist devices: the HeartMate II risk score. *J Am Coll Cardiol.* 2013;61(3):313-321.

24. Adamson RM, Stahovich M, Chillcott S, et al. Clinical strategies and outcomes in advanced heart failure patients older than 70 years of age receiving the HeartMate II left ventricular assist device: a community hospital experience. *J Am Coll Cardiol.* 2011;57(25):2487-2495.

25. Stevenson LW, Pagani FD, Young JB, et al. INTERMACS profiles of advanced heart failure: the current picture. *J Heart Lung Transplant.* 2009;28(6):535-541.

26. Boyle AJ, Ascheim DD, Russo MJ, et al. Clinical outcomes for continuous-flow left ventricular assist device patients stratified by pre-operative INTERMACS classification. *J Heart Lung Transplant.* 2011;30(4):402-407.

27. Aaronson KD, Slaughter MS, Miller LW, et al. Use of an intrapericardial, continuous-flow, centrifugal pump in patients awaiting heart transplantation. *Circulation.* 2012;125(25):3191-3200.

28. Rasmussen TL, Raveendran G, Zhang J, Garry DJ. Getting to the heart of myocardial stem cells and cell therapy. *Circulation.* 2011;123(16):1771-1779.

29. Hajjar RJ, Zsebo K, Deckelbaum L, et al. Design of a phase 1/2 trial of intracoronary administration of AAV1/SERCA2a in patients with heart failure. *J Card Fail.* 2008; 14(5):355-367.

30. Ginsburg R, Bristow MR, Billingham ME, Stinson EB, Schroeder JS, Harrison DC. Study of the normal and failing isolated human heart: decreased response of failing heart to isoproterenol. *Am Heart J.* 1983;106(3):535-540.

31. Kranias EG, Hajjar RJ. Modulation of cardiac contractility by the phospholamban/SERCA2a regulatome. *Circ Res.* 2012;110(12):1646-1660.

32. Jaski BE, Jessup ML, Mancini DM, et al. Calcium upregulation by percutaneous administration of gene therapy in cardiac disease (CUPID Trial), a first-in-human phase 1/2 clinical trial. *J Card Fail.* 2009;15(3):171-181.

33. Jessup M, Greenberg B, Mancini D, et al. Calcium Upregulation by Percutaneous Administration of Gene Therapy in Cardiac Disease (CUPID): a phase 2 trial of intracoronary gene therapy of sarcoplasmic reticulum Ca$^{2+}$-ATPase in patients with advanced heart failure. *Circulation.* 2011;124(3):304-313.

# CHAPTER 12

# A Patient-Oriented Perspective to the 4 Stages of Heart Failure

## FAST FACTS

- A patient-oriented lifestyle and education program can provide a foundation for living with heart failure.

- Pharmacologic and interventional therapies are added as needed to assist the patient in improving quality of life and extending long-term survival.

- The HF-ACTION trial demonstrated that a moderate exercise program was safe for patients with heart failure and associated with improvements in functional capacity.

- Dietary sodium restriction is appropriate for most patients with Stage C or D heart failure.

- Multidisciplinary outpatient monitoring of symptoms, weights, and other physiologic signals may complement traditional clinical management.

- Attention to the Stages of Heart Failure designation can provide a basis for selection of evidence-based therapies.

*"For the secret of the care of the patient is in caring for the patient."*

—Francis Peabody[1]

# Lifestyle Recommendations

## OUTPATIENT COUNSELING AND EDUCATION

Patient education includes symptom recognition, medication instruction, heart physiology basics, causes of heart failure, and diagnostic testing. Written materials to reinforce verbal instruction are often included. Patients or their families should also know where to get additional information if desired. The Internet represents an increasingly accessible medium for obtaining information regarding all aspects of heart failure conditions and treatment (for example, www.heartfailure.org; Figure 12.1). Involvement of the patient's family in education and discussions of prognosis is important, because lack of emotional support is a predictor of subsequent cardiovascular events.[2]

## WORD CHOICE THAT EMPOWERS THE PATIENT

Some of the terminology that is commonplace for physicians can be frightening and intimidating for patients with no medical background. The word "failure" carries a huge burden of connotation that implies a total collapse of the heart, or even worse, a sense of personal failure regarding health. In the Introduction to this book, the word "insufficiency" was suggested as a better description of the actual clinical situation. Heart failure is primarily a mismatch between the needs of the body for circulation and the ability of the heart to pump oxygenated blood. Using "mismatch" implies that there are almost always hygienic and medical interventions to make the situation better, and suggests that balance can be restored.

## EXERCISE

Whenever possible, patients should be encouraged to walk on level ground for 20 to 40 minutes or the equivalent, with rest breaks as needed, 4–5 days per week. Some patients may benefit from a structured cardiac rehabilitation program with supervised exercise. Regular exercise leads to long-term decreases in heart rate and blood pressure. For the patient with heart failure, regular exercise may serve to restore neurohormonal balance[3]—in effect a natural blockade of the aberrant neurohormonal response to long-term heart failure. This "hygienic approach" to neurohumoral withdrawal may contribute to the consistent benefit reported by studies of exercise rehabilitation in patients with heart failure (see HF-ACTION study on next page).

Patients with heart failure often have abnormalities of skeletal muscle physiology that limit their functional capacity, but that may improve with exercise.[3] Belardinelli and coworkers found that heart failure patients improved and maintained their peak oxygen consumption over a 10 year period after initiating a 2-times-a-week aerobic exercise training program at 60% baseline peak $VO_2$.[4] In non-training patients, peak $VO_2$ progressively decreased. Hare and coworkers found that patients who underwent resistance exercise targeting the chest, shoulder, and knee improved muscle strength and endurance. This type of exercise alone, however, was not associated with an improvement in peak $VO_2$.[5]

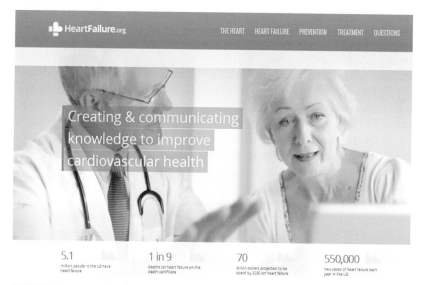

FIGURE 12.1    Example of available Internet resource: www.heartfailure.org.

In addition to improving functional capacity, a moderate exercise-training program may reduce other important endpoints in some groups of heart failure patients. The HF-ACTION trial (Heart Failure: A Controlled Trial Investigating Outcomes of exercise traiNing)[6] randomly assigned 2,331 patients (median age of 59 years, EF $\leq 35\%$) to a treatment arm consisting of usual care plus aerobic exercise training versus a treatment arm of usual care alone, with a median duration of follow-up of 30.1 months. Exercise training consisted of 36 supervised sessions followed by home-based training. After adjustment for prognostic risk factors, there was a statistically significant 15% reduction in cardiovascular mortality or heart failure hospitalization in the exercise-training group.

In the same study, patients in the exercise-training group had a greater improvement in functional capacity compared with patients in the usual-care group at 3 months of follow-up. Exercise-training patients showed improvements in median distance in the 6-minute walk test (20 meters vs. 5 meters; $P < 0.001$), exercise time on the cardiopulmonary exercise test (1.5 minutes vs. 0.3 minutes; $P < 0.001$), and peak oxygen consumption (0.6 vs. 0.2 mL $O_2$/min/kg; $P < 0.001$). Thus, HF-ACTION confirmed that moderate exercise in HF-rEF is safe and is likely associated with benefits in outcome and functional status that would improve quality of life.

## DIET

Dietary instruction, preferably by a dietitian and/or heart failure clinician, is an integral part of treatment for patients with heart failure. Depending on the severity of heart failure, a patient should restrict sodium intake to 1.5–4 grams per day. A patient's total volume of fluid intake is a secondary concern unless the patient has a decreased serum sodium concentration. In this case, a 1- to 2-liter fluid restriction should accompany a restriction of sodium intake. With heart failure due to coronary artery disease, patients should follow a diet that contributes to control of hyperlipidemia. Despite the possibility of the "obesity paradox" (Chapter 3), most clinicians recommend weight loss for patients with a Body Mass Index > 30. If heart failure is advanced, patients may actually lose muscle weight (cardiac cachexia). They may feel too weak or short of breath to prepare and eat regular meals. If patients consistently lose weight, suggest a high calorie, high-protein diet with protein-shake supplements, if needed (e.g., Boost®, Ensure®). Patients may also try eating smaller, more frequent meals. Patients should measure and record weight at regular intervals.

## OTHER RESTRICTIONS FOR OPTIMAL HEART "HYGIENE"

Alcohol depresses myocardial function. In some individuals with "idiopathic cardiomyopathy", cessation of alcohol consumption leads to a marked improvement in myocardial function. In patients with mild to moderate left ventricular dysfunction, allowance of no more than one drink per day may offset the psychological burden imposed by other lifestyle restrictions. In patients with a left ventricular ejection fraction < 30%, however, guidelines recommend total cessation of alcohol ingestion.[7] Similar recommendations apply to patients with a history of use of cardiotoxic recreational drugs.

Smoking cessation is recommended for all patients, but may be difficult. Nicotine patches, use of low doses of oral bupropion (Zyban®, Wellbutrin®), varenicline (Chantix®), or formal smoking cessation programs may help.[8]

The basic recommendations for counseling heart failure patients focus on moderate activity and a healthy diet (List 12.1).

**LIST 12.1   Dietary and Lifestyle Recommendations for Heart Failure Patients**

| ACTIVITY | RECOMMENDATION |
|---|---|
| Exercise | Walking, cycling, etc., 20–30 minutes daily |
| Sodium intake | Restrict to close to 2 to 4 grams per day |
| Fluid intake | In moderation, but less important than sodium intake |
| Calorie intake | Appropriate to achieve ideal body weight |
| Alcohol consumption | Should be discouraged; patients who drink should be advised to consume no more than 1 drink per day (1 drink equals a glass of beer or wine, or a mixed drink or cocktail containing no more than 1 ounce of alcohol) |
| Smoking | Immediate cessation |

# Outpatient Support and Monitoring

Symptoms of heart failure are potentially recurrent and disabling. New paradigms using "low-tech" approaches, including a multidisciplinary heart failure clinic, can complement "high-tech" approaches to reduce the disability associated with chronic heart failure (Figure 12.2). Programs that encourage patient education and appropriate use of medical resources can reduce patient symptoms and possibly improve long-term outcome.

An advanced-practice nurse clinician, as a team member who is focused on clinical issues affecting the heart failure patient, can provide care beyond that usually achieved by a physician alone. In addition, database assessment of group patient outcomes in a clinical practice can identify trends in patient care that require additional attention.[9]

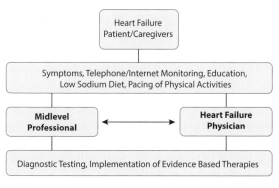

**Heart Failure Clinic**

**FIGURE 12.2   Team approach of the multidisciplinary heart failure clinic.** Comprehensive care is provided by combining high-tech and low-tech approaches to treatment.

Traditionally, telemonitoring intervention requires communication between the data-processing staff, a midlevel professional, and the physician before the patient is contacted to change therapy. Alternatively, an independent advanced-practice nurse clinician may provide more timely feedback to the patient. Ideally, in the future, patients would be empowered to assess and respond to their own physiological information.[10]

## Summary of Therapeutic Approaches to the 4 Stages of Heart Failure

Heart failure is a multifaceted condition with a natural history that progresses from early identification of risk factors to advanced disease. A variety of therapeutic options have evolved that optimize patient function at the various stages. One way to gain perspective on the overall picture is to use the workhorse analogy by Dr. Arnold Katz (Figure 12.3).

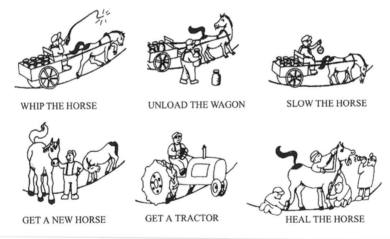

WHIP THE HORSE    UNLOAD THE WAGON    SLOW THE HORSE

GET A NEW HORSE    GET A TRACTOR    HEAL THE HORSE

**FIGURE 12.3** **The workhorse analogy for heart failure treatment.** Dr. Arnold Katz created this analogy to describe options for heart failure therapy. Whipping a tired horse up a steep hill can be viewed as a sick, failing heart. Encouraging the horse to move faster by using the whip (inotrope) can potentially harm the animal. Unloading the wagon (vasodilators) may be beneficial. Delaying the journey by slowing the horse (beta-blockers) can be helpful. Replacing the horse (heart transplant) can be advantageous, as long as there are enough spare healthy "horses." Getting a tractor (left ventricular assist device) is a solution if suitable machines are available. The ideal solution is to learn what helps heal the horse.[11] *Source:* Adapted with permission from Katz AM, *Heart failure: Pathophysiology, molecular biology, and clinical management.* Philadelphia: Lippincott Williams & Wilkins, 2000.

There are different goals and therapeutic approaches for each stage—with some overlap. Thus, it is crucial to maintain a sense of the overall natural history of the disease and the patient position on the spectrum. This has been the impetus for creating a systematic approach to heart failure treatment based on the 4 Stages of Heart Failure (Figure 12.4). Most of the therapeutic recommendations are based on clinical trial results (see Appendix B).

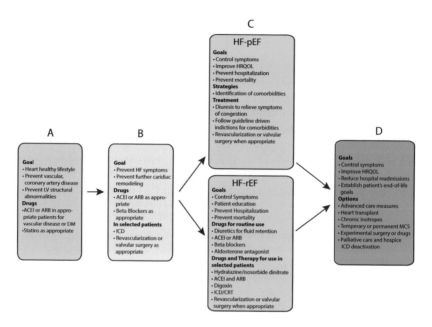

**FIGURE 12.4   Summary of therapies from the 2013 ACCF/AHA Guidelines across the 4 stages of heart failure.** Abbreviations: ACEI, angiotensin-converting enzyme inhibitor; ARB, angiotensin-2 receptor blocker; CRT, cardiac resynchronization therapy; DM, diabetes mellitus; HRQOL, health-related quality of life; ICD, implantable cardioverter-defibrillator; MCS, mechanical circulatory support.[12] *Source:* Adapted from Yancy et al., *J Am Coll Cardiol.* 2013;62(16):e147-e239, with permission.

## Concluding Comments

Heart failure is a common condition of increasing incidence that will affect over 8 million people in the United States by 2030.[13] As heart failure is a cumulative consequence of all insults to the heart and related body systems over someone's life, this book has emphasized an integrated approach to both improve symptoms and prevent progressive stages of structural heart disease. Disease management partnerships between a patient and medical team can promote understanding and compliance with regimens that at times are demanding. The challenge is heightened by the life-threatening potential of heart failure. To meet this challenge, it is hoped that the clinician will heed the call of Hippocrates to console, comfort, and cure.

# References

1. Peabody FW. The care of the patient. *JAMA.* 1927;88(12):877-882.

2. Krumholz HM, Butler J, Miller J, et al. Prognostic importance of emotional support for elderly patients hospitalized with heart failure. *Circulation.* 1998;97(10):958-964.

3. Coats AJ. Exercise training for heart failure: coming of age. *Circulation.* 1999;99(9): 1138-1140.

4. Belardinelli R, Georgiou D, Cianci G, et al. 10-year exercise training in chronic heart failure: a randomized controlled trial. *J Am Coll Cardiol.* 2012;60(16):1521-1528.

5. Hare DL, Ryan TM, Selig SE, Pellizzer AM, Wrigley TV, Krum H. Resistance exercise training increases muscle strength, endurance, and blood flow in patients with chronic heart failure. *Am J Cardiol.* 1999;83(12):1674-1677, A7.

6. O'Connor CM, Whellan DJ, Lee KL, et al. Efficacy and safety of exercise training in patients with chronic heart failure: HF-ACTION randomized controlled trial. *JAMA.* 2009;301(14):1439-1450.

7. Lang RM, Borow KM, Neumann A, Feldman T. Adverse cardiac effects of acute alcohol ingestion in young adults. *Ann Intern Med.* 1985;102(6):742-747.

8. Konstam MA, Dracup K, Baker DW. Heart failure: evaluation and care of patients with left ventricular systolic dysfunction. *J Card Fail.* 1995;1(2):183-186.

9. Rich MW, Beckham V, Wittenberg C, Leven CL, Freedland KE, Carney RM. A multidisciplinary intervention to prevent the readmission of elderly patients with congestive heart failure. *N Engl J Med.* 1995;333(18):1190-1195.

10. Desai AS, Stevenson LW. Connecting the circle from home to heart-failure disease management. *N Engl J Med.* 2010;363(24):2364-2367.

11. Katz AM. *Heart Failure: Pathophysiology, Molecular Biology, and Clinical Management.* Philadelphia: Lippincott Williams & Wilkins, 2000: xvi, 381.

12. Yancy CW, Jessup M, Bozkurt B, et al. 2013 ACCF/AHA guideline for the management of heart failure: A report from the American College of Cardiology Foundation/ American Heart Association Task Force on Practice Guidelines. *J Am Coll Cardiol.* 2013;62(16):e147–e239.

13. Heidenreich PA, Albert NM, Allen LA, et al. Forecasting the impact of heart failure in the United States: a policy statement from the American Heart Association. *Circ Heart Fail.* 2013;6(3):606-619.

# Glossary

## A

**abdominojugular reflux.** Neck vein distention observed when pressing firmly on the upper mid-abdomen.

**aldosterone.** A steroid hormone of the mineralocorticoid family released from the adrenal cortex of the adrenal gland.

**anasarca.** Severe generalized edema.

**angiotensin converting enzyme inhibitor.** A medication class that blocks the angiotensin converting enzyme from producing angiotensin II.

**angiotensin II.** A peptide hormone that causes vasoconstriction and other cellular effects. Angiotensin converting enzyme converts angiotensin I to angiotensin II (the active hormone).

**angiotensin II receptor blocker.** A medication class that blocks the binding of angiotensin II to its receptor.

**apoptosis.** Programmed cell death (in contrast to necrosis).

**autophagy.** An intracellular catabolic mechanism that utilizes lysosomes to degrade unnecessary or dysfunctional cellular components.

## B

**β-adrenergic receptor blocker.** A medication class that blocks the action of catecholamines on the heart and other tissues; also called "beta-blockers."

**bioavailability.** The rate and degree of a substance absorbed by a living organism or made readily available to the physiological active site.

**biomarkers.** A measurable biological molecule found in body fluids or tissues that may be used to indicate a specific biological state or condition.

**biphasic positive airway pressure (BiPAP).** Pressure-controlled ventilation allowing unrestricted, spontaneous breathing during the ventilatory cycle.

**B-type natriuretic peptide.** A 32-amino acid hormone released by ventricular myocytes used to diagnose heart failure. Also, an intravenous vasodilator, nesiritide, for treatment of acute heart failure.

# C

**cardiac output.** The amount of blood ejected by the heart per minute to the systemic circulation. In the absence of significant valvular regurgitation or cardiovascular shunts, this quantity equals the heart rate (bpm) multiplied by the stroke volume.

**cardiogenic shock.** Heart failure with severe systemic hypoperfusion, usually with hypotension and pulmonary edema.

**cardiomegaly.** The medical condition of an enlarged heart stemming from various etiologies.

**Cheyne-Stokes respiration.** A cyclic pattern of breathing with a gradual increase in depth and sometimes in rate to a maximum, followed by a decrease (especially in rate) resulting in apnea; the cycles ordinarily are 30 seconds to 2 minutes in duration, with 5 to 30 seconds of apnea. Related to the abnormal feedback control of respiration in heart failure.

# D

**diastolic dysfunction.** Impaired ventricular filling.

# E

**ejection fraction.** The ratio of the volume ejected during systole, or stroke volume, to the end-diastolic volume for any given beat; calculated as (EDV − ESV)/EDV = SV/EDV, where EDV = end-diastolic volume, ESV = end-systolic volume, and SV = stroke volume. This parameter may also be expressed as a percentage, i.e., ejection fraction × 100.

**epigenetics.** Changes in gene expression due to activation or inactivation of certain base pairs in DNA or RNA via chemical reactions.

# F

**Frank-Starling Law of the Heart.** States that the stroke volume (SV) of the heart increases in response to an increase in left ventricular end-diastolic volume. Named after the cardiac physiologists Otto Frank (1865–1944) and Ernest Starling (1866–1927). The same principle applies to other measures of cardiac function such as cardiac output (SV × heart rate) or stroke work. Cardiac function can be adjusted for body size by dividing by body surface area. In some clinical or research settings, left ventricular end-diastolic or pulmonary capillary wedge pressures are substituted for left ventricular end-diastolic volume.

**fulminant myocarditis.** Widespread myocardial inflammation leading to acute, severe heart failure or cardiogenic shock.

# G

**genotype/phenotype.** The genetic makeup of an individual/the observable physical characteristics of an individual.

# H

**HF-pEF/HF-rEF.** Two classifications of heart failure determined by ejection fraction. Heart Failure with preserved Ejection Fraction (having an EF > 40%) and Heart Failure with reduced Ejection Fraction (having an EF ≤ 40%). In the literature, cutoffs between reduced and preserved ejection fraction range from 40%–55%.

**hypertrophy.** Increase in the size of an organ or tissue due to the enlargement of component cells.

# I

**intra-aortic balloon pump.** An intravascular balloon that is inflated and deflated in the descending thoracic aorta from a percutaneous catheter in the femoral artery that supports the systemic and coronary circulations.

**ischemia.** Tissue blood flow insufficient for cellular function.

# L

**loop diuretic.** A medication class that acts on the ascending loop of Henle of the kidney to increase the urine excretion of sodium, chloride, and water. Specific drugs include furosemide, bumetanide, torsemide, and etacrynic acid.

# M

**mineralocorticoid receptor antagonist.** A medication class that inhibits the physiological action of mineralocorticoids, such as aldosterone.

# N

**neck vein distention.** The visible pulsations of the jugular veins from either side of the neck as a result of increased venous pressure, indicating increased right atrial pressure.

**necrosis.** Unprogrammed cell or tissue death as a result of injury, radiation, or chemicals. Usually involves widespread release of toxic components contributing to additional tissue damage.

# O

**orthopnea.** Difficulty in breathing brought on or aggravated by lying flat.

**oxygen consumption (VO$_2$).** VO$_2$ equals the circulating cardiac output multiplied by the tissue oxygen extraction or $\Delta$AVO$_2$ (difference between the arterial oxygen concentration delivered to the body tissues minus the remaining oxygen concentration in the venous circulation after capillary exchange).

# P

**paroxysmal nocturnal dyspnea.** Dyspnea that appears suddenly at night, usually waking the patient after an hour or two of sleep; caused by pulmonary congestion and edema resulting from left-sided heart failure.

**phenotype.** See genotype/phenotype.

**pheochromocytoma.** A tumor of cells that secrete catecholamines

**phospholamban.** A 52-amino acid membrane protein that regulates the sarcoplasmic reticulum calcium ATPase (SERCA2a) in cardiac and skeletal muscle.

# R

**renin.** A 340-amino acid enzyme secreted by the granular cells of the juxtaglomerular apparatus of the kidney that converts angiotensinogen to angiotensin I, initiating the renin-angiotensin-aldosterone system.

# S

**sarco(endo)plasmic reticulum calcium ATPase2a (SERCA2a).** A calcium ATPase in muscle cells that translocates calcium from the cytosol to the lumen of the sarcoplasmic reticulum via ATP hydrolysis. Sufficient calcium levels in the sarcoplasmic reticulum are needed for muscle contraction.

**stroke volume.** The amount of blood ejected with each heart beat calculated as the difference between ventricular volume at end-filling (diastole) and end-contraction (systole). Also calculated as end-diastolic volume × ejection fraction.

**stroke work.** A measure of the pressure-volume work done by the heart with each contraction; an index of ventricular contractility. Stroke work may be estimated as the stroke volume × (mean arterial − ventricular end-diastolic pressure) or more simply stroke volume × mean aortic pressure.

**stroke work index.** Work of ejection expressed as units of energy/body surface area.

**structural heart disease.** Any detectable physical or biochemical abnormality of the heart's muscular, valvular, or pericardial components.

**systolic dysfunction.** Impaired ventricular contraction.

# T

**tissue oxygen extraction ($\Delta AVO_2$).** The difference between arterial and venous blood oxygen concentration.

# U

**ultrafiltration.** A method of removing isotonic fluid from blood via an extracorporeal circuit that works via convection (vacuum removal through a filter).

# V

**Valsalva.** A maneuver that requires an individual to forcefully attempt exhalation against a closed airway in order to test cardiac function.

**valvuloplasty.** The process of increasing the area of a stenotic heart valve via balloon catheter inflation.

**vasopressin.** A posterior pituitary hormone, also known as antidiuretic hormone, that acts as a vasoconstrictor and signal to increase the retention of free water by the kidney.

# Summary of Clinical Trials of Therapy

## SECTION 1: PHARMACOLOGY TRIALS

### Angiotensin Converting Enzyme (ACE) Inhibitor Trials

#### ATLAS
Assessment of Treatment with Lisinopril and Survival (*Circulation* 1999;100:2312)

**Design:** Patients with moderate to severe CHF were randomized to low-dose lisinopril (2.5–5 mg/d) or high-dose lisinopril (32.5–50 mg/d).

**Results:** Lower incidence of adverse events was found with high-dose lisinopril.

#### SOLVD PREVENTION TRIAL
Studies of Left Ventricular Dysfunction (*N Engl J Med* 1992;327:685)

**Design:** The study included 4228 asymptomatic patients with EF < 35% not receiving drug treatment for heart failure. Patients were randomized to enalapril (2.5–20 mg/d) or placebo.

**Results:** At average follow-up of 37 months, combined endpoint of death or heart failure was lower in enalapril group compared to placebo (30% vs. 39%). Fewer hospitalizations for enalapril group (21% vs. 25% for placebo).

## SOLVD TREATMENT TRIAL

Studies of Left Ventricular Dysfunction (*N Engl J Med* 1991;325:293)

**Design:** This study included 2569 patients with chronic heart failure with EF < 35% not receiving drug treatment for heart failure. Patients were randomized to enalapril (2.5–10 mg b.i.d.) or placebo.

**Results:** The results showed a lower incidence of death or hospitalization due to heart failure in enalapril group compared to placebo (48% vs. 57%).

## V-HeFT II

Veterans Administration Heart Failure Trial II (*N Engl J Med* 1991;325:303)

**Design:** In this study, 804 men with NYHA class II–III heart failure and EF < 45% were randomized to hydralazine/isordil combination (75 mg + 40 mg q.i.d.) or enalapril (10 mg b.i.d.).

**Results:** At 2 years, there was decreased mortality in enalapril compared to hydralazine/isordil group (18% vs. 28.2%). Mortality benefit due to a reduction in sudden cardiac death.

---

# Angiotensin II Receptor Blocker (ARB) Trials

---

## CHARM-ALTERNATIVE

Candesartan in Heart Failure: Assessment of Reduction in Morbidity and Mortality (*Lancet* 2003;362:772)

**Design:** In the study, 2028 patients with symptomatic heart failure, an ejection fraction ≤ 40%, and intolerant to ACE inhibitors were randomized to receive candesartan (target 32 mg once daily) or placebo.

**Results:** The study found reduced cardiovascular death or hospital admission for CHF in candesartan group compared to placebo group (33% vs. 40%).

## ELITE

Evaluation of Losartan in the Elderly (*Lancet* 1997;349:747)

**Design:** In the study, 722 patients with class II–IV CHF and EF < 40% were randomized to captopril (6.25–50 mg t.i.d.) plus placebo or losartan (12.5–50 mg/d) plus placebo.

**Results:** The study found lower mortality (4.8% vs. 8.7%), hospitalization rate (22% vs. 30%), and side effects with losartan.

## ELITE II

Effect of Losartan Compared with Captopril on Mortality in Patients with Symptomatic Heart Failure: Randomised Trial—The Losartan Heart Failure Survival Study ELITE II. (*Lancet* 2000;355(9215):1582-1587)

> **Design:** Preliminary report of 3152 patients with class II–IV CHF and EF ≤40% randomized to captopril (12.5–50 mg t.i.d.) or losartan (12.5–50 mg/d) plus placebo.
>
> **Results:** All-cause mortality showed no statistically significant difference (captopril 16% vs. losartan 18%).

## VALIANT

The Valsartan in Acute Myocardial Infarction Trial (*N Engl J Med* 2003;349:1893)

> **Design:** Patients previously receiving conventional therapy were randomly assigned, 0.5 to 10 days after MI, to receive valsartan (4909 patients), valsartan plus captopril (4885 patients), or captopril (4909 patients).
>
> **Results:** Valsartan is as effective as captopril, with similar mortality rates in each group.

---

# Beta-Blocker Trials

---

## AUSTRALIA/NEW ZEALAND HEART FAILURE RESEARCH COLLABORATIVE GROUP

Australia/New Zealand Heart Failure Research Collaborative Group (*Lancet* 1997;349:375)

> **Design:** A total of 415 patients with class II–III CHF and EF < 45% were randomized to carvedilol (6.25–25 mg b.i.d.) or placebo.
>
> **Results:** The study found an increase in EF (5.3%) and decreased mortality or hospitalization with carvedilol (104 vs. 131).

## CARVEDILOL HEART FAILURE STUDY

U.S. Carvedilol Heart Failure Study Group (*N Engl J Med* 1996;334:1349)

> **Design:** The study included 1094 patients who had symptomatic heart failure for > 3 months and EF < 35% receiving diuretics and ACE inhibitors randomized to carvedilol (12.5–50 mg b.i.d.) or placebo.
>
> **Results:** The study found lower mortality (3.2% vs. 7.8%) and hospitalization due to cardiovascular causes (14% vs. 20%) with carvedilol.

## CIBIS-II

The Cardiac Insufficiency Bisoprolol Study II (*Lancet* 1999;353:9)

**Design:** The study included 2647 patients with class III or IV CHF with LVEF ≤35% receiving standard therapy with diuretics and ACE inhibitors. Patients were randomized to bisoprolol 1.25 mg/d, increased to a maximum of 10 mg/d, or daily placebo.

**Results:** Lower all-cause mortality was found with bisoprolol than placebo (11.8% vs. 17.3%). Fewer sudden deaths occurred among patients on bisoprolol than in those on placebo. Treatment effects were independent of the severity or cause of heart failure.

## COMET

Carvedilol or Metoprolol Evaluation Trial (*Lancet* 2003;362:7)

**Design:** Patients with class II–IV CHF and EF ≤35% received treatment with carvedilol (1511 patients) 25 mg b.i.d. or metoprolol tartrate (1518) 50 mg b.i.d. Mean study duration was 58 months.

**Results:** All-cause mortality was 34% (512 of 1511) for carvedilol and 40% (600 of 1518) for metoprolol. EF treated with carvedilol increased by 9% during follow-up.

## COPERNICUS

Carvedilol Prospective Randomized Cumulative Survival Trial (*Circulation* 2002;106(17):2194)

**Design:** In this study, 2289 patients with symptoms of heart failure at rest and with an ejection fraction <25% were randomized to receive placebo (1133 patients) or carvedilol (1156 patients) for an average of 10.4 months.

**Results:** The study found that carvedilol reduced combined risk of death or hospitalization for a cardiovascular reason by 27%. Risk of death or hospitalization for heart failure was reduced by 31%.

## MERIT-HF

Metoprolol CR/XL Randomized Intervention Trial in Congestive Heart Failure (*Lancet* 1999;353:2001)

**Design:** A total of 3991 patients with class II–IV CHF and EF ≤40% were randomized to metoprolol CR/XL, with a target dose of 200 mg/q.d., or placebo.

**Results:** Lower all-cause mortality was found in the metoprolol CR/XL group than in the placebo group (7.2% vs. 11.0%). Fewer sudden deaths and deaths from worsening heart failure occurred in the metoprolol CR/XL group.

# Calcium Blocker Trials

### PRAISE-2
Prospective Randomized Amlodipine Survival Evaluation 2 Trial (*JACC Heart Failure* 2013;1:308)
>  **Design:** The study included 1654 patients with severe heart failure and EF < 30% who were randomized to amlodipine (10 mg/d target dose) or placebo.
>  **Results:** No evidence of favorable effect of amlodipine on mortality were found when results from patients with nonischemic CMP in both PRAISE and PRAISE-2 trials were combined (hazard ratio: 0.97; 95% CI: 0.83 to 1.13; *P* = 0.66)
>  (See entry in **Section 2: Device- or Procedure-Related Trials.**)

### V-HeFT III
Veterans Administration Heart Failure Trial III (*Circulation* 1997;856:863)
>  **Design:** The study followed 450 patients with CHF and EF < 45% receiving diuretics and enalapril. Patients were randomized to felodipine (5 mg b.i.d.) or placebo.
>  **Results:** Prevention of worsening exercise tolerance and worsening quality of life occurred with felodipine.

# Digoxin Trials

### DIG
Digitalis Investigation Group (*N Engl J Med* 1997;336(8):525-533)
>  **Design:** The study included 6800 patients with heart failure, sinus rhythm, and EF < 45% randomized to digoxin or placebo.
>  **Results:** No difference was found in overall mortality. Lower incidence of death or hospitalization due to worsening heart failure was found with digoxin (27% vs. 35%).

### PROVED
Prospective Randomized Study of Ventricular Failure and the Efficacy of Digoxin (*J Am Coll Cardiol* 1993;22(4):955)
>  **Design:** The study included 88 patients with mild–moderate CHF receiving digoxin (median dose 0.37 mg/d) and diuretics. Patients

were randomized to continue receiving digoxin or digoxin withdrawal for 12 weeks.

**Results:** Patients withdrawn from digoxin had decreased exercise tolerance, deterioration in ventricular function, and more frequent progression of heart failure symptoms (39% vs. 19%).

### RADIANCE

Randomized Assessment of Digoxin or Inhibitors of the Angiotensin-Converting Enzyme (*N Engl J Med* 1993;329:1)

**Design:** The study followed 178 patients in sinus rhythm, class II–III heart failure, EF < 35%, and stable on digoxin, diuretics, and ACE inhibitor were randomized to continue receiving digoxin or digoxin withdrawal for 12 weeks.

**Results:** Worsening heart failure necessitating withdrawal from study occurred more often in placebo group (25%) than in those maintained on digoxin (5%). Ventricular function also deteriorated when digoxin was withdrawn.

## Diuretic/Ultrafiltration Trials

See Diuretic/Ultrafiltration Trials in **Section 2: Device- or Procedure-Related Trials**.

## Mineralocorticoid Receptor Antagonist (MRA) Trials

### EMPHASIS-HF

Eplerenone in Mild Patients Hospitalization and Survival Study in Heart Failure (*N Engl J Med* 2011;364:11)

**Design:** In this study, 2737 patients with NYHA class II HF and EF ≤ 35% were randomly assigned to receive eplerenone (up to 50 mg daily) or placebo, in addition to recommended therapy.

**Results:** Risk of death from cardiovascular causes or hospitalization for heart failure were reduced 37% in eplerenone group. Compared to placebo, eplerenone reduced both risk of death due to cardiovascular causes (13.5% in the placebo arm vs. 10.8% in the treatment arm) and hospitalizations among patients with systolic heart failure and mild symptoms.

## EPHESUS

Eplerenone Post-Acute Myocardial Infarction Heart Failure Efficacy and Survival Study (*N Engl J Med* 2003;348:1309)

**Design:** In this study, 6632 patients after acute MI with LVEF ≤ 40% and heart failure were randomly assigned to eplerenone (25 mg/d initial dose titrated to maximum of 50 mg/d in 3313 patients) or placebo (3319 patients) in addition to optimal medical therapy, continuing until 1012 deaths occurred.

**Results:** Addition of eplerenone to optimal medical therapy reduced mortality 15%.

## RALES

Randomized Aldactone Evaluation Study Investigators (*N Engl J Med* 1999;341:709)

**Design:** In this study, 1663 patients with severe heart failure and left ventricular ejection fraction ≤ 35% who were being treated with an ACE inhibitor, a loop diuretic, and in most cases digoxin were randomized to 25 mg of spironolactone daily and to placebo.

**Results:** A 30% reduction in the risk of death was found in the spironolactone group due to a lower risk of death from progressive heart failure and sudden death. Frequency of hospitalization for worsening heart failure was 35% lower in the spironolactone group than in the placebo group. Side effects included gynecomastia in 10% of men.

# Nesiritide

## VMAC

Vasodilation in the Management of Acute CHF (*JAMA* 2002;287:1531)

**Design:** Randomized, double-blind trial of 489 patients with dyspnea at rest from CHF, 246 of whom had received pulmonary artery catheterization. Patients were treated with intravenous nesiritide, intravenous nitroglycerin, or placebo.

**Results:** Nesiritide improved hemodynamic function in patients with acutely decompensated CHF. Mean PCWP decrease from baseline of −5.8 mm Hg for nesiritide vs. −3.8 mm Hg for nitroglycerin vs. −2.0 mm Hg for placebo.

## Nitrate – Hydralazine

### A-HeFT
African-American Heart Failure Trial (*N Engl J Med* 2004;351:2049)
**Design:** The study included 1050 African-American patients with NYHA class III or IV heart failure with dilated ventricles. Patients were randomized to receive a fixed dose of isosorbide dinitrate plus hydralazine or placebo in addition to standard therapy.
**Results:** Mortality rate were significantly higher in placebo group compared to isosorbide plus hydralazine group (10.2% vs. 6.2%).

# SECTION 2: DEVICE- OR PROCEDURE-RELATED TRIALS

## Bone Marrow or Stem Cell Therapies

### ASTAMI
Intracoronary Injection of Mononuclear Bone Marrow Cells in Acute Myocardial Infarction (*N Engl J Med* 2006;355:1199-1209)
**Design:** In this study, 100 patients with anterior ST-elevation myocardial infarction and percutaneous coronary intervention on left anterior descending artery were randomized to receive intracoronary injection of mononuclear bone marrow cells (mBMC) or not.
**Results:** No differences were seen between groups in measurements of left ventricular function.

### BOOST
Intracoronary Autologous Bone-Marrow Cell Transfer after Myocardial Infarction: The BOOST Randomised Controlled Clinical Trial (*Lancet.* 2004;364(9429):141-148)
**Design:** Patients successfully treated for acute ST-elevation MI via percutaneous coronary intervention (PCI) were randomized to bone marrow cell (BMC) transfer (30 patients) or control group (30 patients). Cardiac MRI performed at 4.8 days after PCI and at 6 months to determine effect on left ventricular systolic ejection fraction.
**Results:** BMC transfer provided early improvement in left ventricular systolic ejection fraction after an acute MI.

# Diuretic/Ultrafiltration Trials

### DOSE
Diuretic Optimization Strategies Evaluation (*N Engl J Med* 2011;364:797)

**Design:** In this study, 308 patients with acute decompensated heart failure were randomized to receive furosemide administered by means of either a bolus every 12 hours or continuous infusion at either a low dose or high dose.

**Results:** No significant differences were found in patient symptoms or renal function change when diuretic therapy was administered via bolus vs. continuous infusion or at high dose vs. low dose. Greater weight loss was observed with high-dose therapy.

### UNLOAD
Ultrafiltration versus Intravenous Diuretics for Patients Hospitalized for Acute Decompensated Congestive Heart Failure (*JACC* 2007;49:675)

**Design:** In this study, 200 patients hospitalized for HF with $\geq 2$ signs of hypervolemia were randomized to ultrafiltration or intravenous diuretics.

**Results:** For decompensated HF, ultrafiltration produced greater weight ($5.0 \pm 3.1$ kg vs. $3.1 \pm 3.5$ kg) and fluid loss (4.6 L vs. 3.3 L) than intravenous diuretics, and reduced 90-day resource utilization for HF.

# Exercise Training

### HF-ACTION
Heart Failure—A Controlled Trial Investigating Outcomes of Exercise Training (*JAMA* 2009;301:1451)

**Design:** In this study, 2331 medically stable patients with HF with LVEF of $\leq 35\%$ were randomized to receive usual care plus aerobic exercise training or usual care alone.

**Results:** Usual care plus exercise training led to greater improvement in KCCQ overall summary score compared with usual care alone (5.21 vs. 3.28) at 3 months, after which no further significant changed in KCCQ score occurred for either group. Improvements persisted over 2.5 year follow-up period.

# Implantable Cardioverter-Defibrillator (ICD) Trials

### CARE-HF
Cardiac Resynchronization-Heart Failure (*N Engl J Med* 2005;352(15): 1539–1549)

**Design:** The study included 813 patients with class III/IV heart failure due to left ventricular systolic dysfunction with EF ≤35% and with cardiac dyssynchrony. Patients presented with LVED of at least 30 mm and QRS interval of 120–149 ms. Patients were treated for 29.4 months; 404 patients received medical therapy alone and 409 received medical therapy and cardiac resynchronization.

**Results:** There were 82 deaths in the cardiac-resynchronization group, as compared with 120 in the medical-therapy group (20% vs. 30%). Cardiac resynchronization reduced the interventricular mechanical delay, the end-systolic volume index, and the area of the mitral regurgitant jet; increased the left ventricular ejection fraction; and improved symptoms and the quality of life.

### COMPANION
Comparison of Medical Therapy, Pacing, and Defibrillation in Heart Failure (*N Engl J Med* 2004;350:2140)

**Design:** The study included 1520 patients with NYHA class III or IV heart failure due to ischemic or nonischemic cardiomyopathies and QRS interval of at least 120 ms. Random assignment received optimal pharmacologic therapy alone or in combination with cardiac-resynchronization therapy using either a pacemaker or pacemaker-defibrillator.

**Results:** Cardiac-resynchronization therapy with a pacemaker or pacemaker-defibrillator reduced rate of hospitalization for heart failure by 34% and 40%, respectively, and reduced rate of mortality by 24% and 36%, respectively, compared to optimal pharmacologic therapy alone.

### MADIT-CRT
Multicenter Automatic Defibrillator Implantation Trial–Cardiac Resynchronization Therapy (*N Engl J Med* 2010;363:2385)

**Design:** In this study, 1798 patients with NYHA class II or III HF and LVEF of ≤30% with intrinsic QRS duration of ≥120 ms or paced QRS duration of ≥200 ms were randomly assigned to received either an ICD alone or an ICD plus CRT.

**Results:** Addition of CRT to ICD therapy reduced the rate of death (186 vs. 236 patients) and of hospitalization (174 vs. 236 patients) for heart failure.

## MADIT II

The Multicenter Automatic Defibrillator Implantation Trial (*N Engl J Med* 2002;346:877)

**Design:** The study included 1232 patients with a prior myocardial infarction and a LVEF of 30% or less.

**Results:** Risk of death was reduced 31% with implantation of defibrillator.

## SCD-HeFT

Sudden Cardiac Death in Heart Failure Trial (*N Engl J Med* 2005;352:225)

**Design:** In this study, 2521 patients with NYHA class II or II CHF (52% ischemic, 48% nonischemic) and LVEF ≤ 35% were randomly assigned to conventional CHF therapy plus placebo (847 patients), conventional therapy plus amiodarone (845 patients), or conventional therapy plus a single-lead ICD (conservatively programmed, shock-only, 829 patients).

**Results:** Amiodarone had no favorable effect on survival rate. Single-lead, shock-only ICD therapy reduced overall mortality rate by 23%.

---

# Mechanical Support Device Trials

---

## HEARTMATE II

Use of a Continuous-Flow Device in Patients Awaiting Heart Transplantation (*N Engl J Med* 2007;357:885)

**Design:** The study examined the effects of implantation of a continuous-flow pump in 133 patients with end-stage heart failure who were on a waiting list for heart transplantation.

**Results:** Survival rate during support was 75% at 6 months and 68% at 12 months. Significant improvement in functional status and quality of life was noted.

## HEARTMATE II IN ADVANCED HF

Advanced Heart Failure Treated with Continuous-Flow Left Ventricular Assist Device (*N Engl J Med* 2009;361:2241)

**Design:** A group of 200 patients with advanced heart failure who were ineligible for heart transplantation was randomly assigned to undergo implantation of a continuous-flow HMII device (134 patients) or a pulsatile-flow device (66 patients). The primary composite endpoint was survival free from disabling stroke and reoperation to repair or replace the device at 2 years post implantation.

**Results:** Use of the HMII reduced the combined endpoint of survival without occurrence of stroke or device failure at 2 years by 62%, compared to treatment using a pulsatile-flow LVAD (62 of 134 vs. 7 of 66 patients). Treatment using a continuous-flow LVAD significantly improved probability of survival compared to a pulsatile-flow LVAD (58% vs. 24% at 2 years).

## REMATCH

Randomized Evaluation of Mechanical Assistance for the Treatment of Congestive Heart Failure (*N Engl J Med* 2001;345:1435)

**Design:** The study included 129 patients with NYHA class IV heart failure who were ineligible for cardiac transplantation. Patients were randomly assigned to receive LVAD (68 patients) or optimal medical management (61 patients).

**Results:** The 2-year risk of death was reduced 48% with LVAD. Use of LVAD resulted in improved quality of live and increased rate of survival compared to optimal medical management alone (52% vs. 25% at one year, 23% vs. 8% at two years).

# Transcatheter Aortic-Valve Replacement

## PARTNER A

Placement of Aortic Transcatheter Valves Trial (*N Engl J Med* 2011;364:2187)

**Design:** In this multicenter study, 699 high-risk patients with severe aortic stenosis were randomized to undergo either transcatheter aortic-valve replacement (TAVR) with balloon-expandable bovine pericardial valve or surgical valve replacement.

**Results:** Death rates were reduced in the transcatheter group compared to surgical group at 30 days (3.4% vs. 6.5%) and at 1 year (24.2% vs. 26.8%).

## PARTNER B

Placement of Aortic Transcatheter Valves Trial (*N Engl J Med* 2010;363:1597)

**Design:** In this study, 358 patients with aortic stenosis not considered suitable for surgery were randomized to undergo standard therapy (including balloon aortic valvuloplasty) or transfemoral transcatheter implantation of a balloon-expandable bovine pericardial valve (TAVI).

**Results:** Mortality rates at 1 year were significantly lower in the TAVI group compared to standard therapy (30.7% vs. 50.7%).